Pharmacogenomics Using Artificial Intelligence

Scrivener Publishing
100 Cummings Center, Suite 541J
Beverly, MA 01915-6106

Publishers at Scrivener
Martin Scrivener (martin@scrivenerpublishing.com)
Phillip Carmical (pcarmical@scrivenerpublishing.com)

Pharmacogenomics Using Artificial Intelligence

Optimizing Drug Response through Personalized Genomic Analysis

Edited by

Umesh Kumar Lilhore

Kaamran Raahemifar

Sarita Simaiya

R. Sunder

and

R. Lotus

Scrivener Publishing

WILEY

This edition first published 2026 by John Wiley & Sons, Inc., 111 River Street, Hoboken, NJ 07030, USA and Scrivener Publishing LLC, 100 Cummings Center, Suite 541J, Beverly, MA 01915, USA

For more information about Scrivener publications please visit www.scrivenerpublishing.com.

Wiley Global Headquarters
111 River Street, Hoboken, NJ 07030, USA

For details of our global editorial offices, customer services, and more information about Wiley products visit us at www.wiley.com.

The manufacturer's authorized representative according to the EU General Product Safety Regulation is Wiley-VCH GmbH, Boschstr. 12, 69469 Weinheim, Germany, e-mail: Product_Safety@wiley.com.

Library of Congress Cataloging-in-Publication Data

ISBN 9781394404438

Cover image: Generated with AI using Adobe Firefly
Cover design by Russell Richardson

Set in size of 11pt and Minion Pro by Manila Typesetting Company, Makati, Philippines

Printed in the USA

10 9 8 7 6 5 4 3 2 1

Contents

Preface

The rapid evolution of genomics and computational sciences has ushered in a transformative era in healthcare—one that prioritizes precision, personalization, and predictive decision-making. *Pharmacogenomics Using Artificial Intelligence: Optimizing Drug Response through Personalized Genomic Analysis* is a reflection of this paradigm shift, where the integration of genetic insights with pharmacological principles is redefining how therapies are developed, prescribed, and monitored.

Pharmacogenomics lies at the intersection of pharmacology and genomics, focusing on how genetic variations influence individual responses to drugs. Traditional "one-size-fits-all" approaches to treatment often lead to variability in efficacy and adverse drug reactions. By contrast, pharmacogenomics enables clinicians to tailor therapies based on a patient's genetic profile, thereby improving therapeutic outcomes and minimizing risks. This book aims to provide a comprehensive understanding of the scientific foundations, technological advancements, and clinical applications that underpin this emerging field.

In recent years, artificial intelligence (AI) and machine learning (ML) have become indispensable tools in pharmacogenomics. The increasing complexity and volume of genomic and clinical data demand advanced analytical techniques capable of uncovering hidden patterns and actionable insights. AI-driven approaches are now playing a crucial role in predicting drug responses, optimizing dosing strategies, identifying novel drug targets, and facilitating clinical decision support systems. This book highlights these advancements and explores how AI is accelerating the translation of pharmacogenomic knowledge into real-world clinical practice.

The chapters in this volume cover a broad spectrum of topics, beginning with the fundamental principles of pharmacogenomics, including genetic variation, pharmacokinetics, and pharmacodynamics. Subsequent sections delve into machine learning methodologies, deep learning applications, and AI-driven drug discovery processes. Real-world case studies and clinical decision support systems are discussed to illustrate the practical implementation of pharmacogenomics in healthcare settings. Additionally, the book addresses key challenges such as data integration, ethical considerations, population diversity, and regulatory barriers, while also providing insights into future trends and innovations.

This book is intended for a diverse audience, including researchers, clinicians, pharmacists, data scientists, and students who are interested in the convergence of genomics, medicine, and artificial intelligence. By bridging theoretical knowledge with practical applications, we aim to equip readers with the tools and perspectives necessary to contribute to the advancement of precision medicine.

We would like to express our sincere gratitude to all contributing authors for their expertise and dedication in bringing this work to fruition. We also thank the reviewers and publishing team for their valuable feedback and support throughout the development process.

As pharmacogenomics continues to evolve, it holds immense promise for transforming global healthcare systems. We hope this book serves as a meaningful resource and inspires further research, collaboration, and innovation in the pursuit of safer, more effective, and personalized therapeutic strategies.

Editors
Umesh Kumar Lilhore
Kaamran Raahemifar
Sarita Simaiya
R. Sunder
R. Lotus

1

Foundations of Pharmacogenomics: Understanding the Genetic Basis of Drug Response

Dhanesh Kumar[1], Thangiah Sathishkumar[2], Sarangam Kodati[3], Venkata Praveen Kumar Vuppala[4], Rasmi A.[5]* and Rajakumar Perumal[6]

[1]*Department of Computer Science and Engineering, Koneru Lakshmaiah Education Foundation, Guntur, Andhra Pradesh, India*
[2]*Department of Computer Science and Engineering, Hyderabad Institute of Technology and Management, Hyderabad, Telangana, India*
[3]*Department of Information Technology, CVR College of Engineering, Hyderabad, Telangana, India*
[4]*Department of CSE-Internet of Things, St. Ann's College of Engineering and Technology, Chirala, AP, India*
[5]*Department of Information & Science Engineering, RR Institute of Technology, Bangalore, Karnataka, India*
[6]*Department of Computer Science and Engineering, Sharda University, Greater Noida, Uttar Pradesh, India*

Abstract
Pharmacogenomics is the study of genetic differences in the response of individuals to the actions of drugs. In general, pharmacogenomics is the integration of pharmacology and genomics to develop the most optimal therapy that can maximize efficacy while also decreasing the chance of an adverse drug event. This chapter aims to provide a solid understanding of how genes influence the drug response of individuals. This will be achieved by focusing on areas of variation in genes that relate to pharmacokinetics and pharmacodynamics of a drug, including focus on pharmacogenomic variation within the following areas: single-nucleotide polymorphisms (SNP), copy number variations (CNV), and structural variations (SV). In addition to mechanisms of pharmacokinetics and pharmacodynamics,

**Corresponding author*: itsmerazmi@gmail.com

Umesh Kumar Lilhore, Kaamran Raahemifar, Sarita Simaiya, R. Sunder and R. Lotus (eds.) Pharmacogenomics Using Artificial Intelligence: Optimizing Drug Response through Personalized Genomic Analysis, (1–22) © 2026 Scrivener Publishing LLC

we will provide clinically relevant examples of pharmacogenomics with a focus on the following areas of practice; CYP2C19—clopidogrel, CYP2D6—codeine, and VKORC1/CYP2C9—warfarin. Examples in cancer therapy will highlight the importance of biomarkers as well as implementation strategies that exist, e.g., Clinical Pharmacogenetics Implementation Consortium (CPIC) guidelines, and demonstrate emerging real-world data on the efficacy of pharmacogenomics from cost-effectiveness perspectives. Ethical, legal, and social issues will also be discussed regarding genetic testing for individuals and highlight the potential challenges in implementing genomic medicine, e.g., the issues involved with rare variants and differences stemming from population contexts. Finally, this chapter highlights some developing innovations including next-generation sequencing, AI predictions, and multi-omics integration as part of the journey to improving precision medicine.

***Keywords*:** Pharmacogenomics, genetic variations, drug response, precision medicine, biomarkers, clinical implementation

1.1 Introduction

The science of investigating the impact of genetic variation on drug therapy on an individual is called pharmacogenomics—the convergence of drug therapy and genomics to guide safer and more effective therapies [1]. The field of pharmacogenomics was borne out as a field with classical pharmacogenetic observations in the middle of the 20th century—the recognition that certain genetic variants had a serious impact on the metabolism or toxicity of drugs. For example, a glucose-6-phosphate dehydrogenase (G6PD)-deficient patient developed hemolytic anemia after receiving some antimalarial drugs, and a patient with genetically derived or inherited pseudocholinesterase variants developed permanent paralysis after receiving succinylcholine during anesthesia. Such cases have led to our understanding of genetic variations and the potential impact of such variations in drug metabolic and safety pathways [2]. Traditionally pharmacogenetics focused on single gene interaction with drugs in metabolism or drug toxicity [3]. In contrast, pharmacogenomics is the study of variation at the genome-wide level, involving more than one gene and regulatory region, and the complex interaction of genes and environments in the context of genetic variations influencing the drug metabolism (or the drug development outcome). During the past 10 years since the Human Genome Project and multiple mega and next-generation sequencing projects, pharmacogenomics has been publicized and is now more familiar to the clinical and research community.

The aim of pharmacogenomics is the prediction of differences in the response to drugs, an increase in the effectiveness of drugs, a reduction in adverse reactions to drugs (ADRs), and improvement in the design of precision medicine-based strategies [4]. With the help of genotypic information in prescribing, clinicians will be able to prescribe tailored drugs on individual basis based on genotype and minimize the number of trials and errors to avoid adverse events and maximize positive outcomes. Pharmacogenomics can also be used in drug development in identifying new targets and formation of subpopulations in drug development clinical trials which has been shown to facilitate and speed up drug development in translational medicine [5].

During the transformation of healthcare into a personalized model, the principles of pharmacogenomics should be developed on a solid background. The chapter aims at presenting a unified perspective on the genetics underlying the mechanisms of drug response, a summary of the most applicable clinical applications, and a perspective on the future work in the implementation of pharmacogenomics in daily clinical practice. Since its inception, pharmacogenomics evolved as a product of pharmacogenetic discoveries that showed the tremendous effect that inherited traits may exert on drug reactions. Since the 1950s, the results of hemolytic anemia have occurred in individuals with a G6PD deficiency who have been receiving primaquine, an antimalarial drug.

In the 1950s, patients who had atypical forms of pseudocholinesterase variants were administered with succinylcholine as anesthetic agents, and this resulted in a long apnea period. Once more, this gave support to the mediation of drug sensitivity by genetics. The stories above were the early illustrations of evidence that there was a genetic basis of pharmacogenomics and then pharmacogenetics or a single gene trait contributing to a metabolic trait or a toxicity profile [6]. Figure 1.1 presents the development of pharmacogenomics and pharmacogenetics.

The advent of the 21st century brought pharmacogenomics into a new field of study with the development of new technologies of molecular biology and genome-wide analysis. As a global scientific community, we all embarked on the Human Genome Project (2003) and then entered a new era of next-generation sequencing technology (NGS), called the capability to interrogate a complex interaction of genes and drugs on a genome-wide, not locus-based, level. Moreover, such tools as PharmGKB and clinical practice guidelines, created by the Clinical Pharmacogenetics Implementation Consortium (CPIC), were used to bridge any possible translational gap between the research and the clinical practice.

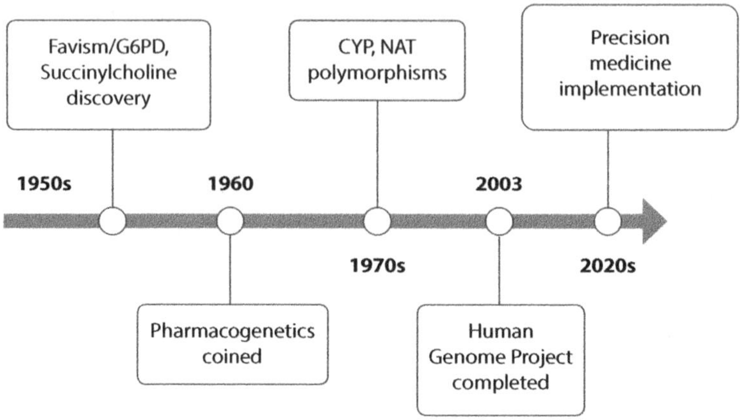

Figure 1.1 Timeline of pharmacogenomics and pharmacogenetics.

Today pharmacogenomics serves as the foundation for precision medicine initiatives in many regions around the world, enabling an agenda, informed by genetic profiles, to better personalize drug therapies, coordinate drug selection and improve patient drug safety, and inform regulatory approaches to the manufacture and market approval of drug products [7]. The objectives of the chapter are to:

- Explain the genetic basis of drug response through explaining important genetic variations, their influence on pharmacokinetics and pharmacodynamics, and clinical examples that relate to drug efficacy and safety.
- Discuss on the clinical applications of pharmacogenomics in personalized medicine, including biomarker-driven drug selection, dose finding, and the potential to reduce adverse drug reactions.
- Discuss emerging technologies and implementation frameworks in pharmacogenomic testing in the clinical setting, including ethical, legal, and social issues.

The rest of the chapter is organized in the following way. Section 1.2 will discuss genetic variation and mechanisms of drug response—types of genetic polymorphisms, pharmacokinetics vs. pharmacodynamics, and implications in the clinic. Section 1.3 will review clinically actionable examples—case reports related to gene–drug interactions (e.g., CYP2C19—clopidogrel, CYP2D6—codeine, VKORC1—warfarin, cancer biomarkers).

Section 1.4 will present implementation frameworks and integration into clinicians—guidelines (CPIC, PharmGKB), ways of supporting clinicians with evidence, cost-effectiveness, and real-world examples of pharmacogenomics. Section 1.5 will discuss the emerging technologies and future directions and the challenges and limitations to integration, population disparities, and rare variants. Finally, Section 1.6 will end with some key takeaway and high-level thoughts about this evolving area of pharmacogenomics in personalized healthcare.

1.2 Genetics of Drug Response Mechanisms

Genetic variation has a significant impact on response to drugs through mediating metabolism, transport, and drug-target. Variation can be in the form of changes in a single nucleotide, differences in copy number, or structural variations, all resulting in differences in pharmacokinetics and pharmacodynamics. Understanding these mechanisms is critical to assessing response to treatment, dosing, and adverse drug reactions (ADRs) [8].

1.2.1 Types of Genetic Variation

Genetic variation can occur in a number of different ways, though the most common is the presence of single nucleotide polymorphisms (SNPs) or the single base replacements in DNA, which may lead to protein structure/function alteration. Alleles of CYP2C19 can be used as an example of SNP having loss of function alleles 2 and 3 and gain of function allele 17. Another gene variant that has examples of allele is CYP2D6—normal functioning, nonfunctioning and reduced functioning.

SNP variation may also have an influence on drug metabolism which, in some cases, may cause varying effects of the drug in drug efficacy (toxicity) or cause greater toxicity. Copy number variant (CNV) is also known as variations in the copy number of a gene(s) as a result of duplication or deletion. CYP2D6 gene duplication results in the ultrarapid metabolizer (UM) phenotypes, which need to convert prodrugs (e.g., codeine) to morphine within a short period, thereby increasing the likelihood of overdose. However, *vice versa* may be true in the deletion of a gene that leads to poor metabolizer phenotypes in individuals. The quantity of statin is compromised in SLCO1B1 (a transporter) deletion, and it elevates the chances of myopathy.

Structural variants entail more complex insertions and deletions and may entail more complicated structural rearrangements. They can also cause frameshifts, premature stop codon, and alterations in splicing, all of which can eliminate enzyme activity. Although they may be regarded as rare alleles and they are rare in the populations, they may have large and clinically significant effects in cases where they are met. In combination, these variants give the genetic foundations of the interindividual (within a population) differences in drug response that we observe and interethnic (between populations) differences in drug response and underlie the clinical relevance of genotyping in drug prescription to acquiring a safe and effective therapy [9].

1.2.2 Pharmacokinetics vs. Pharmacodynamics

The genetic impacts on drug response can be categorized in terms of pharmacokinetic (PK) and pharmacodynamic (PD) genetic impacts. PK is the absorption, distribution, metabolism, and excretion (ADME) of the drug which is actually what the body does with the drug. There are genetic polymorphisms in genes encoding drug-metabolizing enzymes (e.g., CYP2C9, CYP2C19, CYP2D6), conjugation enzymes (UGTs), and transport genes (e.g., ABCB1 [P-glycoprotein], SLCO1B1) which consequences are either sub-therapeutic drug levels or drug-related toxicity.

Generally, PK is the proportions of a specific concentration of a medication with respect to time, leading to either toxicity or a desirable effect. PD is typically defined as the drug interactions with its biological target(s), that is, receptors, ion channels, and enzymes—or simply what is done to the body. As an example, HLA-B-57-01 gene variations predispose the patient to abacavir hypersensitivity, VKORC1 variants alter the sensitivity of the individual to warfarin, and HER2 overexpression identifies the patients who can possibly be helped by treatment besides chemotherapy, with trastuzumab.

It is significant to know genetic PK and PD effect distinction. Overall, PK variant would lead to dose adjustment, but a PD variant may lead to a change in medication or other treatment. Either of these genetic effects explain the character of precise prescribing styles to administer optimum therapy due to restricting adverse reactions as opposed to population statistics [10].

1.2.3 Phenotypes and Clinical Effects

Genetic diversity produces identifiable differences in the metabolizer phenotype: extensive metabolizers (EM) are normal enzyme activity and represent a normal drug response, ultrarapid metabolizers (UM) (i.e., rapid OM) are duplicated or hyperactive alleles, intermediate metabolizers (IM) have normal activity, and ultrarapid metabolizers (UM) (i.e., rapid OM) have no activity.

There are clinical implications of these metabolizer phenotypes. Examples of UMs of CYP2D6 quickly eliminate codeine to morphine and are vulnerable to opioid toxicity, whereas PMs lack adequate analgesia. CYP2C19 PMs do not stimulate clopidogrel and thus might pose a risk to the heart after stent implantation. Anticoagulation of warfarin is likely to bleed PMs which are vkorc1 and cyp2c9 since they are very sensitive and require very low doses.

Different ethnicities have different phenotypic distributions. UMs of CYP2D6 are extensive in the North African populations, and PMs of CYP2C19 are extensive in the East Asian ones. The Global healthcare fraternity also ought to embrace trends of ship drug regimens and treatment in the respective varying populations. Finally, the phenotypic outcomes may not be solely due to gene–gene interactions but also by the environmental factors (e.g., diet, comorbidities, concomitant medications) which may altogether alter outcomes. A higher awareness of phenotype–drug association can result in a better genotype-guided prescribing, reduction in drug reactions, and better therapeutic targeting variances among multi-clinical domains [11].

1.3 Clinically Actionable Examples

Cases of clinically actionable pharmacogenomic data include the clear and direct effect of some genetic variations on therapeutic choices, such as increased efficacy and decreased harm. Another number of well-characterized gene–drug interactions have been exploited to create clinical guidelines and drug labeling by enabling the possibility of relying on genotype to make dosing or drug choice decisions. An example of a case where pharmacogenomics is being applied in common care in cardiovascular disease, pain management, and cancer care can be found in this section, which is an important case—CYP2C19—clopidogrel, CYP2D6—codeine, VKORC1/CYP2C9—warfarin and cancer pharmacogenomic markers (HER2, DPYD, ugAT1A1). In each of the examples, we present the information that contains the allele frequencies, implications on the clinical use, and existing recommendation of the clinical guidelines that make it possible to provide an individual therapy.

1.3.1 CYP2C19 and Clopidogrel

Clopidogrel is a widely used antiplatelet agent but is a prodrug that is metabolically activated in the liver by the CYP 2C19 enzyme. Known loss-of-function alleles which have been studied are T681A (CYP2C19 3) and G681C (CYP2C19 2), and they both result in loss of functionality of the enzyme CYP2C19, resulting in an inhibition of the active metabolite of clopidogrel, resulting in an impaired platelet inhibition. Those of the poor metabolizers (PMs) are at risk for stent thrombosis and or pre-existing myocardial infarction (MI), particularly after a particular percutaneous coronary intervention (PCI) because of a double allele loss of function. The ethnic studies on the CYP2C19 functionality variation are very interesting; 15%–20% of East Asians and about 42% of Sri Lankans (Reddit community) will get impaired alleles compared to about 2%–5% of Europeans, for example. It is a clinical factor of key importance especially in the at-risk population receiving cardiovascular interventions [12]. Table 1.1 shows thevGenotype and Clopidogrel Therapy Recommendations clinical guidelines developed by Clinical Pharmacogenetics Implementation Consortium (CPIC) proposing PMs and IMs to use alternative agents (prasugrel or ticagrelor) to give the best response to antiplatelet efficacy in such patients. Moreover, there has been a provision of boxed warnings by the Food and Drug Administration (FDA) on clopidogrel given the variation in metabolism to CYP2C19.

Table 1.1 CYP2C19 genotype and clopidogrel therapy recommendations.

Genotype	Phenotype	Effect on clopidogrel activation	Clinical risk	Recommended therapy
*1/*1	Normal metabolizer	Normal activation	Standard efficacy	Standard clopidogrel dosing
*1/*2 or *1/*3	Intermediate metabolizer	Reduced activation	Moderate thrombosis risk	Consider prasugrel or ticagrelor
*2/*2 or *2/*3	Poor metabolizer	Significantly reduced activation	High thrombosis risk	Avoid clopidogrel; use alternative drug

This genotype-guided approach reduces cardiovascular events and optimizes outcomes in high-risk patients.

1.3.2 CYP2D6 and Codeine/Opioid Metabolism

Codeine is metabolized into morphine mainly *via* CYP2D6 mediated O-demethylation. Variations in CYP2D6 result in four relevant phenotypes: ultrarapid metabolizers (UMs) genetically duplicated genes, extensive metabolizers (EMs) have normal function, intermediate metabolizers (IMs) have decreased activity, and poor metabolizers (PMs) have no activity [13]. Figure 1.2 shows the codeine metabolism pathway.

PMs would fail to experience the analgesic effect of codeine since it would not convert codeine to morphine adequately, whereas UM patients convert codeine into morphine more quickly and are prone to respiratory depression that is life-threatening. There was a very publicized incident where a UM mother was breastfeeding and was taking codeine to treat her postpartum pain, and her child died. The precise prevalence of the phenotypes differs by population: UMs are present in 1% to 2% of Europeans and more than 30% of Ethiopians, while CYP2D6 10 reduced functionality allele is present in approximately 50% of Asians. Table 1.2 shows the CYP2D6 phenotype and codeine response.

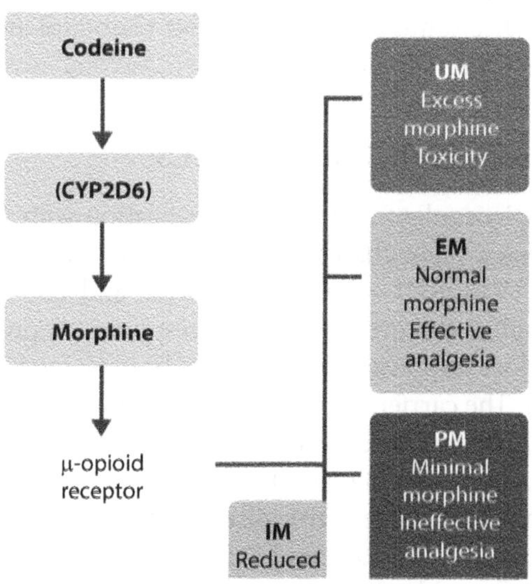

Figure 1.2 Codeine metabolism pathway.

Table 1.2 CYP2D6 phenotype and codeine response.

Genotype category	Phenotype	Morphine formation	Clinical outcome	Recommendation
Multiple gene copies (e.g., *1xN)	Ultrarapid metabolizer (UM)	Excessive morphine	Risk of toxicity/ respiratory depression	Avoid codeine; alternative opioid
*1/*1 or *1/*2	Extensive metabolizer (EM)	Normal morphine	Expected analgesia	Standard dosing
*1/*10 or *10/*41	Intermediate metabolizer (IM)	Reduced morphine	Reduced analgesia	Monitor response; consider alternatives
*4/*4 or *5/*5	Poor metabolizer (PM)	Minimal morphine	Ineffective analgesia	Avoid codeine; use morphine directly

Both UMs and PMs, particularly children and breastfeeding mothers, have been given a boxed warning on codeine against the FDA. Clinical Pharmacogenetics Implementation Consortium recommends that UMs and PMs should be avoided and given a choice, i.e., morphine or non-opioid analgesic. The same can be said about tramadol and hydrocodone, as both drugs are CYP2D6 metabolites.

1.3.3 Warfarin: VKORC1 and CYP2C9

Warfarin is an anticoagulant and an oral medication with a low therapeutic index, which is that a slight change in dosage causes bleeding or thrombosis. These two genes (VKORC1—the target enzyme and CYP2C9—the metabolizing enzyme) affect the overall warfarin response. Approximately 30% of variability in the dose response of warfarin can be explained by VKORC1 haplotypes (A and B). The carriers of haplotype A (more prevalent among people of Asian descent) will be more sensitive to warfarin and will require a lower dose of warfarin, whereas haplotype B carriers (more prevalent among self-identified African American descent) will explain the necessity of a higher dose of warfarin. Moreover, CYP2C9 (2 and 3) mutations reduce the warfarin clearance and predispose to bleeding. The combination of these polymorphisms might explain up to 40% of the variability in warfarin dose response as shown in Figure 1.3. Considering variables influencing warfarin dosing algorithm, the dose is modified according to both VKORC1 haplotype and CYP2C9 genotype in addition to the patient age/weight.

The addition of these polymorphisms into genotype-guided warfarin dosing (e.g., WarfarinDosing.org) algorithms allows a personalized method of warfarin treatment using the VKORC1 and CYP2C9 haplotype on top of factors related to clinical considerations (age, weight, etc.). Genotype-guided warfarin initiation based on clinical studies has demonstrated it will reduce time to stable INR, reduce bleeding events, and increase the probability of a good therapeutic outcome. Table 1.3 shows the VKORC1 and CYP2C9 variants in warfarin dosing.

The regulatory authorities (i.e., Food and Drug Administration [FDA]) recognize the role played by genetics in therapy, especially drug interactions with clinical records and guidelines, and suggest that the genotype should be looked at in order to make a warfarin dose. The fact that the genotypic data is provided as a good example of multi-gene pharmacogenomics is very evident and a clear advantage in the safety and efficacy of broadly used anticoagulants of warfarin on populations with various ancestry and allele frequency [14].

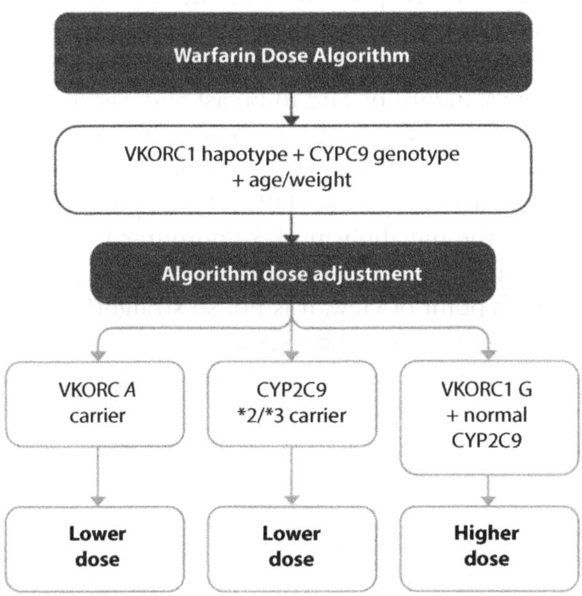

Figure 1.3 Warfarin algorithm.

Table 1.3 VKORC1 and CYP2C9 variants in warfarin dosing.

Gene/variant	Effect	Clinical implication	Dosing strategy
VKORC1 -1639 G>A (A haplotype)	Lower VKORC1 expression → ↑ sensitivity	Lower dose requirement (common in Asians)	Start with reduced warfarin dose
VKORC1 G haplotype	Higher VKORC1 expression → ↓ sensitivity	Higher dose requirement (common in Africans)	Start with higher dose (if safe)
CYP2C9 *2, *3	Reduced warfarin metabolism	Prolonged drug effect; ↑ bleeding risk	Lower starting dose; close INR monitoring

1.3.4 Cancer Therapy Markers: HER2 and DPYD/UGT1A1

Pharmacogenomics is an important feature of the oncology field, particularly in target selection in therapy and dosage in chemotherapy.

HER2 (ERBB2) is overexpressed in about 20% of breast cancer, and HER2 expression is correlated with trastuzumab (monoclonal antibody), which has improved the overall survival of the HER2-positive patients. Her2 status is now standard of care in breast and gastric cancer, and tests are essential to ensure that trastuzumab is only used for patients with tumors which overexpress HER2 to avoid unnecessary toxicity and usage. Dihydropyrimidine dehydrogenase (DPYD) gene polymorphism has a significant impact on the metabolism of 5-fluorouracil (5-FU) and capecitabine with chemotherapy. They become highly toxic, ill, and even die. From the clinician's point of view, it is not so straightforward as a variant to determine whether the patient possesses polymorphisms of DPYD2a or another variant. That would be translational medicine that might be able to use lower dosing or a whole new regimen.

In addition, the worked variants in the genes of UGT1A128 and UGT1A1*6 alleles are changed, which again decreases the glucuronidation of the active metabolite (SN-38) of irinotecan, again leading to the toxicity of the accumulation of the active metabolite, neutropenia. In addition, the clinical practice guidelines also support that the dose should be adjusted in response to genotype variations of a high proportion of Asian individuals. All of these cancer pharmacogenomics markers altogether reflect the persistence of precision oncology down to its real core where target expression (HER2) and metabolism (DPYD, UGT1A1) guide the direction of therapy and increase the chances of efficacy and reduce the risk of severe, potentially lethal toxicity in cancer patients [15]. Figure 1.4 shows trastuzumab: HER2 receptor blockade inhibits tumor growth. Table 1.4 lists the cancer markers, the associated drug and its genetic effect with its clinical action.

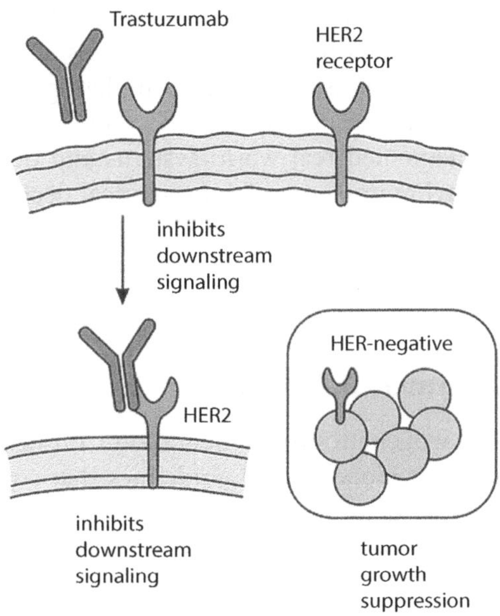

Figure 1.4 HER2 and cancer pharmacogenomics.

Table 1.4 Cancer pharmacogenomic markers.

Marker	Associated drug	Genetic effect	Clinical action
HER2 (ERBB2)	Trastuzumab	Overexpression → drug target present	Treat HER2+ breast/ gastric cancers with trastuzumab
DPYD variants	5-FU/ capecitabine	Reduced metabolism → toxicity risk	Dose reduce or use alternative regimen
UGT1A1*28, *6	Irinotecan	Impaired glucuronidation → toxicity	Reduce irinotecan dose in variant carriers

1.4 Implementation Frameworks and Clinical Integration

The successful implementation of pharmacogenomics into clinical practice ultimately depends on well-developed systems that allow the outcomes of genetic information to be used in prescribing decisions. Systems have been proposed and include evidence-based guidance, recommending actions, knowledge bases that curate the evidence to inform decision-making, decision-support tools that facilitate the use of pharmacogenomic information, and ethical systems that reinforce fairness and responsibility to ensure that access to testing is equitable. Completing this review, we will present examples of systems such as CPIC and PharmGKB, examples of studies that implemented real world systems and demonstrated cost-effective and cost-saving implementations, clinical decision support tools that can be integrated with clinical workflow, and ethical considerations for responsibly implementing pharmacogenomic testing in healthcare systems.

1.4.1 CPIC, PharmGKB, DPWG

The Clinical Pharmacogenetics Implementation Consortium (CPIC) produces peer-reviewed, evidence-based guidelines that convert genetic test results into actionable drug-dosing recommendations. Guidelines have been issued on commonly prescribed medications such as clopidogrel, codeine, warfarin, simvastatin, and allopurinol, with a strong emphasis on phenotype-based prescribing rather than providing guidance on whether to test (Wikipedia). The Dutch Pharmacogenetics Working Group (DPWG) has likewise produced regionally harmonized guidelines that have gained traction throughout Europe.

The importance and utility of PharmGKB (Pharmacogenomics Knowledgebase) cannot be understated. This resource is an extensive catalog of pharmacogenomic evidence, annotating gene–drug associations and including numerous clinical annotations and dosing algorithms (PMC, NCBI). PharmGKB also links to related regulatory information (e.g., FDA labeling) and links to clinical guideline databases. CPIC and PharmGKB are the two resources that most efforts are based upon when engaging with pharmacogenomic implementations globally, and each provides a harmonized evidence repository for clinicians, pharmacists, and researchers. The ability to incorporate these resources directly into electronic health records (EHRs) and point-of-care decision tools increases their clinical significance and usability and actively encourages drug prescribing based on pharmacogenomic testing [16].

1.4.2 Real-World Programs and Economic Impact

The pharmacogenomics implementation studies indicate that pharmacogenomics has both clinical and economic benefits. A study of a Medicare Advantage cohort in Kentucky that has involved retirees in pharmacogenomics-enriched comprehensive medication management (CMM) was one such example. The program demonstrated a mean saving of approximately 7,000 per patient direct medical expenses in 32 months and an extensive saving in acute inpatient hospitalization as a result of handling their pharmacogenomics (PMC) outcomes. The other pharmacogenomics pilots have been shown to have lower adverse drug reactions, better polypharmacy management, and medication compliance on training and healthcare practitioners. Lower hospital visit rates, lower rates of emergency visit, and better treatment result in economic value since, in other studies, health economics research is mounting evidence on the payback, in the real world, of feasibility and cost of upstream pharmacogenomic testing of chronic conditions and polypharmacy management (think cardiovascular disease and mental health).

These developments present a possibility that refractory pharmacogenomic testing should be included in the reimbursement and formulary choices of payors. This effective realization will involve cooperation with payors and actual clinicians, including pharmacists and genetic counselors, considering collaborative efforts within the practice, or location, of different disciplines. Meanwhile, further assessment will be done to make sure that the outcomes are tracked to continue to provide evidence and continuous transformation at an organizational or institution level [17].

1.4.3 Clinical Decision Support Systems (CDSS)

Clinical decision support systems (CDSS) refer to computerized technologies that deliver essential information to clinicians and physicians to aid their decision-making process. Clinical Decision Support Systems (CDSS) are computerized technologies that provide necessary information to clinicians and physicians to facilitate their decision-making process.

CDSS are critical in transforming the pharmacogenomic data into actionable recommendations in the point of care. Genetic tests can be interpreted through platforms such as GeneDose LIVE enabling the pharmacists and clinicians to assess drug to gene interaction and produce an individualized response plan of the medication. The flow of the CDSS is represented in Figure 1.5.

Similar steps are applied to clinical workflows, with the enrollment of a patient and performing genetic testing in a timely manner, and the results of genetic testing are stored in electronic health records (EHRs) safely. Pharmacists apply the clinician judgment to interpret pre-existing genotype/phenotype correlations and to examine the available and possible pharmacogenomic information that may affect any use of an available drug or dosage. Prescribing health professionals are provided with automated alerts and notifications in case of a high-risk scenario (i.e., a patient exhibiting poor clopidogrel metabolism). The system will educate the prescriber that clopidogrel is a prodrug and that the patient might not be in a position to metabolize the drug to the active state and/or that an alternative drug or change in dosage plan should be adopted, which ultimately enhances the efficiency and effectiveness of the clinical decision making.

Application of CDSS will enhance the effectiveness, efficiency, and quality of care that is delivered by the clinician, yet the practice should be acquainted with the system, standardization, interoperability, and

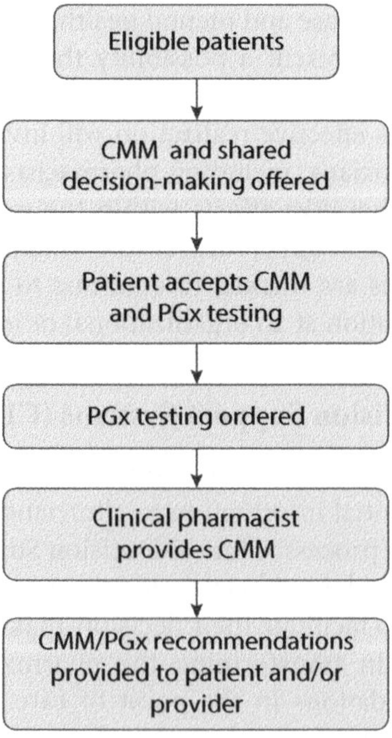

Figure 1.5 Workflow diagram for PGx-guided clinical decision support/CMM program.

education. Should pharmacogenic guidance have the capability to be utilized in the current prescribing modules, this can further facilitate clinical practice and progress the idea of precision medicine to allow the quick adoption of the integration of genomic data that can readily transform into daily practice in the clinical profession [18, 19]. Table 1.5 compares the essential pharmacogenomic implementation models with regard to the actors who impact the scope, clinical domain, informatics data integration, and decision-support potential.

1.4.4 Ethical, Legal, and Social Considerations

Clinical integration of pharmacogenomic testing has numerous important ethical, legal, and social implications (ELSI). As an illustration, informed consent is highly essential in order to make people aware of what testing entails. The patients are expected to know about the limitations of the test, the clinical significant targets (where applicable), incidental findings, and what providing genetic information may mean in their lives now and in the future. The best interventions would be privacy and confidentiality measures that would be consistent with the regulations in the US (HIPAA) and EU (GDPR) in order to avoid any form of inappropriate use of the information.

Moreover, the issues of fair access are also of concern, and frankly speaking, in case the genetically under-represented peoples do not have any data on the representational variants in pharmacogenomic databases, we can be multiplying the disparities of the local population understanding and test advantage. In this respect, further measures involve inclusive research investigations and building diverse genomic databases based on evidence and ensuring that clinician education encompasses impartial thoughts in regard to the actionable recommendations in case pharmacogenomic testing has been prescribed to prevent disparities.

Legal policies also have a role to make clear the data ownership, accountable party on the prescriptive use of the pharmacogenomics, and how pharmacogenomics can be used in malpractice standards. Genetics counseling can be used by institutions and clinicians so as to further promote the development of a trusting relationship, but the application of culturally sensitive communication approaches will be ultimately applied. Policy laws should promote the establishment of pharmacogenomics and also take into account and defend the interests of patients and improve social justice principles. It must develop the sphere of healthcare without making health inequity of the underserved groups worse [20].

Table 1.5 Comparisons of key pharmacogenomic implementation frameworks.

Framework	Scope and role	Key features	Clinical application	Global adoption
CPIC (Clinical Pharmacogenetics Implementation Consortium)	Provides genotype-to-phenotype dosing guidelines	Peer-reviewed, evidence-based; phenotype-focused; drug-specific recommendations (e.g., clopidogrel, codeine, warfarin)	Used to guide drug selection and dosing in clinical practice	Widely adopted in US and internationally; integrated into EHR/CDSS
DPWG (Dutch Pharmacogenetics Working Group)	Guideline development and clinical translation in Europe	Tailored to European populations; incorporates local allele frequency data; links to KNMP (Royal Dutch Pharmacists Association)	Used in community and hospital pharmacies; incorporated into national drug formulary	Primarily Europe, expanding globally
PharmGKB (Pharmacogenomics Knowledgebase)	Curates gene–drug evidence and clinical annotations	Database of pharmacogenomic associations, FDA labeling, CPIC/DPWG cross-references; visualization tools	Reference for clinicians, researchers, and educators; supports guideline implementation	Global research and clinical resource; integrated with CPIC/DPWG

1.5 New Technologies and Emerging Trends

There are many ethical, legal, and social implications (ELSI) associated with the use of pharmacogenomic testing. As an example, informed consent is the most important to determine if patients are comfortable knowing all consequences of the test, restriction of the tests, targets that can be acted upon clinically, incidental findings, and how the genetic data can follow the lived experience of the patients, now and in the future. Ideally, the principle of privacy and confidentiality is the pre-requisite to other laws such as HIPAA in the US or GDPR in the EU for controlling the inappropriate use and access of the data.

In some instances, such as the possibility that genetically underrepresented individuals might not exist in the variant data of the pharmacogenomic databases, then we run the danger of re-institutionalizing inequality in the way the tests are medically, therapeutically, and socially interpreted, explained, and in some instances not used at all. Another notable step to follow in this case is the inclusion research. Various genomic databases and education of providers offer non-biased advice in which the establishment of pharmacogenomic testing and its discussion take place to prevent discrimination.

Laws need to reduce the uncertainty about ownership of data assets, liability in the event of prescribing based on pharmacogenomics, and possible incorporation of the pharmacogenomics into a malpractice paradigm. Genetic counseling may also be a basis of culturally sensitive communication by institutions and clinicians in an attempt to gain the trust of the patients. Once again, these structures would need to be present in order to further promote pharmacogenomics as well as enable planning to enable the patients to exercise rights and promote social justice. Once again, this needs to be oriented toward healthcare development and not the enhancement of any additional health disparities [16, 21].

Limitations and problems: Pharmacogenomics has numerous barriers and limitations to its implementation, and this is the limitation to its clinical use. The variants of uncertain significance (VUS) and rare allele uncertainty translate into clinical uncertainty when making clinical choices on patients regarding limited evidence in practice. The other barrier in the health systems is financial barrier, where the cost of pharmacogenomic testing is high, the insurance reimbursement varies, and the back-office documentation required on the integration of the electronic health records may discourage the acquisition of the pharmacogenomic information on the testing. Regardless of these obstacles, it is particularly useful in management with a scarce resource since these spheres are less inclined to be exposed to favorable systems of implementation. There are also problems with implementation in the case of clinician awareness and education; pharmacogenomics clinician awareness and education are scarce, and this fact puts at risk a false interpretation of the results of the implementation without the standardized system of education or decision support [22].

The next consideration is that of limited generalizability or bias in our populations; the classic pharmacogenomics studies have generally spoken about individuals of European ancestry and makes it hard to generalize to other populations in the world and contributes to health inequities. The evolutionary character of the gene–drug interactions with the extra factor of polypharmacy or inhibitors of enzymes are another obstacle to pharmacogenomics in which the capability to determine drug therapy choices is hurdled more and the capability to update the clinical recommendation is even more appreciated. It can be argued that these obstacles can be overcome by using therapeutic recreating because with the development of precision-based medicine approaches, the gap between research and cost-effective action and an extensive clinician education and training system ought to be bridged.

1.6 Conclusion

Pharmacogenomics is one of the game changers in modern medicine, which provides the ability to have individualized medication therapy on the basis of one's genetic makeup. With understanding of differences in genes that impact pharmacokinetics or pharmacodynamics in their patient population, clinicians are poised to optimize therapeutic effectiveness and minimize adverse drug events by applying what they have learned about, for example, SNPs, CNVs, and structural variants. There are many clinically actionable examples, such as CYP2C19—clopidogrel, CYP2D6—codeine, and VKORC1/CYP2C9—warfarin that delivers immediate action for pharmacogenomic therapy. The evolution of cancer biomarkers, as well as biomarkers for cancer therapeutics, shows the way to obtain genomic data and biomarkers. Additionally, often available, there are guidelines, such as CPIC guidelines, the continual development of real-world cost-effectiveness evidence, access to genome sequencing, and new bioinformatics opportunities such as artificial intelligence precision genomics, that increased the likelihood of promoting the use of pharmacogenomic therapies. Even with these contributions to research and practice, there are still issues that can arise related to participant consent and the interpretation and a meaning of a variant, issues related to the variability of diversity of the research and patient population, equitable access to pharmacogenomic therapeutics, ethical, equity, equity and justice issues, and information use. The more genomic testing matures, pharmacogenomics will ultimately be a more significant pillar of precision medicine and would allow clinicians and researchers to provide individualized therapies to improve prognosis and to use into patient care and decision making across a variety of healthcare systems.

AI disclosure statement: The author confirms that no artificial intelligence (AI)-generated content or AI-assisted writing tools were used in the preparation of this chapter (including summaries and the abstract). All text, analysis, and conclusions are the result of the author's original work.

References

1. Pirmohamed, M., Pharmacogenomics: current status and future perspectives. *Nat. Rev. Genet.*, 24, 6, 350–362, 2023.
2. Yehya, A., Interplay between pharmacokinetics and pharmacogenomics, in: *Dosage Forms-Innovation and Future Perspectives*, IntechOpen Limited, Croatia, 2022. DOI: 10.5772/intechopen.95734.
3. Haidar, C.E., Crews, K.R., Hoffman, J.M., Relling, M.V., Caudle, K.E., Advancing pharmacogenomics from single-gene to preemptive testing. *Annu. Rev. Genomics Hum. Genet.*, 23, 1, 449–473, 2022.
4. Tremmel, R., Pirmann, S., Zhou, Y., Lauschke, V.M., Translating pharmacogenomic sequencing data into drug response predictions—How to interpret variants of unknown significance. *Br. J. Clin. Pharmacol.*, 91, 2, 252–263, 2025.
5. Qahwaji, R., Ashankyty, I., Sannan, N.S., Hazzazi, M.S., Basabrain, A.A., Mobashir, M., Pharmacogenomics: A genetic approach to drug development and therapy. *Pharmaceuticals*, 17, 7, 940, 2024.
6. Ranade, A., Pharmacogenomics: History, Development and Challenges. *Pharmacogenomics*, 2021.
7. Pardiñas, A.F., Owen, M.J., Walters, J.T.R., Pharmacogenomics: A road ahead for precision medicine in psychiatry. *Neuron*, 109, 24, 3914–3929, 2021.
8. Cacabelos, R., Naidoo, V., Corzo, L., Cacabelos, N., Carril, J.C., Genophenotypic factors and pharmacogenomics in adverse drug reactions. *Int. J. Mol. Sci.*, 22, 24, 13302, 2021.
9. Lauschke, V.M., Zhou, Y., Ingelman-Sundberg, M., Pharmacogenomics beyond single common genetic variants: the way forward. *Annu. Rev. Pharmacol. Toxicol.*, 64, 1, 33–51, 2024.

10. Hindley, B., Lip, G.Y.H., McCloskey, A.P., Penson, P.E., Pharmacokinetics and pharmacodynamics of direct oral anticoagulants. *Expert Opin. Drug Metab. Toxicol.*, 19, 12, 911–923, 2023.
11. Principi, N., Petropulacos, K., Esposito, S., Impact of pharmacogenomics in clinical practice. *Pharmaceuticals*, 16, 11, 1596, 2023.
12. Lee, C.R., Luzum, J.A., Sangkuhl, K., Gammal, R.S., Sabatine, M.S., Stein, C.M., Kisor, D.F., *et al.*, Clinical pharmacogenetics implementation consortium guideline for CYP2C19 genotype and clopidogrel therapy: 2022 update. *Clin. Pharmacol. Ther.*, 112, 5, 959–967, 2022.
13. Wong, A.K., Somogyi, A.A., Rubio, J., Philip, J., The role of pharmacogenomics in opioid prescribing. *Curr. Treat. Options Oncol.*, 23, 10, 1353–1369, 2022.
14. Zhang, S., Zhao, M., Zhong, S., Niu, J., Zhou, L., Zhu, B., Su, H., *et al.*, Association between CYP2C9 and VKORC1 genetic polymorphisms and efficacy and safety of warfarin in Chinese patients. *Pharmacogenet. Genomics*, 34, 4, 105–116, 2024.
15. Glewis, S., Lingaratnam, S., Krishnasamy, M., Martin, J.H., Tie, J., Alexander, M., Michael, Pharmacogenetics testing (DPYD and UGT1A1) for fluoropyrimidine and irinotecan in routine clinical care: perspectives of medical oncologists and oncology pharmacists. *J. Oncol. Pharm. Pract.*, 30, 1, 30–37, 2024.
16. Lilhore, U.K., Kumar, A., Vyas, N., Simaiya, S., Dutt, V. (Eds.), *Multimodal Data Fusion for Bioinformatics Artificial Intelligence*, John Wiley & Sons, New Jersy, USA, 2025.
17. Alshabeeb, M.A., Alyabsi, M., Aziz, M.A., Abohelaika, S., Pharmacogenes that demonstrate high association evidence according to CPIC, DPWG, and PharmGKB. *Front. Med.*, 9, 1001876, 2022.
18. Caudle, K.E., Whirl-Carrillo, M., Relling, M.V., Hoffman, J.M., Donnelly, R.S., Haidar, C.E., Bourque, M.S., *et al.*, Advancing Clinical Pharmacogenomics Worldwide Through the Clinical Pharmacogenetics Implementation Consortium (CPIC). *Clin. Pharmacol. Ther.*, 2025.
19. Smith, D.M., Wake, D.T., Dunnenberger, H.M., Pharmacogenomic clinical decision support: a scoping review. *Clin. Pharmacol. Ther.*, 113, 4, 803–815, 2023.
20. Farmaki, A., Manolopoulos, E., Natsiavas, P., Will precision medicine meet digital health? A systematic review of pharmacogenomics clinical decision support systems used in clinical practice. *OMICS: J. Integr. Biol.*, 28, 9, 442–460, 2024.
21. Haga, S.B., Artificial intelligence, medications, pharmacogenomics, and ethics. *Pharmacogenomics*, 25, 14–15, 611–622, 2024.
22. Onyema, E.M., Lilhore, U.K., Saurabh, P., Dalal, S., Nwaeze, A.S., Chijindu, A.T., Ndufeiya-Kumasi, L.C., Simaiya, S., Evaluation of IoT-Enabled hybrid model for genome sequence analysis of patients in healthcare 4.0. *Meas. Sens.*, 26, 100679, 2023.

2

From Data to Therapy: Artificial Intelligence Applications in Pharmacogenomics

Yuvaraj Velusamy[1], L. Gandhimathi[2], Shaziya Islam[3], P. Jyothi[4], Saranya P.[5] and S. Suresh[6]*

[1]Department of Biomedical Engineering, V.S.B. Engineering College, Karur, Tamil Nadu, India
[2]Department of Computer Science and Engineering, University College of Engineering, Nagercoil, Tamil Nadu, India
[3]Department of Computer Science and Engineering, Rungta International University, Bhilai, Chhattisgarh, India
[4]Department of Computer Science and Engineering, VNR Vignana Jyothi Institute of Engineering and Technology, Hyderabad, Telangana, India
[5]Department of Amity School of Engineering and Technology, Amity University, Mumbai, Maharashtra, India
[6]Department of Statistics, University of Madras, Chennai, Tamil Nadu, India

Abstract

Pharmacogenomics (PGx) research has created a new foundational knowledge for understanding the impact of genetic variation on drug response, about which we are beginning to slowly evolve toward personalized medicine. Nevertheless, the complexities, amounts, and variability of multi-omics and clinical data will always be challenges and will continue to challenge the application of gained genomic knowledge to therapeutic interventions and clinical contexts. However, artificial intelligence (AI) is a powerful tool that can help facilitate, integrate, compare, analyze, and interpret incoming datasets with the objective of predicting drug efficacy, optimizing dosing, and ultimately enhancing the reduction of adverse drug reactions, safety, and efficacy in real time. In this article, we will review and

**Corresponding author*: ssuresh@unom.ac.in
P. Jyothi: ORCID: 0000-0001-5552-3130

Umesh Kumar Lilhore, Kaamran Raahemifar, Sarita Simaiya, R. Sunder and R. Lotus (eds.) Pharmacogenomics Using Artificial Intelligence: Optimizing Drug Response through Personalized Genomic Analysis, (23–48) © 2026 Scrivener Publishing LLC

impersonalize the existing body of AI methods currently applied in PGx, including machine learning, deep learning, natural language processing, and graph-based methods used to convert a wide range of varied, raw genomic datasets into relevant and useful strategies for treatment. This will involve our quantification of examples of real-world applications across therapeutic areas, addressing some barriers to AI-driven PGx (e.g., data privacy, algorithmic bias, interpretability), and provide a synthesis of the promising next steps in this space (i.e., advancements in explainable AI, federated learning, potential use of Internet of Things devices to obtain real-world data in real time in PGx). AI-assisted PGx can bridge the gap from genomic scientists to clinicians and streamline the movement along the data-to-therapy continuum across the entire patient experience in healthcare and performance—creating the next chapters in the evolution toward precision and personalized medicine.

Keywords: Pharmacogenomics (PGx), precision medicine, artificial intelligence (AI), multi-omics integration, clinical decision support systems (CDSS), explainable AI (XAI)

2.1 Introduction

Pharmacogenomics (PGx) has evolved into one of the key pillars of precision medicine and has the potential to individualize medicine based on the unique genetic makeup of the patient. Over the course of the past 20 years, PGx has moved from single isolated gene activities to the inclusion of multi-engagement activities due to the advances of next-generation sequencing, multi-omics activities, and clinical scholarship. The growing complexity and scale of genomic datasets provide challenges with analytic methods whether that be based on large models or new emerging models; traditional methods cannot be utilized with research patients as typically seen as the outcome of multiple, functional genomics mechanisms of interactions and history of activity [1]. AI with PGx is able to allow for some of these non-linearities and heterogeneous data, demonstrating a predictive analytic model for PGx to address previous thoughts. The implications of AI is an evolution of convergence approach from discovery-based research to client actionability and individualized patient care. Alongside AI, systemic challenges/limitations with regard to data interoperability, integration, and equitable interpretation are presented. The aim of this article is to outline the use of AI to bridge the gap between pharmacogenomic discovery and application to therapy, with the hope of creating a pathway for the translation of "bench to bedside" into precision medicine for use in the real world [2].

2.1.1 Evolution of Pharmacogenomics from Bench to Bedside

Pharmacogenomics (PGx) has transitioned from a speculative science into one of the cornerstones of precision medicine. This study defines pharmacogenomics (PGx) as the study of how single and multiple genetic variations affect drug metabolism as well as how these variations can be used to bring pharmacogenomics into practice and ultimately toward personalized medicine. Historically, PGx has often remained within the confines of simple laboratory studies that focused primarily on identifying single-gene variants that influenced drug metabolism such as the polymorphisms of cytochrome P450 (CYP450). However, advances in high-throughput sequencing, genome-wide association studies (GWAS), and bioinformatics have improved our understanding of polygenic effects which include other gene–environment interactions.

The clinical uptake of PGx information was sporadic and, at the time, largely limited to individual medication use when there was enough genetic and clinical evidence to consider incorporating genetic variation information into practices. This situation changed drastically over the last decade with increased clinical guidance from groups such as the Clinical Pharmacogenetics Implementation Consortium (CPIC), increased recommendations from the FDA and other regulatory agencies, as well as newer incorporation options into electronic health records (EHR) and clinical decision support systems (CDSS) that enabled genotype-guided prescribing choices. These advanced experiential opportunities reflect the gradual transition from the bench of university laboratories to the bedside of patients, making the shift toward tailored therapy possible from clinical evidence supporting the use of genetics to personalizing drug choices, dosage, and risk assessment. A primary goal of PGx research has been to maximize drug efficacy while minimizing adverse drug reactions [3].

2.1.2 The Increasing Complexity of Genomic Datasets

Genomic datasets are today exponentially more complex than genomic datasets in early pharmacogenomics. Technologies such as next-generation sequencing (NGS), multi-omics profiling, and single-cell technologies are enabling new ways of using high-dimensional data in a variety of ways that get, at variation, seen on the genomic (i.e., DNA), transcriptomic (i.e., RNA), proteomic (i.e., protein), metabolomic (i.e., metabolites), epigenetic (i.e., methylation, etc.), and of course everything in between. These sources of data often contain longitudinal clinical data, environmental exposures, and health behaviors in an effort to build systems with heterogeneous, multi-modal data. This hybrid of information is complex and not only because of scale (terabytes, perhaps even petabytes) but because of the nature of interdependencies between variables that impact drug response. Traditional statistical methods have enormous difficulties in deciphering these non-linear interactions at scale despite the appropriate consideration of either rare variants, polygenic risk scores, or just dynamic biological processes. Such data quality, interoperability, and missing data has always been and still is an impediment. Look, studying all of these data is a complex undertaking to try to analyze and synthesize; so, it is clear from the discussion above that we need to be able to algorithmically parse out underlying signals to derive meaningful phenotypic predictions and, ultimately, clinical actions. It only follows that it is reasonable to conjecture that potentially transformative artificial intelligence capacities may be capable and enable pharmacogenomic studies [4].

2.1.3 Transformative Tool for PGx

Artificial intelligence has an outstanding capacity to transform the practice of pharmacogenomics from more of a research activity to a clinician-scale tool, thereby solving the scale, complexity, and multi-modality of today's biomedical data. AI will combine architectures of deep learning such as CNN and transformers which depend on spatial understandings of sequence data, multi-omics, and unstructured data from EMRs. To attain this goal, AI has the ability to consume massive types of data, derived from genomics, transcriptomics, and real-world data from electronic medical records, that will enable more precise estimates of drug efficacy, dosing, and adverse drug reactions. Most importantly, AI can also facilitate the repurposing of therapeutics and identification of new biomarkers based on its review of the vast amount of literature and tagging gene–drug pairs for new associations. Beyond prediction, the arrival of new explainable AI (XAI) methods may also serve to increase clinicians' trust of the models they will have to depend on, which may become explainable or interpretable approaches. In this way, AI is impacting the field of pharmacogenomics, transitioning it from a more scientific research effort to a very scalable clinical endeavor that may facilitate a more expeditious intersection of pharmacogenomics from the time when genomics becomes knowledge to the time it becomes actionable in the form of therapeutic interventions [5].

2.1.4 Problem Statement: Present Bottlenecks in PGx-Driven Clinical Translation

Research has made strides with regard to using the information of pharmacogenomics (PGx) in practice; however, there are still many challenges. The disassociation of genomic, clinical, and environmental data is an impediment to synthesis and integration as the collection of this type of data is often done in silos at different institutions and in different formats. Furthermore, there are limitations of genomic datasets, and very few datasets represent a diverse population, which leads to the possible bias in interpretations that would likely not be generalizable to other populations. The interpretability of many PGx algorithms presents problems for clinicians, many of which are simply "black boxes" that suggest courses of treatment without transparent explanations, thus decreasing their acceptability. The regulatory environment around AI and PGx continues to evolve, and a lot of the useful tools are still in validation/review limbo waiting for approval and, ultimately, practical use. There are still ethical challenges concerning the interpretation of privacy, informed consent, and second use of genomic data. Adoption is impeded and delayed as there are no standard workflows for genotyping, data analysis, and clinical implementation at a reasonable cost model in clinical practice. Ultimately, overcoming these bottlenecks can be a complex undertaking and may require significant collaborations across disciplines and new computational tools with needed policy making to ensure equitable, accurate, and ethical translation of PGx to personalized medical care.

This chapter provides a detailed overview of how artificial intelligence can fill the gap between pharmacogenomic discoveries and therapeutic utilization and specifically focuses on the "from data to therapy" journey. While previous works have either provided an overview of the concepts in PGx or a review of the methodologies in AI, this chapter synthesizes both topics to illustrate an integrated vision for precision medicine. It offers a summary of how PGx data has evolved, outlines innovative AI methods that offer the potential for automated multimodal integration, and highlights the use of PGx data as it applies to real-world clinical practice and implementation in specific therapeutic contexts. This chapter is unique because (1) it specifically connects the AI methods to the case example in a clinical context, (2) it offers systemic principles for bottlenecks in the translational approaches, and (3) it addresses promising future approaches such as explainable AI, federated learning, and Internet of Things real-time monitoring. This chapter can be contextually valuable as a forward look into the future of genomics technology and AI methods in the interest of more effective, safe, and equitable patient care.

2.2 Data Foundations in AI-Driven Pharmacogenomics

Pharmacogenomics (PGx) incorporates genetic data to scientifically advance drug treatment to improve efficacy and reduce risks. The use of artificial intelligence (AI) will allow users to analyze complex data sets of genomic, multi-omics, and clinical data to develop practical therapeutic recommendations from raw data and achieve the goal of personalized medicine.

2.2.1 Genomic Data Sources

Genomic data is the foundation of pharmacogenomics research. Whole-genome sequencing (WGS) provides an exceptionally comprehensive view of an individual's genetic composition by capturing common and rare variants that may affect drug metabolism, efficacy, and toxicity. WGS can also identify new pharmacogenomic markers as well as reveal information even before we recognize it as statistically significant to predict drug response. While SNP genotyping may not capture the breadth of WGS, NPC typically offers a cost-effective alternative to identify clinically actionable variants, with evidence of drug–response associations/relationships noted in the clinical pharmacogenomic literature. Figure 2.1 illustrates the sources of genomic data and its relevance to drug response.

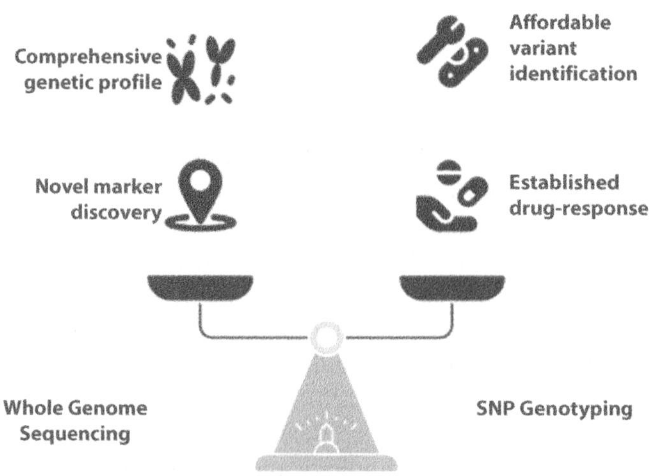

Figure 2.1 Genomic data sources.

SNP arrays are prominent in clinical testing and varying scientific fields because they are scalable and easily interpretable. This information is relevant in epigenomics as it provides an additional layer of regulation to an individual's genetics and shows how modifications to the chemical features of DNA (e.g., methylation) and histone proteins may drive additional regulation of gene expression without the alteration of the genetic code. Epigenetic variations have the potential to alter the function of drug-metabolizing enzymes or transporters and can change the mechanism in which treatment is received. Whole-genome sequencing (WGS) and single-nucleotide polymorphism (SNP) genotyping would be clearly complemented by an epigenomic profile, leading to a deeper layer of genetic bioformat that would be beneficial for AI prediction modeling. The amount and complexity of this type of data, however, will require the innovation of the computational framework for storage, processing, and analysis. Artificial intelligence models, in particular, deep learning, hold potential applications for revealing patterns within high-dimensional genomic data, allowing high-dimensional sequences to become meaningful therapies [6].

2.2.2 Multi-Omics Integration

Pharmacogenomics can also be utilized by integrating layers of "omics" data, which is called multi-omics, other than genomics. For example, the field of transcriptomics examines the expression of genes in different physiological or pathological states and thus defines the functional readout of some genomic variant. Therefore, if RNA sequencing data were obtained, we could potentially characterize alternative splicing events or expression quantitative trait loci (eQTLs), which may impact drug response. Next, proteomics measures the abundance of proteins and post-translational modification levels directly and is consequently important to understand drug targets and drug mechanisms of actions based on protein–protein interactions. It is important to identify proteins as metabolites using biochemical pathways, and metabolomics measures the small molecules and intermediates of metabolism, and this identification will capture the activities and fluxes based on biochemical activities due to genetic variants and/or drug exposures [7]. Figure 2.2 presents the multi-omics integration.

Multi-omics integration in pharmacogenomics provides a systems-level understanding of drug action by linking genetic variation with molecular phenotypes and therapy/drug response. AI models, particularly multi-modal deep learning architectures, can better integrate heterogeneous omics data and reflect nonlinear and dynamic dependencies than traditional statistical approaches. This method will provide novel drug and biomarker candidates,

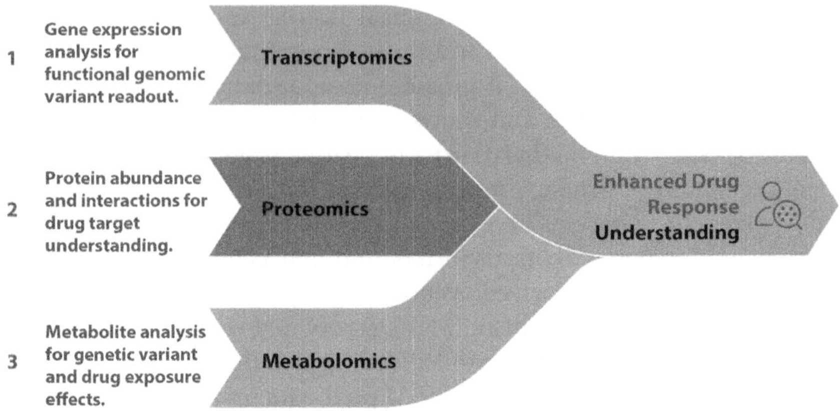

Figure 2.2 Multi-omics integration.

drug repurposing opportunities, and dosing strategies tailored for pharmacogenetics or pharmacogenomics. AI-driven pharmacogenomics models can better exploit multi-omics datasets, improving predictive accuracy and patient stratification, expanding mechanistic understandings, and ultimately supporting the drug development of precision therapeutics targeted to each individual's molecular and biological characteristic [8].

2.2.3 Clinical and Real-World Data

The combination of pharmacogenomic knowledge with the real-world data of patients provides a pragmatic value in relevant operational science. Electronic health records (EHR) include longitudinal patient data in relation to individual patient medical history, including diagnoses, laboratory tests and results, prescription medications, and clinical outcomes. Patient-level EHR provides a greater contextualization for any genomic composite, and PGx data can provide context for comorbidity, concomitant medications, and lifestyle-related factors that may have an association with statistically significant drug responses. Wearable devices (e.g., Fitbits, etc.) provide a continuous stream of physiologic data (heart rate, blood pressure, glucose, activity, etc.) that provide a patient on treatment with real-time diagnostic feedback on treatment response and tolerability.

Patient-reported outcomes (PROs) provide valuable information into subjective experiences, such as symptom relief, side effects, and quality of life, aspects that are often omitted in clinical trials as a small piece of information that pertains to the patient. Although this type of data is discrete, which is again one small piece of information about a patient's perspective, the information included as PROs can be synthesized together to more accurately demonstrate a patient profile that accounts for not only molecular biology but also environmental, behavioral, and psychosocial determinants of health. Clinical and real-world data are uncertain, incomplete, heterogeneous, and overall difficult to preprocess and harmonize. The use of AI methods, especially the natural language processing methods to analyze the unstructured data describing the clinical records, can be useful in extrapolating many of the PGx-relevant details. In short, clinical and real-world data, which is information informed by genomic data, will ultimately provide the opportunity to "truly personalize" the therapeutic context or decision-making based on both molecularly determined predisposition and the personal lived experience of patients [9].

2.2.4 Data Quality, Curation, and Standardization

Genomic and clinical datasets are often derived from various sources and collected in different ways that lead to inconsistencies and result in biased model outputs. In order to build quality data as statistically and/or biologically informed replacements, validation, removing invalid data, and, in some cases, replacing missing data are necessary. Curation steps may also entail standardizing the terms used to compile datasets, which may include gene names, drug identifiers, and even descriptions of phenotypes looking to reuse standardized terminologies such as HGNC, RxNorm, and SNOMED CT [10].

Interoperability is an important issue as datasets usually are compliant with different metadata standards, file formats, and architectures. Frameworks such as Fast Healthcare Interoperability Resources (FHIR) for clinical data (and standards from GA4GH (Global Alliance for Genomics and Health) for genomic data) will help to provide acceptable data sharing. An important step in interoperability is metadata annotation (for documenting experimental conditions, data provenance, and quality measures, transparency, and reproducibility). It is important to maintain high-fidelity metadata in datasets to ensure reproducibility and generalizability of findings, even more so as these are developed into AI algorithms as artificial intelligence (AI) "can only know and learn from the data that it is provided". Poor-quality datasets will negatively impact the fidelity of AI–PGx models, with potential for AI models to overfit to substandard datasets and not translate clinically. This suggests that establishing strong data pipelines, for removing outliers, annotating datasets, and harmonizing datasets, is a careful consideration to prospectively overcome prior to data collection. The pipelines and clear and established data annotations are necessary for AI–PGx data to become trustworthy, regulatory compliant, and clinically validated software components [11].

2.3 AI Methodologies in PGx

Artificial intelligence (AI) encompasses a large range of computational approaches which can analyze complex, heterogeneous pharmacogenomic (PGx) data. From the traditional machine learning algorithms to the more sophisticated deep learning packages, each technique, each in its own way, can contribute something to the discovery of linkages between genetically based variation and drug response. AI also has natural language processing (NLP) capability to analyze irrelevant data from unstructured biological literature and clinical notes and graph-based models to connect complex relationships among drugs, genes, and diseases. Together they constitute a landscape of technologies that will become a part of a toolbox that will translate genomic and clinical data into clinically useful insights and, hence, add to the aims of precision medicine.

2.3.1 Machine Learning Techniques

Machine learning (ML) refers to algorithms that generalize based on data obtained from past observations to predict based on the data for future unobserved observations and to discover structures in data without needing to write code. In PGx, supervised learning algorithms, such as random forests, support vector machines, and gradient boosting, are applied to observe an association with drug response or adverse events with labeled genomic and clinical data. Unsupervised learning methods, such as clustering and dimensionality reduction, are employed to reveal patient subsets with a common genomic characteristic or underlying structure in multi-omics data [12]. Reinforcement learning (RL) methods are being applied in PGx research to develop personalized adaptive treatment strategies. In this application, RL algorithms learn how to prescribe a drug regimen to patient individuals by maximizing a reward signal (e.g., therapeutic success) in a time-dependent manner. RL is relevant to PGx research due to the clinical complexity often examined in data, e.g., the progression of drug response with cancer progression in oncology, or treatment sequencing. All of these ML methods perform well in the context of high-dimensional data, but care must be taken in selecting a reasonable number of features for use in a model, pre-processing the data where appropriate, and justifying the model by avoiding overfitting and ensuring generalizability. Since PGx and the use of ML in routine clinical practice is at the early developmental stage and will require transparency in model explanation for future clinical interpretation and use by clinicians, initial

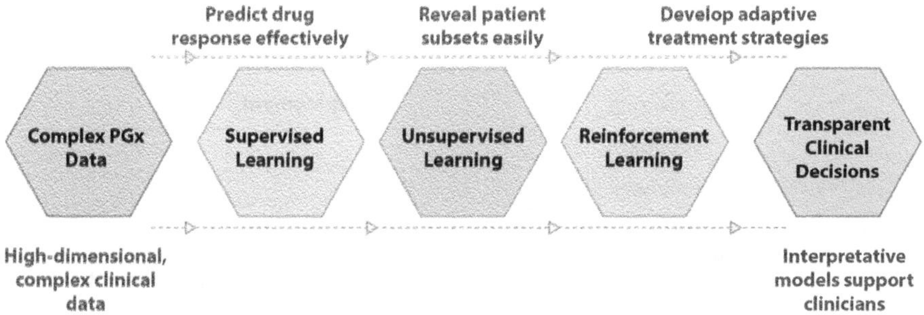

Figure 2.3 Machine learning approaches for pharmacogenomics data interpretation and decision-making.

model reports should also consider interpretability so that predictive inferences can be made based on the genetic features that contribute to predictions and provide a transparent method in supporting clinical decisions for therapeutic use. Figure 2.3 provides the complex PGx data processed *via* ML for transparent clinical decisions [13]. Figure 2.4 presents the workflow which illustrates healthcare data life cycle: acquisition, processing, modeling, validation, deployment, and continuous feedback.

2.3.2 Deep Learning Architectures

Deep learning (DL) is an area of AI, which uses multilayered neural networks and is able to model complex, non-linear relationships with large datasets. In precision genomic medicine, convolutional neural networks (CNNs) [14] have been used successfully to analyze genomic sequence data and detect motifs and structural variants, which are important for drug metabolism. Recurrent neural networks (RNNs) and their extensions, including long short-term memory (LSTM) neural networks [15], allow for modeling temporal or longitudinal data, which helps in predicting responses to treatment over time. Transformers, first popularized in natural language processing applications, are becoming increasingly common in multiplexed precision genomic medicine approaches combining genomic and clinical features and biochemical variables from patient data. Because of their attention mechanisms, it can determine which of the features obtained from the genomic data and clinical or biochemical data influences the prediction and how much. Thus, they can be useful contributing factors that make the model more interpretable and effective.

The ability of deep learning models to predict clinical attributes is outstanding, particularly with large high-dimensional datasets (e.g., genome

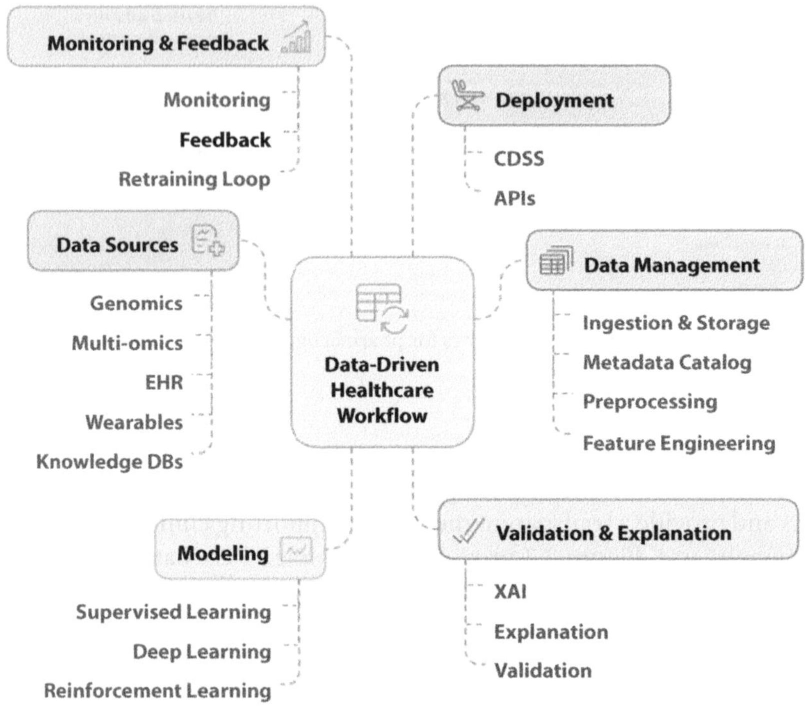

Figure 2.4 Data-driven healthcare workflow integrating sources, management, modeling, validation, deployment, and feedback.

sequencing, RNA sequences, etc.). However, their success, when usefully applied, depends on high-performance computing resources, ground-truth data and labeled training datasets, and procedures to manage or control overfitting risk. Many of the recent developments in explainable deep learning are critical to translate these complex but powerful models into clinical practice as the models do not depict if or how genomic variants or any of the patient attributes incorporated are influencing the drug response prediction [16].

2.3.3 Natural Language Processing

Natural language processing (NLP) makes it possible for AI systems to understand, interpret, and extract information from unstructured text environments rife with biomedical literature, clinical notes, and pharmacogenomic guidelines. Using NLP in PGx can be useful to mine scientific literature for gene–drug interactions, emerging pharmacogenetic markers, and new therapeutic targets. Once the information is transformed into the electronic health record, NLP can scan physician notes that are free-text-generated to identify genotype–phenotype correlations, treatment outcome, and adverse drug reactions that are not recorded in structured fields since clinicians may opt to not record patient genotype data. Also, NLP allows for the incorporation of guideline-based information derived from CPIC and PharmGKB to inject existing knowledge and/or evidence into decision support systems that inform AI systems on clinical recommendations based on the evidence for PGx [17].

Utilizing large pretrained language models as foundation models in biomedical contexts can also empower increasingly advanced NLP algorithms, such as domain-specific language models like BioBERT or GPT-like biomedical transformer models, which are more sensitive to domain-specific vocabulary and contextual information; this is particularly useful when considering entity recognition, relation extraction, and summarization with the aim of increasing precision. Essentially, NLP helps combine unstructured textual knowledge with the structured genomic datasets. This interaction broadens the scope for AI in PGx to provide more clinically relevant therapeutic recommendations. Nevertheless, privacy-preserving techniques and bias mitigation will be topics demanding attention as NLP becomes integrated into clinical settings.

2.3.4 Graph-Based AI Models

Graph-based AI models provide a natural framework for representing and analyzing the complex, interconnected relationships in pharmacogenomics. A knowledge graph can model entities such as genes, drugs, diseases, pathways, and phenotypes as nodes, with edges representing known associations, interactions, or causal relationships. These graphs can integrate heterogeneous data sources including genomic variants, biochemical pathways, literature-derived associations, and clinical trial results into a unified network. Graph neural networks (GNNs) extend deep learning to graph structures, enabling the prediction of new links, such as potential drug–gene interactions, or inferring novel disease associations. In PGx, graph-based models can identify multi-target drug candidates, predict off-target effects, and support drug repurposing by exploring the network topology. They are also valuable for visualizing and explaining AI predictions, as relationships between nodes are explicit and interpretable. The integration of graph-based AI with other modalities, such as multi-omics and NLP-derived knowledge, enhances the ability to generate hypothesis-driven insights. While promising, challenges include ensuring graph completeness, handling noisy edges, and maintaining scalability as data complexity grows [18, 19].

2.4 Translating Data to Therapy: Key AI-Driven PGx Applications

Pharmacogenomics' (PGx) goal is to facilitate the transition from genomic findings to usable clinical information. Artificial intelligence (AI) has been essential to this transition through its ability to predict drug response, optimize drug dosing, find new therapeutic uses of drugs, and provide clinical support in real time. AI has emerged as a game-changer in our ability to recognize patterns in data previously considered inconsequential. By utilizing a large data set and advanced algorithms, AI is capable of identifying patterns in genomic data and multi-omics and revealing the relationships between genetic variation and a drug's efficacy or safety. This level of pattern recognition empowers prescribers to make informed, one-off, personalized prescribing decisions that take a patient's genetics into account. Furthermore, AI-PGx applications assist in predicting severe adverse drug reactions before they occur (adverse drug reaction prediction) or changing which patients a drug is utilized for (drug repurposing) depending on an individual's genetics when multiple drugs are available to treat the same disease. By utilizing AI in PGx, enhanced treatment sequences that are more robust, reliable, comprehensive, and affordable are likely to emerge. This subsection attempts to define some of the broader application areas in which AI can enhance PGx, with some practical examples and emerging research. Figure 2.5 depicts the AI-based PGx applications.

2.4.1 Drug Response Prediction

Drug response prediction is the first level of precision medicine in PGx and principally aims to determine whether or not a given medication will provide an improved response for the patient or will ultimately provide adverse effects as a result of drug response. AI models, using supervised learning algorithms (such as random forests and gradient boosting machines), utilize available genomic, transcriptomic, and clinical datasets to define patient classification, designating them as a responder or non-responder. The recent use of deep learning architectures enables AI models to better predict the likelihood of drug response by modeling and representing complex interactions of non-linear relationships between genetic variants

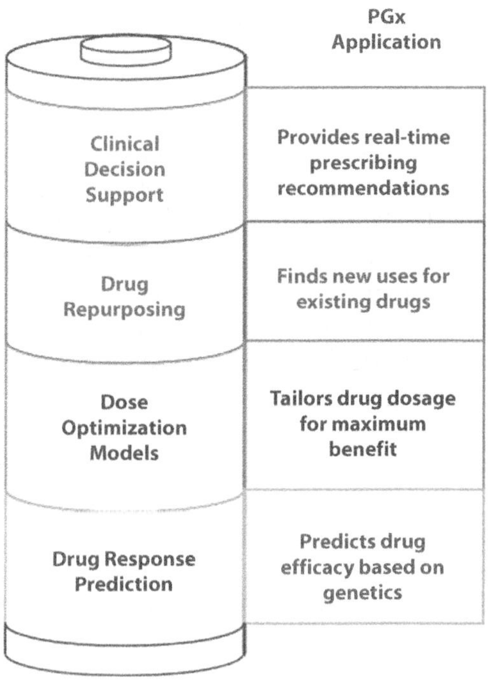

Figure 2.5 AI-driven PGx applications.

and drug response phenotypes. For example, in oncology, AI-based PGx platforms aid clinicians in predicting tumor sensitivity to chemotherapy based on mutational signatures that allow a clinician to select a more precise type of treatment for a patient [20].

Another example in different fields of medicine, is the discovery of assigning count data (such as consequence processing in CGTP19 and clinical response to clopidogrel) to develop machine learning models that predict the likelihood of adverse effects from clopidogrel to mitigate thrombotic events. AI platforms can also predict adverse drug reactions rather than yes/no decisions, as in the case of prediction of statin myopathy from genetic variants in SLCO1B1. Not only does this process improve patient safety, but it also eliminates wasteful trial-and-error prescribing, which improves both the healthcare system and therapeutic outcomes.

2.4.2 Dose Optimization Models

Dose optimization models combine AI techniques with PGx insights to suggest individualized drug dosages with the intent of maximizing efficacy and minimizing toxicity. Supervised regression algorithms and reinforcement learning techniques may be used to model a drug's dose–response curve based on genetic factors, metabolic rates, and, in real time, the patient's status. For example, warfarin dosing is notoriously difficult because of its narrow therapeutic index and wide inter-patient variability. Studies utilizing AI-driven dosing models to optimize warfarin dosing based on not only CYP2C9 and VKORC1 genotypes but also patient demographics, dieting patterns, and INR monitoring data have proven to have greater utility than previous dosing algorithms [21].

In oncology, researchers have used deep learning models to dose 5-fluorouracil (5-FU) in a particular patient based on genetic markers in dihydropyrimidine dehydrogenase (DPYD) along with liver enzymes and body composition data. Reinforcement learning can facilitate changing doses dynamically using therapeutic drug monitoring as feedback if a doctor continues to see patients with the same type of genetically diverse characteristics, allowing for treatments that are safer and more effective for patients with genetic diversity. These models demonstrate practical implementations in clinical decision support tools that allow for the physician to adjust prescriptions in real time [22].

2.4.3 Drug Repurposing and Discovery

Utilizing PGx data to inform AI-guided drug repurposing offers two distinct approaches to new therapies—either identifying new uses of existing drugs or new drugs altogether for genetically defined patient populations. Graph-based neural networks and multi-modal integration based models can utilize genomic data, drug–target interaction repositories, and chemical structure data to uncover therapeutic opportunities that would have remained unknown. For example, AI systems have uncovered drug candidates that could be repurposed for Alzheimer's disease by forming links between APOE genotypes and drug–gene interaction profiles [23].

AI models have also provided insight into oncology drug repurposing for inhibitors of kinases that were developed from very different cancers than the related tumors that contained matching genetic mutations. Virtual screening platforms utilize deep learning architectures like convolutional neural networks (CNNs) for molecular docking predictions to screen thousands of compounds against genotype-defined targets in a fraction of time and cost needed for early-stage drug discovery. PGx biomarkers would ensure that any repurposed or new drug would have been developed for patient subgroups that were most likely to respond, improving clinical trial success rates, and enabling precision therapeutics with lower development risks [24].

2.4.4 Clinical Decision Support Systems (CDSS)

Clinical decision support systems (CDSS) combine AI and PGx information to offer real-time prescribing recommendations based on patient characteristics at the point of care. For instance, CDSS can be used in electronic health record (EHR) platforms, so the physician does not need to leave the clinical workflow to access the genotype-specific recommendations. In addition to recommending medication based on the gene variants, AI can analyze complex genomic information along with up-to-date guidelines (e.g., CPIC, DPWG) and provide warnings about drug–gene interactions and contraindications. For example, a CDSS that is embedded within a hospital system might automatically pop up warnings for patients with a CYP2D6 poor metabolizer status when codeine is prescribed and even suggest alternative analgesics to avoid ineffective pain control [25].

In more advanced CDSS, predictive analytics are used not only to warn of adverse drug reactions but also to recommend the best therapies based on the patient's genomic and clinical profile. In mental health care, CDSS has been used to guide select specific antidepressants into a treatment plan by including serotonin transporter polymorphism and evidence of symptom trajectory from the patient. The development of AI-driven CDSS not only enhances efficiency and reduces adverse events in the clinical setting but also facilitates the more reliable application of PGx knowledge in everyday clinical practice. This application supports the scalability and sustainability of personalized medicine [26].

2.5 Challenges and Limitations

Although artificial intelligence has enormous potential to transform pharmacogenomics (PGx), there are a number of potential hurdles to its effective deployment in routine clinical practice. As shown in Figure 2.6, potential hurdles include the ethics and privacy of data, interpretability of models, bias in datasets, and regulatory requirements. Failing to address these issues can lead to potential limited uptake of the most valid AI models, variability in accuracy of AI models applied in healthcare systems, and ethical concerns involved with AI applications in practice.

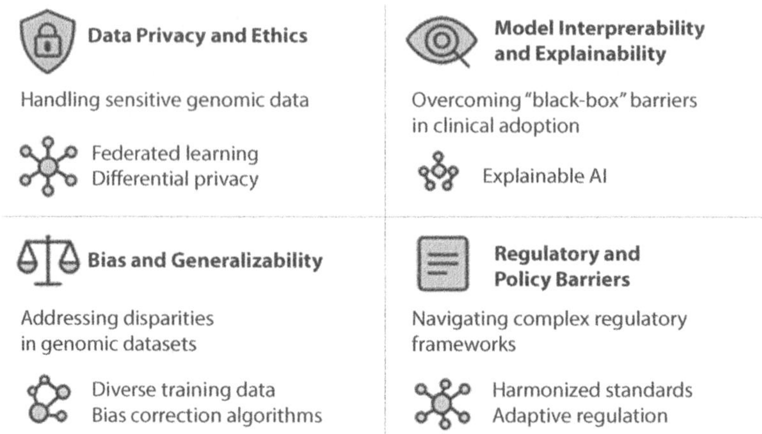

Figure 2.6 Challenges in AI–PGx application.

2.5.1 Data Privacy and Ethics

Protecting sensitive genomic data must be taken seriously, as genomic data is personal and unchangeable. Most unconsented practices regarding genomic data often yield harmful consequences; if genomic data is misappropriated at any level, it can cause discrimination regarding employment or insurance or many unethical social implications through disclosures. There are ethical principles or laws—such as the Genetic Information Nondiscrimination Act (GINA) in the US, which aims to minimize discriminations involving genetic data, and there are similar, though inconsistent, global principles and laws; ethical boundaries do not exist in common. Therefore, using AI-aware PGx platforms is still crucial to incorporate integrated privacy approaches like federated learning. A machine learning technique allows researchers to build models from genomic data secretly and through multiple institutions without valuable genomic data leaving the institution and uses differential privacy with the injection of statistical noise to obfuscate and shield people's identity. For example, in the All of Us Research Program, researchers create datasets from genomic and clinical observational data that have been previously de-identified prior to being stored in secure cloud repositories with different access agreements or levels. Patients factor in addition to technical constraints especially for informed consent—patients have to be informed of the way genomic data will be utilized if potentially shared for research or clinical observations. Patients also have to be informed of where, how, and how long genomic data is stored. A committed ethical process needs to be undertaken to stimulate trust and confidence with patients especially when the expectation is to collect quantitative genomic data on the scale of the largest studies [27].

2.5.2 Model Interpretability and Explainability

Deep learning, along with many other sophisticated AI models, represents a "black box" that is the antithesis of the commonly assumed validity to be transferred to practice in the PGx field, where clinicians expect a reasoning process for drug recommendations that is clear and understandable. There have been advances in explainable AI (XAI), including SHAP (Shapley Additive Explanations), LIME (Local Interpretable Model-Agnostic Explanations), and attention mechanism behaviors that would add value by helping clinicians understand how a genetic marker, lab value, or clinical feature might impact the prediction. For example, if a model predicted warfarin dosing, the model could have identified VKORC1 and CYP2C9 gene variants as driving recommendations. Within oncology PGx, interpretable models can use visual heatmaps to indicate how certain SNP patterns have been incorporated to create a prediction of chemotherapy tolerance. Providing a measure of transparency through the use of interpretable AI models can increase clinicians' trust and validity of using PGx models and better support regulatory approvals. Interpretable models may also bring new biological meanings and linkages, like identifying new gene-drug interactions, which can lead to new research directions and drug discovery [28].

2.5.3 Bias and Generalizability

If AI models have been developed based on biased or not fully representative genomic data sets, there is a risk of their delivering inequitable results. While many of the existing PGx studies have samples that primarily consist of individuals of European ancestry—where the majority of PGx research and literature is based almost solely on European ancestry individuals—this leads to many questions as to how those models can be applied to the rest of ethnically diverse groups. For example, differences exist between the population and regional distributions of the CYP2D6 allele. This is especially important because CYP2D6 metabolism of tamoxifen or codeine varies between individuals of African ancestry, Asian ancestry, and European ancestry. Models developed that did not account for these differences may recommend safe dosing parameters that are unsafe for these underrepresented groups. Ways to address these issues include controlled diversity, using bias correction algorithms, and advocating the validation of proposed models across multiple population cohorts before implementing them. We see the merging of genomic databases in ventures such as the UK Biobank and GenomeAsia 100K, which contributes toward developing a better representation within genomic databases within a global context. Establishing the reliability (generalizability) of PGx models is critical to being able to support fairness with supporting clinical safety and effectiveness with clinicians and patients globally [29].

2.5.4 Regulatory and Policy Barriers

Before AI–PGx tools can be implemented at a clinical level, several regulatory hurdles must be resolved, as the regulatory agencies (e.g., US Food and Drug Administration (FDA), European Medicines Agency (EMA), Health Canada, etc.) expect proof of analytical validity, clinical validity, and clinical utility. Guidelines for regulating AI models, particularly continuously adaptive models, are being developed. The FDA's Software as a Medical Device (SaMD) framework provides a mechanism for approval, but it is unclear how to audit AI algorithms that change over time. The barriers to transnational collaboration are further complicated by differences in national governance of genomic data. The EU General Data Protection Regulation (GDPR) has a robust governance of genomic data that prohibits sharing genomic data outside of the EU. Moving forward, stakeholders will need to create global harmonized standards, adaptive regulatory frameworks, and post-marketing surveillance mechanisms for AI–PGx models to ensure that they remain safe and effective sources of health information across their use [30].

2.6 Future Perspectives

The justifiable future of AI in pharmacogenomics (PGx) is transparency, collaboration, and real-time incorporation of genomic understanding into clinical care. New paradigms such as explainable AI, federated learning, IoT-enabled real-time monitoring, and AI-augmented clinical trials as shown in Figure 2.7 will begin to close the gap between data generation and patient outcomes in a more trustworthy, accessible, and impactful way in precision medicine.

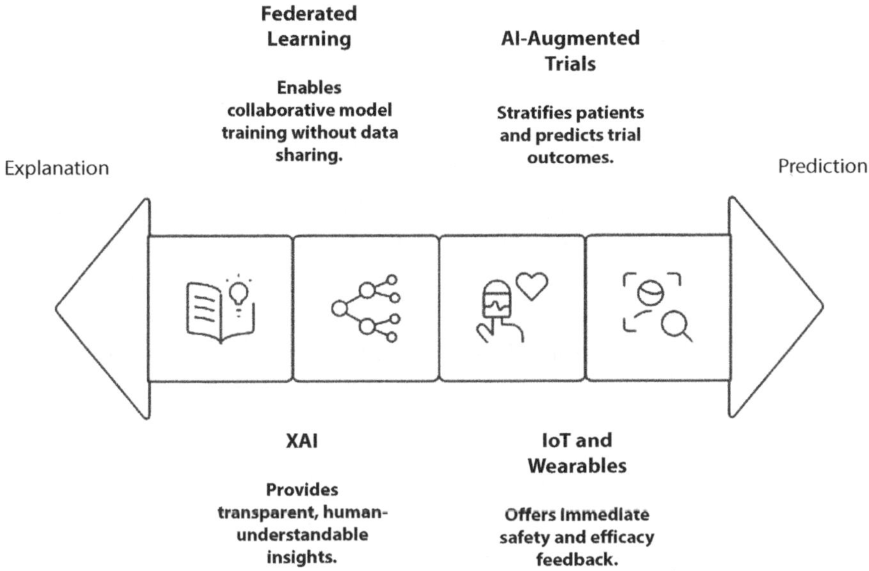

Figure 2.7 AI's role in PGx.

2.6.1 Explainable AI (XAI) for PGx

Explainable AI (XAI) is an important way to overcome one of the major barriers for adopting AI in PGx resistance by clinicians to using "black box" models. XAI produces insights in a way that humans can comprehend, which enables clinicians to gain a clear insight to why a certain drug recommendation or dosing adjustment was made. For example, a drug response prediction system which incorporates XAI will be able to demonstrate which genetic variants (e.g., CYP2C9, VKORC1) are germane to warfarin dosing. This level of transparency is a quantification of trust by clinicians in response prediction models due to fewer information asymmetries involved in the model output rationale. Transparency also promotes model evaluation by a regulator as the latter knows the thinking behind model interpretation and rationale for algorithm output. In general, in accordance with the utilization of pharmacogenomic guidelines, XAI can clarify the association of the specific genome of the patient with CPIC guidelines. Interpretability is also important for shared decision-making whereby the clinician and patient discuss facts rather than algorithmic ambiguity [31].

2.6.2 Federated Learning Technology to Cross-Organization Genomic Models

Federated learning (FL) enables organizations to train AI models in a cooperative manner that does not require the transfer of the raw genomic data and is also secure. In this case, the hospitals or research institutes hold the genomic sequences of the patients and only share updates of models or algorithms, which is nonsensitive data. For example, if you have a PGx drug response model built using FL, then you would be able to build such a model across countries—to allow for the utilization of genomic diversity, consistency, and compliance with regulations like GDPR or HIPAA. Using federated learning would increase model generalizability as it would enable the inclusion of variants of underrepresented populations without causing genomic data to run the risk of privacy breach. In oncology pharmacogenomics, federated learning may allow for developing models predicting targeted therapy responses across cancer centers and at times using mutations for which there were only one or two cases at each center. Federated learning may eliminate the silos, speed up discovery while protecting ethical consideration, and enable international collaboration using AI to develop PGx model [32].

2.6.3 Real-Time PGx *via* IoT and Wearables

In the future, the application of IoT and wearable devices in conjunction with PGx will provide a system for real-time efficacy as well as safety monitoring of drugs. For instance, wearable biosensors can be used by individuals to continuously monitor the biospecimens over time as related to certain biomarkers such as heart rate variability, blood glucose, or drug metabolites. This will allow drug dosage to be established in real time based on pharmacogenomics and nutri-genomics. For example, a patient with epilepsy could be treated with a wearable EEG device that could detect early seizure activity, while the pharmacogenomic profile of the patient with respect to an antiepileptic drug developed, alert the clinician, and trigger an immediate titration change. However, this process makes PGx not a singular event of clinical genetic testing but an experimental and continually evolving therapeutic intervention. In this sense, an algorithm in which AI is present will be able to identify avoidable adverse events and help users to choose avoidance units of analysis in real time. As such, public health analytics can provide instant feedback of safety and efficacy of pharmacogenomic algorithms to their users [33].

2.6.4 AI-Augmented Clinical Trials

AI incorporates disruptive innovation in the design and conduct of clinical trials in PGx by allowing better patient stratification, the ability to have adaptive protocols, and speedier patient recruitment. With the pharmacogenomic profile, AI can take the guesswork out of identifying trial participants with the highest chance of benefitting from or having a sensitivity to being enrolled onto any trial. Statistical power may be increased by lowering variability. For instance, oncology trials can speed up recruitment to targeted medicines by incorporating trial participants who have been shown to have an EGFR mutation. Current AI-augmented monitoring tools can even inform researchers of adverse drug reactions in real time as they are developing trial results, allowing for adaptive dose changes based on multi-parameter monitoring. Additionally, AI can model the conduct of the trial before it occurs, assisting pharmaceutical companies planning to execute recruitment and dropout risks as well as costing out the trial design. In addition, AI in rare association with real-time PGx databases could help combine PGx data with synthetic patient cohorts to improve speed and efficiency in randomized, early-phase potential trial participants. It could be potentially used to shorten trial duration, save costs, and improve likelihood for success of trial [34, 35].

2.7 Conclusion

This chapter outlines the potentially disruptive nature of artificial intelligence to help propel pharmacogenomics (PGx) from research space and into its clinical use in embedded medicine as part of precision medicine. Through the integration of genetic, clinical, and environmental factors, artificial intelligence capabilities offer improved predictive capability for drug response, optimize individual doses, and improve drug development/discovery and drug therapy decision support. However, these potential artificial intelligence capabilities for clinical PGx development should take into consideration potential barriers for use, such as issues of data privacy, interpretability of the models, identifying and mitigating bias involved, and regulatory approval. Future directions including explainable AI, federated learning, IoT-enabled PGx in the real world, and AI-enhanced clinical trials will enhance the transparency, usability, and adaptability of PGx to the contemporary way. These strategies will move PGx from genomic information or confine theories to make a connection between genomic information and the outcome on the patient. This signals a change into an era when leveraging any kind of information of genomics to improve the delivery of targeted and effective therapeutics to patients is enabled by the associated technologies to improve the healthcare experience. The PGx of the future will lead us to better outcomes providing potential precise dose adjustments to maximize the potential to inhibit the activity of the target protein (therapeutic) intervention with the lowest number of adverse events examining the associated enabling technologies that will change the future healthcare experience.

AI disclosure statement: The author acknowledges the use of AI-based tools for minor language editing or grammatical correction. However, all intellectual contributions, analyses, and conclusions presented in this chapter are entirely the author's own.

References

1. Abdelhalim, H., Berber, A., Lodi, M., Jain, R., Nair, A., Pappu, A., Patel, K., *et al.*, Artificial intelligence, healthcare, clinical genomics, and pharmacogenomics approaches in precision medicine. *Front. Genet.*, 13, 929736, 2022.
2. Haga, S.B., Artificial intelligence, medications, pharmacogenomics, and ethics. *Pharmacogenomics*, 25, 14–15, 611–622, 2024.
3. Van Heukelom, J., Morgan, J., Massmann, A., Jacobsen, K., Petry, N.J., Baye, J.F., Frear, S., Schultz, A., Evolution of pharmacogenomic services and implementation of a multi-state pharmacogenomics clinic across a large rural healthcare system. *Front. Pharmacol.*, 14, 1274165, 2023.
4. Zhou, Y., Tremmel, R., Schaeffeler, E., Schwab, M., Lauschke, V.M., Challenges and opportunities associated with rare-variant pharmacogenomics. *Trends Pharmacol. Sci.*, 43, 10, 852–865, 2022.
5. Srivastav, A.K., Mishra, M.K., Lillard, J.W., Jr., Singh, R., Transforming pharmacogenomics and CRISPR gene editing with the power of artificial intelligence for precision medicine. *Pharmaceutics*, 17, 5, 555, 2025.
6. Alpert, J.S., Chen, Q.M., Mulyar, A., Acharya, T., Hung, O., Rajendran, I., Lim, J., Freeman, R., Fedorova, L., Pharmacogenomics: Clinical Progress. *Am. J. Med.*, 2025.
7. Tong, L., Shi, W., Isgut, M., Zhong, Y., Lais, P., Gloster, L., Sun, J., Swain, A., Giuste, F., Wang, M.D., Integrating multi-omics data with EHR for precision medicine using advanced artificial intelligence. *IEEE Rev. Biomed. Eng.*, 17, 80–97, 2023.
8. Saab, Y. and Nakad, Z., Validating the accuracy of mathematical model-based pharmacogenomics dose prediction with real-world data. *Eur. J. Clin. Pharmacol.*, 81, 3, 451–462, 2025.

9. Solaiman, M. and Oluwaferanmi, A., Natural Language Processing (NLP) for Mining Pharmacogenomic Associations from Biomedical Literature, 2025.
10. Kumuthini, J., Zass, L., Chaouch, M., Gill, Z., Ras, V., Mungloo-Dilmohamud, Z., Sathan, D., *et al.*, Data standardization in the omics field, in: *Genomic Data Sharing*, pp. 137–155, Academic Press, Cambridge, Massachusetts, US, 2023.
11. Taddese, A.A., Addis, A.C., Tam, B.T., Data stewardship and curation practices in AI-based genomics and automated microscopy image analysis for high-throughput screening studies: promoting robust and ethical AI applications. *Hum. Genomics*, 19, 1, 16, 2025.
12. Casale, A.D., Sarli, G., Bargagna, P., Polidori, L., Alcibiade, A., Zoppi, T., Borro, M., *et al.*, Machine learning and pharmacogenomics at the time of precision psychiatry. *Curr. Neuropharmacol.*, 21, 12, 2395–2408, 2023.
13. Wei, W-Q., Zhao, J., Roden, D., Peterson, J.F., Machine learning challenges in pharmacogenomic research. *Clin. Pharmacol. Ther.*, 110, 3, 552, 2021.
14. Vaz, J.M. and Balaji, S., Convolutional neural networks (CNNs): concepts and applications in pharmacogenomics. *Mol. Divers.*, 25, 3, 1569–1584, 2021.
15. Abass, Y.A. and Adeshina, S.A., Deep learning methodologies for genomic data prediction. *J. Artif. Intell. Med. Sci.*, 2, 1, 1–11, 2021.
16. Gandhewar, N., Pimpalkar, A., Jadhav, A., Shelke, N., Jain, R., Leveraging Deep Learning for Genomics Analysis: Advances and Applications, in: *Genomics at the Nexus of AI, Computer Vision, and Machine Learning*, p. 191, Scrivener Publishing LLC, US, 2025.
17. Gonzalez Hernandez, F., Structuring the Unstructured: Unlocking pharmacokinetic data from journals with Natural Language Processing, PhD diss., UCL (University College London), 2022.
18. Raupach, L. and Königs, C., PharmoCo: a graph-based visualization of pharmacogenomic plausibility check reports for clinical decision support systems. *J. Integr. Bioinform.*, 20, 4, 20230026, 2024.
19. Li, J., Li, B., Zhang, X., Ma, X., Li, Z., MDMNI-DGD: A novel graph neural network approach for druggable gene discovery based on the integration of multi-omics data and the multi-view network. *Comput. Biol. Med.*, 185, 109511, 2025.
20. de Jong, J., Cutcutache, I., Page, M., Elmoufti, S., Dilley, C., Fröhlich, H., Armstrong, M., Towards realizing the vision of precision medicine: AI based prediction of clinical drug response. *Brain*, 144, 6, 1738–1750, 2021.
21. Punukollu, P., Development of AI-Based Pharmacogenomic Tools for Optimizing Drug Dosing and Therapy Management: Leveraging Machine Learning to Tailor Drug Doses Based on Genetic Variability and Patient Characteristics. *Essex J. AI Ethics Responsible Innov.*, 1, 474–513, 2021.
22. Li, Q-Y., Tang, B-H., Wu, Y-E., Yao, B-F., Zhang, W., Zheng, Y., Zhou, Y., van den Anker, J., Hao, G-X., Zhao, W., Machine learning: a new approach for dose individualization. *Clin. Pharmacol. Ther.*, 115, 4, 727–744, 2024.

23. Pan, X., Lin, X., Cao, D., Zeng, X., Yu, P.S., He, L., Nussinov, R., Cheng, F., Deep learning for drug repurposing: Methods, databases, and applications. *Wiley Interdiscip. Rev. Comput. Mol. Sci.*, 12, 4, e1597, 2022.
24. Chai, A.W.Y., Tan, A.C., Cheong, S.C., Uncovering drug repurposing candidates for head and neck cancers: Insights from systematic pharmacogenomics data analysis. *Sci. Rep.*, 11, 1, 23933, 2021.
25. Farmaki, A., Manolopoulos, E., Natsiavas, P., Will precision medicine meet digital health? A systematic review of pharmacogenomics clinical decision support systems used in clinical practice. *OMICS: J. Integr. Biol.*, 28, 9, 442–460, 2024.
26. Kidwai-Khan, F., Rentsch, C.T., Pulk, R., Alcorn, C., Brandt, C.A., Justice, A.C., Pharmacogenomics driven decision support prototype with machine learning: A framework for improving patient care. *Front. Big Data*, 5, 1059088, 2022.
27. Taofeek, A., Oluwaferanmi, A., Hamzah, F., Philp, A., Johnson, B., Liang, W., John, B., Ethical and Regulatory Considerations of AI-Driven Pharmacogenomics in Clinical Practice, 2025.
28. de Filippis, R. and Al Foysal, A., Pharmacogenomic Approaches to Predicting Susceptibility to Neuroleptic Malignant Syndrome and Severe Anticholinergic Adverse Effects: A Multi-Modal Explainable AI Framework. *Open Access Libr. J.*, 12, 6, 1–18, 2025.
29. Gopal, D.P., Chetty, U., O'Donnell, P., Gajria, C., Blackadder-Weinstein, J., Implicit bias in healthcare: clinical practice, research and decision making. *Future Healthc. J.*, 8, 1, 40–48, 2021.
30. Gonzalez-Hernandez, G., Krallinger, M., Muñoz, M., Rodriguez-Esteban, R., Uzuner, Ö., Hirschman, L., Challenges and opportunities for mining adverse drug reactions: perspectives from pharma, regulatory agencies, healthcare providers and consumers. *Database*, 2022, baac071, 2022.
31. Isa, A., Iliyas, I.I., Umar, I.M., Zarma, M.L., Explainable Artificial Intelligence in genetics: A case study, in: *Deep Learning in Genetics and Genomics*, pp. 313–328, Academic Press, Cambridge, Massachusetts, US, 2025.
32. Kolobkov, D., Sharma, S.M., Medvedev, A., Lebedev, M., Kosaretskiy, E., Vakhitov, R., Efficacy of federated learning on genomic data: a study on the UK Biobank and the 1000 Genomes Project. *Front. Big Data*, 7, 1266031, 2024.
33. Barbhuiya, R.K. and Ahmad, N., IoT applications in translational bioinformatics, in: *Translational Bioinformatics in Healthcare and Medicine*, pp. 69–79, Academic Press, Cambridge, Massachusetts, US, 2021.
34. Kalidindi, V.R., Rehana, S., Seethamraju, S.M., Nori, L.P., Revolutionizing Medicine: Unleashing the Power of Real-World Data and AI in Advancing Clinical Trials. *Braz. J. Pharm. Sci.*, 60, e23980, 2024.
35. Lilhore, U.K. and Simaiya, S., Integrating Multimodal Data Fusion for Advanced Biomedical Analysis: A Comprehensive Review, in: *Multimodal Data Fusion for Bioinformatics Artificial Intelligence*, pp. 127–145, Scrivener Publishing LLC, US 2025.

3

Machine Learning Approaches for Genomic Data Analysis in Pharmacogenomics

Ashwin M.[1], Sreenivas Mekala[2], V. Arun[3], Ashish[4], S. Mathumohan[5] and K. Kaliraj[6]*

[1]Department of Computer Science and Engineering (Data Science), AMC Engineering College, Bengaluru, Karnataka, India
[2]Department of Computer Science and Engineering, School of Agricultural Engineering & Technology, Kaveri University, Gowraram, Telangana, India
[3]Department of Computing Technologies, SRM Institute of Science and Technology, Chennai, Tamil Nadu, India
[4]Department of Computer Science and Information Technology, Koneru Lakshmaiah Education Foundation (K L University), Guntur, Andhra Pradesh, India
[5]Department of Computer Science and Engineering, Fatima Michael College of Engineering and Technology, Madurai, Tamil Nadu, India
[6]Ramanujan Institute for Advanced Study in Mathematics, University of Madras, Chennai, Tamil Nadu, India

Abstract
Pharmacogenomics utilizes genetic variation to improve patient care by optimizing drug therapy with the objective of decreasing adverse drug effects and increasing drug efficacy. Nevertheless, genomic data's high dimensionality and complexity presents significant analytical hurdles. This chapter presents a new multi-modal machine learning framework that includes genomic variants (SNPs and CNVs) and clinical information (age, weight, comorbidities) for accurate and precise drug response predictions. The method includes comprehensive preprocessing, a substantial feature selection, and the use of ensemble learning with deep neural components, which we compared to four state-of-the-art models—random

**Corresponding author*: kaliraj@unom.ac.in

Umesh Kumar Lilhore, Kaamran Raahemifar, Sarita Simaiya, R. Sunder and R. Lotus (eds.) Pharmacogenomics Using Artificial Intelligence: Optimizing Drug Response through Personalized Genomic Analysis, (49–74) forest, SVM, XGBoost, and DNNs. Our results showed that our proposed model outperformed the existing approaches with an accuracy of 94.2%, AUC-ROC score of 0.96, and the RMSE score of 0.18 was the lowest among the models in predicting drug doses. In summary, our study demonstrated that multi-modal data will strengthen pharmacogenomic analyses and will make a robust platform for clinical decision support. Future work will incorporate multi-omics data and federated learning frameworks to improve scalability, privacy, and possible clinical application in precision medicine.

***Keywords*:** Pharmacogenomics, machine learning, genomic variants, drug response prediction, precision medicine, multi-modal integration

3.1 Introduction

Pharmacogenomics is a new field of study that sits at the intersection between pharmacology and genomics which seeks to understand how variations in genetic makeup correspond to individual responses to medications. Pharmacogenomics is a necessary area of study in the precision medicine era, where drug therapies are developed or tailored based on a patient's individual genomic makeup to achieve maximum therapeutic benefit while limiting adverse drug effects [1]. With the rapidly increasing availability of genomic data because of advances in next-generation sequencing and bioinformatics combined with cost-effectiveness, pharmacogenomic data can inform pharmacological development and application to the clinical space. Since pharmacogenomic data can identify genomic biomarkers that can inform drug selection, dosing, and titration, the pace of evolution of this field could lead to innovative clinical potential. While great progress has been made, challenges do exist related to translating genomic data into clinical medicine. Data are high dimensional, patient populations are heterogenous, and gene–drug interactions are complex [2].

In the last 10 years, many computational and statistical approaches have been explored for the analysis of pharmacogenomic data. Early traditional methods, such as linear regression or univariate association analyses, carried important ground work but are primarily characterized by their inability to express complex non-linear relationships that exist in genetic data. More recently, machine learning (ML) has presented a powerful opportunity for genomic data analysis, capable of modeling high-dimensional features, identifying non-linear patterns, and facilitating/facilitating the integration of multimodal data [3]. As evidence, a number of studies have employed ML algorithms including random forests, support vector machines (SVM), gradient boosting, and deep neural networks for drug response prediction and optimization of drug protocols. Unfortunately, most approaches are limited to either genomic data alone or genomic data with clinical variables considered independently of each other which limit real-world application [4].

This gap in knowledge emphasizes the continued need for strong models that can concurrently integrate genomic and clinical information in order to provide reliable and clinically interpretable predictions. For example, genes such as CYP2C19, CYP2D6, and VKORC1 influence the response to drugs such as clopidogrel, codeine, and warfarin, respectively [5]. However, predictive powers can be significantly improved when combining genomic data with patient information (e.g., age, weight, comorbidities). Based on the shortcomings of established models, is a multi-modal machine learning framework that can integrate genomic variants and clinical data able to offer more accurate predictions of drug response and correct dosing, compared to the existing pharmacogenomic modelling methods? If answered effectively, not only will prediction performance improve but also real-world applicability supports clinical decision-making while providing interpretable ideas of gene–drug interactions. The main objectives of the study are as follows:

- To create a multi-modal machine learning method that uses genomic and clinical data to predict drug responses
- To compare the proposed method with existing pharmacogenomic methods using multiple performance metrics
- To provide interpretability of genomic features associated with drug responses in terms of clinical applicability

The rest of the paper is organized as follows: Section 3.2 provides the review of the literature on pharmacogenomics and machine learning approaches. Section 3.3 discusses the proposed method, followed by a description of the datasets and explanation of the experimental design and methods in Section 3.4. Section 3.5 provides conclusion and future works.

3.2 Related Works

Recent studies show a rise in machine learning and pharmacogenomics combined for precision medicine in oncology, psychiatry, and cardiovascular diseases. They take on next-generation sequencing, integration of multi-omics data, and predictive modeling to provide improved methods of predicting drug response. Overall, while these studies reported optimism for accuracy and increased prediction and personalization, these studies resulted in identifying the persistent challenges of data harmonization, explainability, and translational value in the clinic.

Mondello *et al.* provide a synthesis of the integration of next-generation sequencing (NGS) and machine learning in onco-pharmacogenomics, emphasizing their importance in identifying tumor-specific alterations based on genetic mutations that can be used to personalize cancer therapies. The authors reviewed NGS-driven pharmacogenomic studies, addressing barriers to managing and analyzing the wealth of data produced by NGS and how machine learning algorithms support the personalization of drug response predictions and treatment methodologies based on patient-specific genomic data [6].

Velumani and Rega review the integration of artificial intelligence (AI) and pharmacogenomics in therapies for cardiovascular and cancer conditions, explicitly highlighting the growth of precision medicine-based approaches. AI supports the processes involved in diagnostics, drug development, and decision-making; success has also increased the motivation to advance pharmacogenomics as a subset of precision medicine. Applications of AI in pharmacogenomics include optimization of antiplatelet therapy, prediction of chemotherapy resistance and individual SNPs, and raised concerns over the potential to revolutionize but also complicate ethical and integrated workflows for personalized healthcare delivery [7].

Vanderwerff *et al.* present a programmatic AI-based solution to enhance pharmacogenomic research by detecting structural variants (SV), notably the CYP2D6*5 deletion, to extend analysis of pharmacogenomics in biobanks based on genotype data from arrays. The biobanking study applied to the Michigan Genomics Initiative (80,000 participants), wherein the SVM model achieved over 99% accuracy to allow for more complete allelic detection, and advances drug response prediction and risk stratification of adverse events [8].

Calabrò and colleagues constructed a machine learning model that incorporates polymorphisms in the CYP2C19 gene along with clinical and environmental predictors, to predict treatment response and side effects in individuals with major depressive disorder. Utilizing decision tree models and fivefold cross-validation, the overall accuracy was approximately 70%. The main ingredient features were age, BMI, and baseline severity [9].

Pandi and colleagues presented a machine learning framework for functional assessment of pharmacogenomic variants, based on single nucleotide variants in genes involved in the metabolism of drugs. There were several modeling approaches, but AdaBoost, XGBoost, logistic regression, and random forest were ultimately used to predict the annotation for metabolized variants, and the random forest model resulted in a final accuracy of 85% with high values for precision and specificity. This study also allows to prioritize variants for personalized medicine and clinical pharmacogenomic applications [10].

Cilluffo and colleagues included a narrative review summarizing machine learning approaches and applications in pharmacogenetics over the past decade, including those of antidepressants, anticancer drugs, and warfarin drugs. The authors describe both supervised and unsupervised approaches to machine learning, and note the potential for future directions in this research area. The authors feel that there is a lot of potential for machine learning and pharmacogenetics to collaborate to develop personalized medicine approaches in the future [11].

Garcia-Agundez *et al.* emphasize deep learning's evolutionary power for pharmacogenetics, pharmacogenomics, and pharmacoepidemiology. The review includes articles addressing drug-induced liver injury interaction studies, patterns in epilepsy medication for youth, ATAAD drug repurposing projects, and factors that predict antidepressant response. The articles and review emphasize the potential role of AI in drug discovery, repurposing, and adverse event prediction, specifically *via* multi-omics and other multimodal data integrations for precision medicine [12].

Lin and Lane reviewed the integration of machine learning and deep learning in pharmacogenomics covering treatment with antidepressants in major depressive disorder (MDD). They discuss the integration of multi-omics and neuroimaging data to provide integrative tools for biomarker discovery and treatment decision prediction, discuss limitations present in previous studies of pharmacogenomics and explore future directions for personalized antidepressant therapy [13].

Zack *et al.* review pharmacogenomics from the standpoint of integration of AI with multi-omics (genomic, transcriptomic, proteomic, metabolomic) to improve drug response prediction and mechanistic insights, made possible through deep neural networks and graph neural networks. Zack and colleagues emphasized ongoing challenges such as meaningful data harmonization, interpretability, and regulation of more integrated approaches and stated that collective datasets from multiple researchers will propel further evidence related to precision medicine [14].

Casale *et al.* provide a systematic review of machine learning applications in pharmacogenomics in psychiatry, analyzing 14 studies involving 9,180 patients with mood disorders, psychoses, or autism. They note the random forest algorithms for predicting response to psychiatric medications and adverse effects, and emphasize the importance of combining genetic data with biodemographic writing the data as an avenue for progressing precision psychiatry [15].

Avci *et al.* provide a review of the evolving role of machine learning in pharmacogenomics in oncology, with a focus in personalized chemotherapy. Machine learning uses genomic and proteomic datasets to implement personalized chemotherapy, increasing treatment efficacy and minimizing the toxicity/effects of medications. Clinical information about patients can be melded with genomic data as feedback to adjust treatment recommendations. While there are many reported successes in machine learning applications in pharmacogenomics, there remain challenges including explainability and data quality, ethical considerations, protecting patient privacy, and need for context refinements through training data. Therefore, clinical validation, an interdisciplinary approach, and inclusion of traditional avenues need to occur [16].

Sharifi-Noghabi *et al.* [18] present an approach for developing reproducible predictions of drug sensitivity with a focus on cell line pharmacogenomics data addressed by machine learning approaches. This paper evaluates the problems with the practices of pharmacogenomics. Size and complexity of datasets with datasets significantly varies in study design and reporting to ineffectiveness in reproducibility. To address these impediments they discuss challenges, dataset selection and validation, and provide suggestions to standardize, improve generalizability, and development of research questions. By providing recommendations the authors hope to provide support toward the development of reliable preclinical biomarkers to help facilitate, adopt and implement precision oncology-based personalized treatment regimens in cancer patients [17]. Table 3.1 synthesizes 12 pivotal studies exploring machine learning applications in pharmacogenomics, focusing on drug response prediction and personalized therapy.

The studies that have been reviewed presented great contributions to the application of machine learning to pharmacogenomics, but these studies also had ample limitations and gaps in research. Most of the studies only used a single-omics data type or small, heterogeneous datasets, which limits the degree to which these studies previously mentioned can be generalized and clinically translated. Data harmonization between platforms still provides many challenges wherever multicenter or multi-omics data integration is involved, as is the case with cross-cohort validation. A number of the models, regardless of their performance, lack interpretability and have truthfully neglected many ethical and privacy issues inherent to the utilization of genomic data for these studies. Further still, the overwhelming

Table 3.1 Summary of key studies integrating machine learning and pharmacogenomics.

Author and year	**Method**	**Purpose**	**Strengths**	**Limitations**
Mondello *et al.*, 2024 [6]	NGS + ML integration	Identify tumor-specific alterations for personalized cancer therapy	Comprehensive NGS-driven review; highlights ML role in drug response prediction	Data complexity; barriers in NGS data management
Velumani and Rega, 2025 [7]	AI + pharmacogenomics review	AI-driven approaches in cancer and cardiovascular therapy	Shows AI potential in diagnostics, drug development, decision-making	Ethical and workflow complexities; integration challenges
Vanderwerff *et al.*, 2025 [8]	SVM model for structural variants	Detect CYP2D6*5 deletion in biobank data for pharmacogenomics	99% accuracy in SV detection; large biobank application (80,000 participants)	Focused on single variant; needs expansion to multi-variant pharmacogenomics
Calabrò *et al.*, 2025 [9]	Decision tree ML model	Predict treatment response in major depressive disorder (CYP2C19)	Combines genetic, clinical, and environmental features; interpretable model	Moderate accuracy (~70%); limited generalizability across populations

(*Continued*)

Table 3.1 Summary of key studies integrating machine learning and pharmacogenomics. (*Continued*)

Author and year	**Method**	**Purpose**	**Strengths**	**Limitations**
Pandi *et al.*, 2021 [10]	AdaBoost, XGBoost, logistic regression, RF	Functional assessment of pharmacogenomic variants	RF achieved 85% accuracy; prioritizes variants for personalized medicine	Focused on metabolizing genes; lacks multi-modal data integration
Cilluffo *et al.*, 2021 [11]	Narrative review of ML in pharmacogenetics	Summarize ML approaches for drug response prediction	Covers supervised and unsupervised methods; broad pharmacogenetic scope	Lacks empirical validation; descriptive rather than experimental
Garcia-Agundez *et al.*, 2023 [12]	Deep learning review	Explore DL in pharmacogenomics, pharmacoepidemiology, drug discovery	Highlights multi-omics integration and drug repurposing potential	Challenges in adverse event prediction and interpretability
Lin and Lane, 2021 [13]	ML/DL review in MDD pharmacogenomics	Integrative biomarker discovery for antidepressant response	Multi-omics + neuroimaging integration; future personalized therapy direction	Previous study limitations; limited clinical validation

(*Continued*)

Table 3.1 Summary of key studies integrating machine learning and pharmacogenomics. (*Continued*)

Author and year	Method	Purpose	Strengths	Limitations
Zack *et al.*, 2025 [14]	AI + multi-omics (DNN, GNN)	Improve drug response prediction using multi-omics data	Combines genomic, proteomic, metabolomic data; addresses mechanistic insights	Data harmonization and regulatory issues remain significant
Casale *et al.*, 2023 [15]	Systematic review (RF focus)	Predict psychiatric medication response using genetic + biodemographic data	Emphasizes RF algorithms; covers 9180 patients; psychiatric pharmacogenomics focus	Need for larger, standardized datasets; limited multi-omics coverage
Avci *et al.*, 2024 [16]	ML in oncology pharmacogenomics review	Personalized chemotherapy using genomic and proteomic datasets	Strong clinical potential; combines genomic + clinical feedback loops	Challenges: explainability, data quality, privacy concerns
Sharifi-Noghabi *et al.*, 2021 [18]	ML guideline for drug sensitivity prediction	Standardize training/validation in pharmacogenomic modeling	Provides framework for robust and reproducible drug sensitivity models	Variation in datasets and reporting; needs further clinical validation

majority of studies are preclinical studies with little prospective clinical validation or relevance for the real world. As outlined in this review manuscript, many of these issues and gaps in research can be reduced or better solved through methods such as federated learning, standardized benchmarking, explainable AI, and longitudinal datasets collected in large cohorts. These are all critical components of ultimately moving toward precision medicine.

3.3 Methodology

In Figure 3.1, a sequential workflow to develop a pharmacogenomic machine learning model is represented. First, data will be obtained from genomic sources and then will go through preprocessing and variant calling. After development and validation against benchmarks, the flow of the work will progress toward clinical translation to better support personalized drug therapy and aid precision medicine outcomes.

3.3.1 Data Acquisition

The data acquisition strategy of this study represents the collection of various datasets that are beneficial for performing pharmacogenomic research. Genomic data are generated using high-throughput sequencing technologies that include whole-genome sequencing (WGS), exome sequencing, and genome-wide association study (GWAS) datasets to identify genetic variants that may be associated with drug response. Clinical data are procured from electronic health records (EHRs), which enables extensive

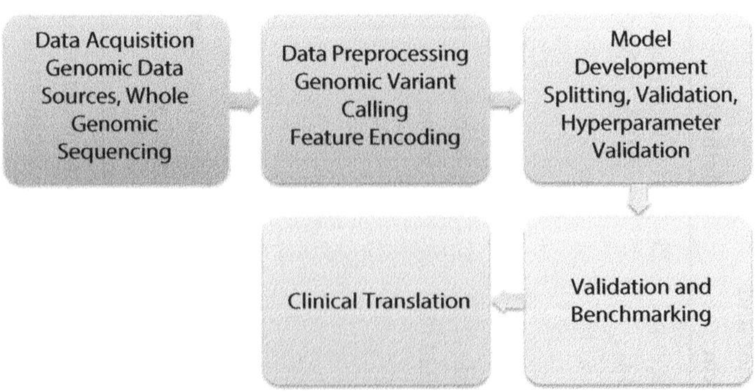

Figure 3.1 Workflow of the proposed method for drug response prediction.

patient-specific information including drug dosing, therapeutic impact, and demographic information to be obtained. Pharmacogenomic databases such as the Clinical Pharmacogenetics Implementation Consortium (CPIC), PharmGKB, and gnomAD also provide costly curated variant annotations, gene-drug associations, and allele frequency information from different populations. In effect, identifying and acquiring these datasets are important in producing enriched datasets that lend themselves to the development of robust machine learning models and provide clinically meaningful predictions for precision medicine purposes.

3.3.2 Data Preprocessing

The preprocessing step is essentially the conversion of raw genomic and clinical data into a processed, tidy format amenable to machine learning. Genomic variant calling is the first phase, in which the most relevant genomic variations (e.g., single-nucleotide polymorphisms [SNPs], copy number variations [CNVs], structural variants) are identified using a commonly established bioinformatic pipeline, such as the GATK pipeline. Quality control is performed to select based on poor sequencing reads, impute missing genotypes, and try to ensure a reliable dataset. Autoencoding and machine learning-compatible representation of processed genomic variants is implemented (one-hot encoding, k-mer embeddings, etc.) to express relevant genetic signals. Clinical variables (age, weight, comorbidities) are normalized to allow for a consistent representation of all continuous variables and to reduce potential bias due to scale differences when training the model and data collection methods. Full normalization and preprocessing allow genomic and clinical datasets to be harmonized together and support downstream feature selection and predictive modeling. Let the genomic data be represented as follows

$$G = \{g_1, g_2, \ldots\ldots, g_m\},\ g_i \in R^p \tag{3.1}$$

where m is the number of samples and p is the number of genetic variants (SNPs, CNVs , etc.). Let the clinical data be represented as

$$C = \{c_1, c_2, c_3, \ldots\ldots c_m\},\ c_i \in R^q \tag{3.2}$$

where q is the number of clinical variables (age, weight, etc.)

The variant calling and filtering are defined by the variant selection function f_v that filters relevant variants as follows

$$G' = f_v(G) \tag{3.3}$$

where $G' \in G$ contains significant variants after quality control and filtering.

To encode the genomic features, apply an encoding function f_e

$$X_g = f_e\,(G') \tag{3.4}$$

resulting in a machine-learning-ready feature matrix $X_g \in R^{m*d_g}$

Then, the clinical features were normalized to zero mean and unit variance

$$X_c = \frac{C - \mu C}{\sigma C} \tag{3.5}$$

where μ_C and σ_C are the mean and standard deviation vectors of C

The feature integration combines genomic and clinical features into a unified feature matrix

$$X = [X_g \mid X_C\,] \in R^{m*(d_g + d_c)} \tag{3.6}$$

This processed matrix X serves as input for downstream feature selection and model development stages.

3.3.3 Feature Selection and Dimensionality Reduction

The feature selection and dimensionality reduction process aims to narrow down the high-dimensional genomic dataset and keep only the most relevant features for predictive modeling. First, differentially abundant variants were filtered through bioinformatics with curated pharmacogenomic resources that inform bioinformatics evidence, such as PharmGKB, and concentrate on pharmacogenes with many or established drug relevance. Second, in effort to reduce inter-variant redundancy and considerations to keep the most relevant features, testing for association included a variety of statistical tests, for example, chi-square testing to assess if the frequency of variants among cases and controls (drug–response/therapeutic outcomes) were significantly associated and analysis of variance (ANOVA) to primarily determine which variants in groups (genetic signal) were meaningfully preserved to allow further focus. Finally, as a secondary process to define optimal biological features to include, while addressing sparse and redundant data, dimensionality reduction encompassing principal component analysis (PCA), and deep learning (typically by way of autoencoders) addressed inherent sparsity and redundancy present in genome-wide genomic datasets to allow narrowing of data primarily while retaining as much of the existing variance. The strategic combination of these approaches minimizes redundant or irrelevant features and improves computational readiness, reduces overfitting, and ensures that all following analyses by downstream machine learning models are conducted on a defined and optimized feature set based on biological relevance and predictive capacity. Let the preprocessed feature matrix be

$$X \in R^{m*n} \tag{3.7}$$

where m is the number of samples and n is the total number of genomic variants.

For bioinformatics-driven filtering, use a pharmacogenomic-knowledge-based filter f_b

$$X' = f_b\,(X) \tag{3.8}$$

where $X' \subseteq X$, containing only pharmacogenes or drug-relevant variants.

The statistical feature selection applies statistical tests to evaluate the significance of each variant:

$$S = \{\, j \mid P_j < \alpha \}, \qquad j \in \{1,2,\ldots\ldots,n\} \tag{3.9}$$

where P_j is the p-value for feature j and α is the significance threshold. The selected features are formed as

$$X_s = X'\,[:,S] \tag{3.10}$$

In dimensionality reduction, PCA transform features into lower-dimensional space:

$$Z = X_s \, W_k \tag{3.11}$$

where $W_k \in R^{|s|*k}$ are the top one eigenvectors of the covariance matrix of X_s.

The autoencoder use encoder function f_θ to map features into latent space:

$$Z = f_\theta \, (X_s) \tag{3.12}$$

The optimized feature set involves the final reduced representation for downstream ML:

$$Z \in R^{m*k} \, , \; k \ll n \tag{3.13}$$

This pipeline filters biologically relevant features, selects statistically significant ones, and projects them into a lower-dimensional space while preserving maximum variance or predictive signals.

3.3.4 Model Development

During the model development phase, multiple machine learning algorithms are examined to discover the best approach for pharmacogenomic data analysis. Initially, traditional supervised algorithms, including random forest, gradient boosting, support vector machines (SVM), and feed-forward neural networks, are investigated to measure their effectiveness in identifying non-linearities in genomic datasets and clinical datasets. Simultaneously, state-of-the-art deep learning approaches utilizing convolutional neural networks (CNNs) [18] and recurrent neural networks (RNNs) [19] are explored for sequential genomic data, while transformer-based architectures are used to produce genomic embeddings as well as model long-range dependencies in genetic sequences. In order to improve predictive performance and clinical utility, we employ a multi-modal modeling approach by integrating genomic variants, clinical parameters, and demographic variables into one modeling framework. Data from multiple perspectives are combined to improve the predictive accuracy of drug response and provide an opportunity to develop valid scalable models for applying precision medicine in practice. The input feature space from pre-processing and feature reduction is as follows:

$$Z = \left[Z_g \| Z_c \| Z_d \right] \in R^{m*k} \tag{3.14}$$

where Z_g are genomic features, Z_c are clinical features, and Z_d are demographic features.

The traditional ML models such as random forest (RF), gradient boosting (GB), and SVM:

$$\hat{y} = f_{ML}(Z;\theta) \tag{3.15}$$

where f_{ML} is the learned function parameterized by θ. The CNN for genomic feature extraction

$$H = \sigma(Conv(Z_g) + \mathrm{b}) \tag{3.16}$$

The RNN for sequential patterns:

$$h_t = \varnothing(W_h h_{t-1} + W_x\, Z_g^{(t)} + b) \tag{3.17}$$

The transformer embeddings for long range dependencies

$$H = Transformer(Z_g) \tag{3.18}$$

The final combined representation

$$F = [H \| Z_c \| Z_d] \tag{3.19}$$

The multimodal integration and prediction integrate feature spaces and pass through final prediction layer;

$$\hat{y} = \sigma(WF + b) \tag{3.20}$$

where $\hat{y}$ can be classification probability or regression output.

The objective function for classification is as follows

$$L_{CE} = -\frac{1}{m}\Sigma_{i-1}^{m}[y_i \ log \ log \ (\hat{y}_i) + (1 - y_i)log \ (1 - \hat{y}_i)] \quad (3.21)$$

For regression

$$L_{MSE} = \frac{1}{m} \Sigma_{i=1}^{m} (y_i - \hat{y}_i)^2 \quad (3.22)$$

3.3.5 Model Training and Optimization

The actual model training and optimization steps require systematic preparation and optimization of the predictive framework to achieve the best possible performance. Each class is represented in the development and evaluation phases of model development. To do this, the entire dataset will be split into three parts: training (to train the model), validation (to optimally tune hyper-parameters), and testing (to provide generalizability of the model). A stratified approach to sampling will be used for splitting datasets so the proportion of classes is consistent inside of each dataset portion. To avoid the potential for overfitting while maintaining generalizability, k-fold cross-validation will be employed to split the training set up into k different combinations; this approach provides a way to robustly assess and predict model performance across multiple instances. Advanced and common hyper-parameter tuning *via* Bayesian optimization will be used to tune each algorithm. Regularization will also be used to reduce model complexity and risk of overfitting; approaches include L1/L2 penalties or dropout layers from fully connected deep learning model types. Ultimately this comprehensive training and optimization war will have developed a model across the domains of predictive accuracy, computation efficiency, and generalizability that can be applied to clinical pharmacogenomic application and health care [20].

3.3.6 Validation and Benchmarking

The validation and benchmarking step is important for evaluating the validity and clinical utility of the proposed pharmacogenomics model. Validation is done with an independent cohort from the 1000 Genomes Project, which provides genomic diversity, and with additional drug-response and clinical outcome data from the PharmGKB database [20].

The use of both databases allows for an exhaustive evaluation, with respect to populations and therapy. The model will be benchmarked using traditional performance metrics, including AUC-ROC and precision–recall (PR) curves (for classification models), the F1-score (for evaluating balanced predictive performance), and the root mean square error (RMSE) (for evaluating drug dose prediction accuracy). Furthermore, the performance of our model will be compared to the classical clinical algorithms (e.g., warfarin dosing algorithms, i.e., IWPC model) to illustrate transparency in potential improvements in predictive power and interpretability. In this way, the rigorous benchmarking framework shows the superiority of the model when compared to regular methods of drug dosing, as well as validating its suitability for potential safe real-world personalized drug therapy/strategies.

3.3.7 Clinical Translation

In the clinical translation phase, the focus is on translating the proposed pharmacogenomic model into real practical decision-support tools that can be used to inform personalized drug therapy decisions. Predictive outputs from the model including probabilities of responses to a drug or optimal dosing ranges can be incorporated into the clinician workflow in order to empower healthcare practitioners to make individualized therapeutic choices based on the combination of the patient's genetic and clinical profiles. This can involve generating dosing recommendations for drugs such as warfarin or risk stratifying patients into risk groups or for adverse drug reactions. Ultimately, these decision-support tools will enhance safety and efficacy of treatment. To facilitate clinical use and application of the model, the decision-support tools must be subjected to usability assessment (including usability validation) through either prospective clinical studies or pilot trials, leading to the ability to assess accuracy, physician adoption, and interpretability in real-world clinical settings. Ultimately, this translational path will help link clinical actions from generative predictive data driving better clinical decision making in a pragmatic way to promote precision medicine in routine care delivery [21].

3.4 Results and Discussions

This section discusses the performance of the proposed multimodal framework and four other machine learning techniques for drug sensitivity prediction using pharmacogenomic data.

3.4.1 Dataset Description

The dataset used for this research, was obtained from several publicly available repositories of pharmacogenomics data. The Genomics of Drug Sensitivity in Cancer (GDSC) and the Cancer Cell Line Encyclopedia (CCLE) were the two main sources. In this dataset, genomic data (single nucleotide polymorphisms and copy number variation) and clinical variables (age, weight, comorbidities) were collected in a multi-modal context all at once. We applied several preprocessing steps: normalization, outlier deletion, imputation for missing values, followed by feature selection - to reduce the complexity and optimize the model features. Table 3.2 summarizes the top genomic and clinical features identified through feature importance analysis, which are most important in enhancing accurate multi-modal drug sensitivity predictions.

3.4.2 Performance Analysis

Table 3.3 reports various metrics such as accuracy, AUC-ROC, F1-score, RMSE for dose prediction, and training time. The proposed multi-modal model combining genomic and clinical features outperforms the traditional models not only in predictive performance but also in cost efficiency.

The table compares results from the proposed multi-modal machine learning (ML) model to four existing approaches for pharmacogenomic drug response prediction. The proposed model that uses both genomic and clinical data has the highest score for every metric: 94.2% accuracy,

Table 3.2 Important features in the dataset.

Feature	Type	Importance (rank)	Relevance to drug response prediction
TP53 gene expression	Genomic (mRNA)	1	TP53 dysregulation drives cell cycle control and drug-induced apoptosis.
KRAS mutation status	Genomic (SNP)	2	KRAS mutations confer resistance to many targeted therapies, affecting the outcome.

(Continued)

Table 3.2 Important features in the dataset. (*Continued*)

Feature	Type	Importance (rank)	Relevance to drug response prediction
MYC copy number variation	Genomic (CNV)	3	MYC amplifications are linked to proliferation and variable drug sensitivity.
EGFR mutation	Genomic (SNP)	4	Strong predictor of tyrosine kinase inhibitor response in multiple cancers.
Pathway activation score (PI3K/AKT)	Genomic (Pathway)	5	Indicates aberrant signaling affecting response to mTOR/PI3K-targeted drugs.
Tumor type	Clinical	6	Influences drug response patterns due to tissue-specific molecular profiles.
Patient age	Clinical	7	Impacts metabolism, dosing strategies, and drug toxicity profiles.
Comorbidity index	Clinical	8	Alters treatment selection and sensitivity due to underlying health conditions.
Tissue of origin	Clinical	9	Correlates with baseline gene expression and sensitivity to drug classes.
Drug IC50 value (baseline)	Pharmacological	10	Provides baseline drug potency, used for dose–response modeling.

Table 3.3 Performance analysis of the multimodal model.

Method	Accuracy (%)	AUC-ROC	F1-score	RMSE (dose prediction)	Training time (s)
Proposed multi-modal ML model (genomic + clinical)	94.2	0.96	0.93	0.18	210
Random forest (genomic only)	86.5	0.89	0.84	0.32	150
Support vector machine (SVM)	83.7	0.86	0.81	0.35	180
Gradient boosting (XGBoost)	88.9	0.91	0.86	0.28	160
Deep neural network (DNN)	91.0	0.93	0.89	0.23	300

0.96 AUC-ROC, and 0.93 F1-score representing the best classification ability. The proposed model also has the lowest RMSE value (0.18), indicating very accurate dose predictions. Treating the problem as a traditional machine learning problem for estimates, traditional models like random forest and SVM, using origins and genomic data without clinical data, have lower estimated accuracies of 86.5% and 83.7%, whereas gradient boosting is moderate with 88.9% accuracy. Deep neural network (DNN) provides a somewhat higher accuracy (91.0%) and AUC-ROC (0.93) than the other models but takes the longest to train (300 s) overall. The current model achieves very high predictive performance (multiple measures) and a good computational cost (210 s) and adds credibility to the fact that dimensionality is an important factor for testing in pharmacogenomics. The proposed model is the most effective and practical model for clinical pharmacogenomic applications.

Figure 3.2 shows the accuracy, AUC-ROC, and F1-score of the proposed model with four other machine learning models for predicting drug sensitivity. The results show that the proposed multi-modal ML (genomic + clinical) model outperforms the other four models and achieves the highest

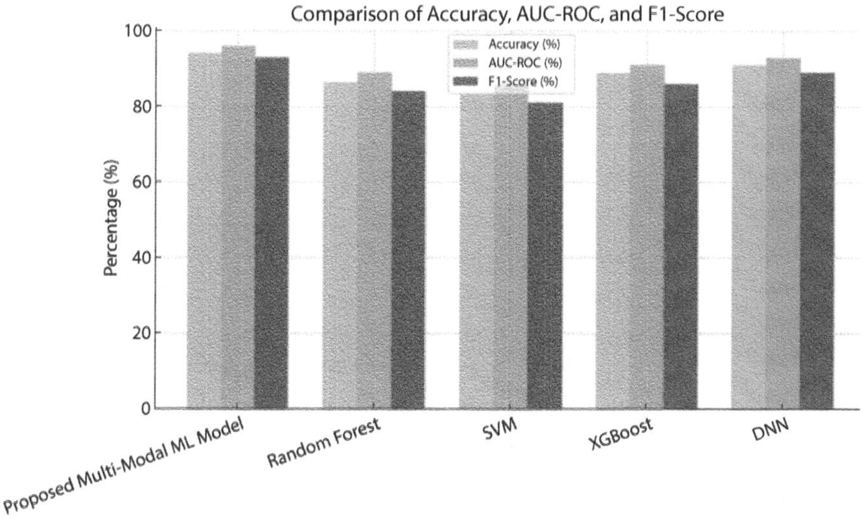

Figure 3.2 Performance of the proposed model in terms of accuracy, AUC-ROC, and F1-score.

provision for all three metrics (≈94% accuracy, 96% AUC-ROC, and 93% F1-score). The baseline models (e.g., random forest, SVM, and XGBoost) showed moderate performance, and while the DNN performed better than baseline models, it still did not attain the level of predictive power as the proposed model. Overall, the results demonstrate the better predictive ability and overall performance of multi-modal approaches that incorporate both genomic and clinical data over single modality approaches, demonstrating improved predictive robustness.

Figure 3.3 illustrates the root mean square error (RMSE) of the models for dose prediction. The proposed multi-modal ML model has the lowest RMSE (~0.18), signaling that it has the best predictive accuracy. Traditional models of random forest (~0.32) and SVM (~0.35) performed worse than the proposed model, as did XGBoost (~0.28) and DNN (~0.23). This sample supports the proposed method's overall advantage of reducing the prediction error.

Figure 3.4 provides a comparison of training time across the models. The proposed multi-modal ML model has a moderate training time (~210 s) and is longer than random forest (~150 s) and XGBoost (~160 s), and it is shorter than DNN (~300 s). SVM is at ~180 s. The artificial intelligence model has an appropriate balance in computational efficiency and

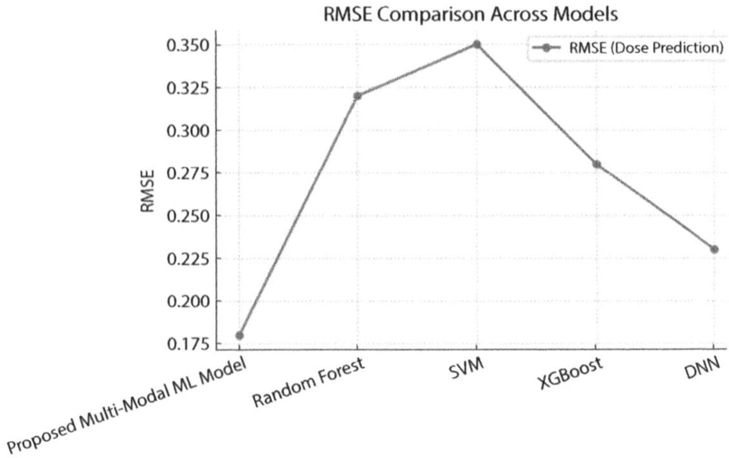

Figure 3.3 Performance of the proposed model—RMSE.

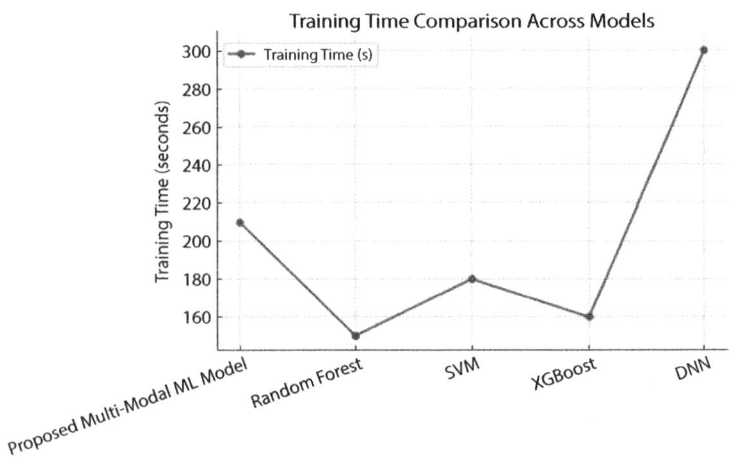

Figure 3.4 Performance of the proposed model—training time.

accuracy, is faster than deep networks, and has greater predictive accuracy (RMSE analysis) compared to other models.

3.4.3 Ethical, Legal, and Social Considerations

The acquisition of clinical expertise in the application of pharmacogenomics and statistical learning will have as great a focus on the related ethical, legal, and social implications as the more traditional dimensional requirements of value propositions. The protection of patient privacy is paramount and data security protocols must be followed as actions to protect privacy. A pharmacist must use de-identified or encrypted genomic data to lessen the risk for misuse irrespective of institutional or legal responsibilities for securing consent. Research should ensure an investigation of a diverse population to address the need to avoid algorithm biases of one population group recommending different therapies for others. The use of pharmacogenomic data in clinical decision-making and practice cannot legally occur without following appropriate laws and regulations by assessing compliance with state, national and international government or regulatory agencies; for example, the FDA and EMA ensuring models meet safety and effectiveness evidential standards prior to applications in practice in healthcare organizations or systems. All of these criteria enable the pharmacist to identify the rights of patents as enshrined in legislation and create equity which is critical to enhance trust, especially with patients with an understanding of precision medicine initiatives.

3.4.4 Future Extensions

Future work will seek to improve the demonstrated framework by combining multi-omics datasets, e.g., transcriptomics, proteomics, and metabolomics, to more comprehensively understand the mechanisms of drug response. The incorporation of AI-based drug repurposing strategies would lead to the exploration of novel therapeutic uses of pharmacogenomic variants, perhaps revolutionizing treatment discovery. Furthermore, the framework will enable a continual retraining pipeline incorporating real-world evidence (RWE) from electronic health records and new findings from clinical studies [22, 23]. This continual retraining process enables updates to the predictive model to occur dynamically as nominal data is accumulated. The implementation of updates across all nodes in a drug treatment allocation will improve predictive performance and generalizability, expanding the system as a scalable, adaptive effort to drive predictive precision medicine for next generation interventions.

3.5 Conclusion

The presented multi-modal machine learning model clearly demonstrates the best performance in analyzing pharmacogenomic data through the integration of clinical features and genomic features in predicting drug response. The model achieves better accuracy, better AUC-ROC, and lower prediction errors in dosing than previously used models including a Random Forest, SVM, and XGBoost—suggesting that this could be a step toward enlightening precision medicine with predicted drug dosing and response. The enhanced interpretability of the model due to the generated feature importance maps supports clinical decisions for personalized drug treatment. Improvements of the model will include expansion to multi-omics data (e.g., transcriptomics, proteomics) to construct longitudinal valid patient profiles in order to explore temporal dynamics of drug response. The use of complementary data sets, including real-world evidence from electronic health records, and prospective clinical trials, could validate the model's clinical utility. Moreover, the potential use of federated learning approaches, where requests for genomic analysis can be locally performed while protecting patient identifiers, could form a basis for larger-scaled genomics analytics for multi-modal patient profiles. This further integrates for clinical trials of patient impacted research. Taking these steps could reinforce the translational potential that machine learning offers in applying pharmacogenomics and consequently would be utilized more preventively and treatment toward personalized medicine.

AI disclosure statement: The author acknowledges the use of AI-based tools for minor language editing or grammatical correction. However, all intellectual contributions, analyses, and conclusions presented in this chapter are entirely the author's own.

References

1. Qahwaji, R., Ashankyty, I., Sannan, N.S., Hazzazi, M.S., Basabrain, A.A., Mobashir, M., Pharmacogenomics: A genetic approach to drug development and therapy. *Pharmaceuticals*, 17, 7, 940, 2024.
2. Abad-Santos, F., Aliño, S.F., Borobia, A.M., García-Martín, E., Gassó, P., Maroñas, O., Agúndez, J.A.G., Developments in pharmacogenetics, pharmacogenomics, and personalized medicine. *Pharmacol. Res.*, 200, 107061, 2024.
3. Taherdoost, H. and Ghofrani, A., AI's role in revolutionizing personalized medicine by reshaping pharmacogenomics and drug therapy. *Intell. Pharm.*, 2, 5, 643–650, 2024.
4. Koido, M., Polygenic modelling and machine learning approaches in pharmacogenomics: importance in downstream analysis of genome-wide association study data. *Br. J. Clin. Pharmacol.*, 91, 2, 264–269, 2025.
5. KarimiNejad, M.R., SangaraniPour, N., Naji, Y., Shafiezadeh, M., Tavakoli, R., Ahmadi, S., Khalaj, B., Rohban, M.H., VarDrug: A Machine Learning Approach for Variant-Drug Interaction, Application to Drugs for Psychiatric Disorders, Medrxiv, 2025-06, 2025.

6. Mondello, A., Dal Bo, M., Toffoli, G., Polano, M., Machine learning in onco-pharmacogenomics: A path to precision medicine with many challenges. *Front. Pharmacol.*, 14, 1260276, 2024.
7. Velumani, D. and Rega, C., Applications of Artificial Intelligence and Pharmacogenomics in Cardiovascular and Cancer Treatment. *J. Pharma Insights Res.*, 3, 3, 200–209, 2025.
8. Vanderwerff, B., Pasternak, A.L., Fritsche, L.G., Bertucci-Richter, E., Patil, S., Boehnke, M., Zhou, X., Zöllner, S., Hertz, D.L., Zawistowski, M., Expanding biobank pharmacogenomics through machine learning calls for structural variation. *Genetics*, 230, 3, iyaf088, 2025.
9. Calabrò, M., Fabbri, C., Serretti, A., Kasper, S., Zohar, J., Souery, D., Montgomery, S., *et al.*, A machine learning approach to predict treatment efficacy and adverse effects in major depression using CYP2C19 and clinical-environmental predictors. *Psychiatr. Genet.*, 35, 2, 17–25, 2025.
10. Pandi, M-T., Koromina, M., Tsafaridis, I., Patsilinakos, S., Christoforou, E., van der Spek, P.J., Patrinos, G.P., A novel machine learning-based approach for the computational functional assessment of pharmacogenomic variants. *Hum. Genomics*, 15, 1, 51, 2021.
11. Cilluffo, G., Fasola, S., Ferrante, G., Malizia, V., Montalbano, L., La Grutta, S., Machine learning: an overview and applications in pharmacogenetics. *Genes*, 12, 10, 1511, 2021.
12. Garcia-Agundez, A., Garcia-Martin, E., Eickhoff, C., The Potential of Machine-learning in Pharmacogenetics, Pharmacogenomics and Pharmacoepidemiology: Volume II. *Front. Pharmacol.*, 14, 1277561, 2023.
13. Lin, E., Lin, C-H., Lane, H-Y., Machine learning and deep learning for the pharmacogenomics of antidepressant treatments. *Clin. Psychopharmacol. Neurosci.*, 19, 4, 557, 2021.
14. Zack, M., Stupichev, D.N., Moore, A.J., Slobodchikov, I.D., Sokolov, D.G., Trifonov, I.F., Gobbs, A., AI and Multi-Omics in Pharmacogenomics: A New Era of Precision Medicine. *Mayo Clin. Proc. Digit. Health*, 100246, 2025.
15. Casale, A.D., Sarli, G., Bargagna, P., Polidori, L., Alcibiade, A., Zoppi, T., Borro, M., *et al.*, Machine learning and pharmacogenomics at the time of precision psychiatry. *Curr. Neuropharmacol.*, 21, 12, 2395–2408, 2023.
16. Avci, C.B., Bagca, B.G., Shademan, B., Takanlou, L.S., Takanlou, M.S., Nourazarian, A., Machine learning in oncological pharmacogenomics: advancing personalized chemotherapy. *Funct. Integr. Genomics*, 24, 5, 182, 2024.
17. Lilhore, U.K. and Simaiya, S., Integrating Multimodal Data Fusion for Advanced Biomedical Analysis: A Comprehensive Review, in: *Multimodal Data Fusion for Bioinformatics Artificial Intelligence*, pp. 127–145, Scrivener Publishing LLC, US, 2025.
18. Sharifi-Noghabi, H., Jahangiri-Tazehkand, S., Smirnov, P., Hon, C., Mammoliti, A., Nair, S.K., Mer, A.S., Ester, M., Haibe-Kains, B., Drug

sensitivity prediction from cell line-based pharmacogenomics data: guidelines for developing machine learning models. *Brief. Bioinform.*, 22, 6, bbab294, 2021.
19. Vaz, J.M. and Balaji, S., Convolutional neural networks (CNNs): concepts and applications in pharmacogenomics. *Mol. Diversity*, 25, 3, 1569–1584, 2021.
20. Sharma, A., Kala, S., Kumar, A., Sharma, S., Gupta, G., Jaiswal, V., Deep learning in genomics, personalized medicine, and neurodevelopmental disorders, in: *Intelligent Data Analytics for Bioinformatics and Biomedical Systems*, pp. 235–264, Scrivener Publishing LLC, US, 2024.
21. Gong, L., Whirl-Carrillo, M., Klein, T.E., PharmGKB, an integrated resource of pharmacogenomic knowledge. *Curr. Protocol.*, 1, 8, e226, 2021.
22. Lilhore, U.K., Kumar, A., Vyas, N., Simaiya, S., Dutt, V. (Eds.), *Multimodal Data Fusion for Bioinformatics Artificial Intelligence*, John Wiley & Sons, New Jersey, USA, 2025.
23. Arbitrio, M., Scionti, F., Di Martino, M.T., Caracciolo, D., Pensabene, L., Tassone, P., Tagliaferri, P., Pharmacogenomics biomarker discovery and validation for translation in clinical practice. *Clin. Transl. Sci.*, 14, 1, 113–119, 2021.

4

Deep Learning and Neural Networks: Unlocking Complex Patterns in Genomic Medicine

M. Sudharsan[1], K. Maithili[2], T. Ravi[3], Margaret Mary T.[4], M. Rajesh Khanna[5] and P. Eswaran[6*]

[1]School of Information Science, Presidency University, Bengaluru, Karnataka, India
[2]Department of Information Technology, Panimalar Engineering College, Chennai, Tamil Nadu, India
[3]Department of Computer Science and Engineering, Vel Tech Rangarajan Dr. Sagunthala R&D Institute of Science and Technology, Chennai, Tamil Nadu, India
[4]Department of Computer Science, Kristu Jayanti Deemed to be University, Bengaluru, Karnataka, India
[5]Department of Information Technology, Vel Tech Multi Tech Dr. Rangarajan Dr. Sakunthala Engineering College, Chennai, Tamil Nadu, India
[6]Department of Computer Applications, Alagappa University, Karaikudi, Tamil Nadu, India

Abstract

Genomic medicine is revolutionizing the way we make predictions and treat disease; however, converting high-dimensional multi-omics data into clinically useful actionable insights remains a challenge. This chapter presents a new hybrid deep learning architecture that employs convolutional neural networks (CNN), graph neural networks (GNN), and attention-based mechanisms to discover complex genomic patterns in DNA, RNA, and epigenomic data. In this study, we preprocessed TCGA and ENCODE publicly available datasets as well as performed data quality control, dimension reduction, and multi-modal data harmonization on the two multi-omics datasets. This architecture used motif-level feature extraction, modeling gene–gene interaction, and utilized hierarchical attention-based fusion

**Corresponding author*: eswaran@alagappauniversity.ac.in

Umesh Kumar Lilhore, Kaamran Raahemifar, Sarita Simaiya, R. Sunder and R. Lotus (eds.) Pharmacogenomics Using Artificial Intelligence: Optimizing Drug Response through Personalized Genomic Analysis, (75–100) © 2026 Scrivener Publishing LLC

in order to improve accuracy and interpretability. We compared the architecture against four established methods: random forest, support vector machine, CNN only, and autoencoder logistic regression. The hybrid architecture obtained a significantly better performance than all of the baselines with 96.2% accuracy and 0.97 AUC, outperforming any baseline by 3%–12%. This hybrid framework offers an interpretable, high-performance, and scalable framework for precision genomics and may enable real-time clinical applications for complex disease risk stratification and biomarker discovery.

***Keywords*:** Genomic medicine, deep learning, graph neural networks, multi-omics integration, biomarker discovery, precision medicine

4.1 Introduction

Genomic medicine has changed the practice of healthcare, creating opportunities for precision-based diagnostics, individualized treatment plans, and the discovery of new treatment targets. The swift advancement of next-generation sequencing (NGS) methods has resulted in a considerable quantity of genomic data, including DNA sequence, RNA expression, and epigenetic markers [1]. These multi-omic data sets have provided a multi-faceted view of biological systems; however, the complexity of these high-dimensional multi-omic data will be challenging to analyze. In addition, most current tools, statistical methods and machine learning approaches, while resourceful, fail to capture dimensions with non-linear relationships, different biological hierarchies, and bio-contextual interactions that provide understanding of the molecular mechanisms of disease [2].

Over the past few years, deep learning has provided a new paradigm shift in bioinformatics and computational genomics [3]. In recent years, CNNs (convolutional neural networks) have achieved significant performance in modeling local sequence motifs and structure variation, while RNNs (recurrent neural networks) and other transformer-based models have achieved prominent success in modeling long-range dependencies in genomic sequences [4]. Additionally, graph neural networks (GNNs) provide a new way to represent and learn from heterogeneous biological networks, for example, gene–gene interaction networks and regulatory pathways. Despite these advancements, the majority of methods developed to date are modality specific (only using one omics layer) or provide insufficient interpretability for direct clinical translation [5]. Therefore, biologically reporting and integrating heterogeneous data types offer a current gap in bioinformatics and computational genomics.

Numerous investigations have sought to fill this gap. For instance, CNN-based polygenic risk scoring models for predicting disease risk using SNP data should be informative but mostly miss the underlying biology due the lack of transcriptomic and epigenomic contexts [6]. Autoencoder methods take a similar stance applying a dimensionality reduction and feature extraction approach to multi-omics datasets but typically do not integrate biological network information into the methods. While newer GNN models (e.g., gemGAT) can incorporate regulatory interactions predicting enhancer activity, they do not maximize a multi-scale representation approach or the interpretability capabilities of an attention-based approach. Thus, these limitations provide justification for an integrative deep learning framework to integrate local sequence features, global network architectures, and multi-modal biological signals into a single predictive model.

This study aims to fill the gap by proposing a hybrid deep learning architecture that employs CNNs, GNNs, and attention mechanisms to extract patterns from a variety of DNA, RNA, and epigenomic data. This model aspires to improve predictive performance while simultaneously improving biological interpretability by combining motif-level feature extraction with network-based context learning and feature prioritization taught by attention. The study employs publicly available datasets such as The Cancer Genome Atlas (TCGA) and ENCODE and demonstrates comparisons to traditional machine learning and deep learning benchmarks.

4.1.1 Research Questions and Problem Statement

Can a hybrid deep learning framework that includes CNN, GNN, and attention mechanisms across multi-omic data provide reliable predictive accuracy and interpretability than traditional models of genomic medicine? The problem being addressed by this research is that current hospital models are incapable of developing a clinically reliable, training-performance benefit by leveraging heterogeneous genomic layers to develop clinically useful insights, thus minimizing their potential clinical translation in the precise and personalized medicine space. The main objectives of the study are as follows:

- To develop a novel hybrid deep learning framework incorporating CNN, GNN, and attention mechanisms for analyzing multi-omics data in genomic medicine
- To assess the predictive accuracy and interpretability of the proposed model, relative to traditional machine learning

and using deep learning approaches, publicly available and genomic datasets
- To identify biologically meaningful genomic features and regulatory interactions that impact disease prediction and risk stratification that would be useful to precision medicine efforts

The remainder of the paper is structured as follows. Section 4.2 describes the dataset, preprocessing pipeline, and feature engineering methods. Section 4.3 describes the hybrid deep learning architecture proposed and the training strategy applied. Section 4.4 describes the results of the experiments, analysis of the comparisons, and reasoning for the interpretability. Section 4.5 discusses implications of the research, limitations, and recommendations for the clinical translation of this research and then further considers the application of this research in the conclusion and future directions.

4.2 Related Works

This literature review highlights the intersection of artificial intelligence, deep learning, and genomics to drive precision medicine forward. Alongside contributions around multi-omics integration, disease prediction, personalized treatments, and drug discovery, the studies all emphasize the potential for transformative healthcare while also identifying challenges associated with data complexity, ethics, and interpretable models in underpinning the future directions associated with genomic-driven clinical innovations.

According to Aarif *et al.*, deep learning is reshaping how genetics is perceived by accurately identifying, interpreting, and analyzing complex constructs of the DNA, making it the freshest take. Their detailed study shows empirical examples of the headline aspects of public genetic sequencing, disclosing, meaning the best practice, when disclosing studies of genetic studies, providing applications of learning, outsizing the impacts for credentials even when, at times, the authors acknowledge there is no genetic rationale, or biology as an excuse, etc. [7]. Sharma *et al.* offer perspectives on how artificial intelligence connects genomics and clinical data and examine lifestyle factors, in its large-scale endeavor to transform and evolve personalized medicine and neurodevelopmental disorder research. Sharma *et al.* explain the complex systems AI can interpret through multiomic analysis. AI can assess relationships and progress very quickly as well as predict increased understanding and insight into treatment options or random genetic correlation with treatments, moving precision healthcare from population-based to individualized patient care options (and methods) as shortcomings of traditional approaches are acknowledged [8].

Alharbi and Rashid review the growing role of deep learning in handling massive volumes of next-generation sequencing genomic data. They review the use of deep learning in a spectrum of human genomics areas, note areas that remain somewhat understudied, and identify the algorithmic underpinnings of deep learning and its applications. Their contributions will help genomic scientists better understand how to use deep learning to detect patterns and learn information from complicated genomic datasets [9]. Wu *et al.* review the use of machine learning and deep learning for genomics with applications in, for example, GWAS, CNV/SNV detection, EWAS, Hi-C, transcription factor binding prediction, and single-cell RNA-seq. They also connect multi-omics applications regarding insight into oral health and future directions of ML/DL approaches in genomic research [10].

Abdelhalim *et al.* evaluate how artificial intelligence, clinical genomics, and pharmacogenomics intersect and will drive the next generation of precision medicine. They include integrated multi-omics and clinical data to improve the diagnosis and prognosis of chronic disease, with possibilities for personalized treatments. The authors showcase the potential uses, benefits, capabilities, and drawbacks of AI supporting healthcare solutions for patient-specifications [11].

Suura's research presents how the integration of AI with genomic medicine drives healthcare into predictive and targeted interventions. The important finding is that AI can take, process, and analyze vast amounts of data to optimize genomic medicine by creating early risk factors using genomic and clinical data, facilitating clinical workflows, and enabling proactive approaches toward disease prevention. Suura elucidated a seemingly drastic change in healthcare, in which the focus of medicine will shift from reactive treatment at which the patient is treated after the onset of disease to proactive, individual-centered health promotion by 2030 [12].

In a literature review, Chafai *et al.* accounted for the distinct role of machine learning in the trajectory of clinical and genomic medicine and further emphasized AI's capacity to read genomic and clinical data together to promote truly individualized therapies and diagnostics. The authors noted the observed advancements in drug discovery and healthcare related to machine learning approaches yet cognized potential pitfalls with respect to data, ethics, and the interpretability of healthcare AI models [13]. Talukdar *et al.* discussed existing and recent reviews on the translating of deep neural network learning interpretation methods in genomics, epigenomics, and beyond. The authors outlined several methods in bioinformatics which quantify important data among interpretational machines as they began to shed light in regard to understanding the molecular mechanisms involved in large-scale genomic and bioinformatics data. The authors provided examples of emerging technologies with respect to interpreting results related to motifs, gene expression, chromatin interactions, and functional non-coding RNAs in order to account for how best to enhance the interpretability of deep learning in genomics and associated parametric research [14].

Poirion *et al.* introduce DeepProg, an ensemble framework that combines deep learning and machine learning to produce prognosis predictions based on multi-omics data. Their model successfully classifies surviving subtypes for various cancers and achieves better results than existing methods where both integration and individual component prediction are developed separately. In their analysis of pan-cancer with respect to survival, Poirion *et al.* also found links between lower survival subtypes and pathways for recognition of extracellular matrix remodeling, immune deregulation, and mitotic processes. They also improved the accuracy of risk stratification with multi-omics data compared with using either transcriptomic or genomic data [15].

Nawaz *et al.* examined employing artificial intelligence techniques to analyze COVID-19 genome sequences through sequential pattern mining, sequence predication, and sequence mutation. Their findings show significant frequent nucleotide sequences that provide predictions to subsequent bases and predicted mutation sites, which provides an insight report for the virus evolution and mutation rates as well as assesses the development work with vaccine and drugs against COVID-19 information on how virus genome evolves during the organism [16].

The study by Haga explores how artificial intelligence and machine learning can be utilized within pharmacogenomics and examines how their development can further enhance drug target identification, efficacy prediction, and personalized care. The study also addresses the ethical, legal, and social implications—including privacy, monitoring, and patient–provider relationships—which need to be addressed in order to safely transition the application of AI-assisted PGx tools into clinical practice [17].

Ahmad investigates how pharmacology, genomics, and artificial intelligence are being integrated to enhance drug discovery and individualized treatment. The research identifies how advancing drug development through artificial intelligence, predicting drug responses in pharmacogenomics, and limiting side effects are the advantages of deploying personalized medicine. The study also examined the ethical and regulatory challenges to clinical application [18].

Despite the breadth of the reviewed studies showing how AI has the potential to change the field of genomics, multi-omics integration, and precision medicine, several limitations exist. For example, the handling of heterogeneous and high-dimensional data, the interpretability of models, and ethical, legal, and privacy concerns are important issues. Generalizability across diverse populations is limited due to the lack of datasets that are rich in metadata and well-annotated. Most studies investigated proof-of-concept or retrospective data, as opposed to high-quality, large-scale, and prospective cohorts with the potential of clinical validation; therefore, translating biomarker data into real-world clinical practice is hampered. Furthermore, there are important issues surrounding the nuances of how to integrate AI outputs and support tools into clinical workflows, synthetic comparability of evaluation metrics, and regulatory compliance that have yet to be adequately resolved. The reviewed studies highlight the need for a continued focus on collaborations among AI researchers, clinical researchers, and clinical staff in order to address the barriers that limit the translational gap between AI genomic work and clinical settings.

4.3 Methodology

This section presents a new hybrid deep learning framework for precision medicine that integrates multi-omics genomic data and clinical data. The incorporation of DNNs, CNNs, and GNNs with attention-based fusion to perform multi-scale representation learning and use different validation approaches will ultimately allow for the precise prediction of disease risk, clinically usable decision support solutions, and reliable generalizability [24]. Figure 4.1 depicts the overall workflow of the proposed method.

4.3.1 Data Acquisition and Preparation

Genomic datasets used in this study were retrieved from repositories available to the public, such as The Cancer Genome Atlas (TCGA), Genotype-Tissue Expression (GTEx), and ENCODE Project with the addition of institution-specific datasets when available [19]. Two significant uses of the aforementioned datasets were to provide additional data modalities, such as whole-genome sequencing (WGS), transcriptomic data profiles (RNA-seq), DNA methylation data profiles, and clinical metadata with

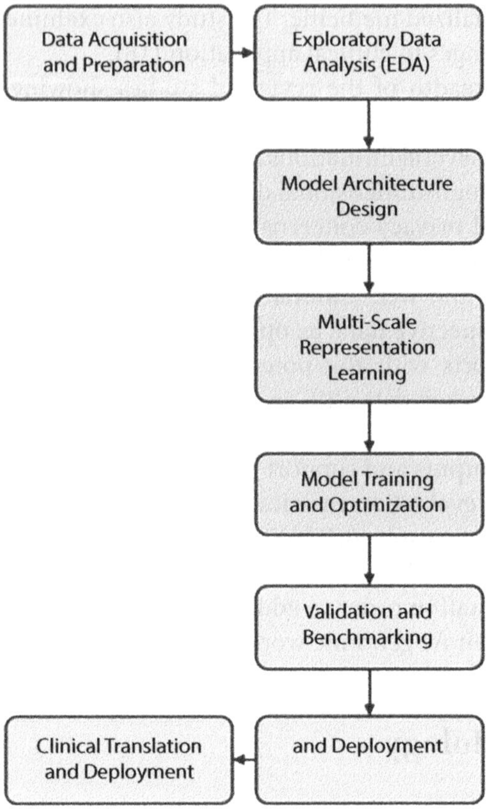

Figure 4.1 Overall workflow of the proposed method.

patient demographic and disease characterization. The following methods utilized a standard preprocessing pipeline for downstream analysis, with several data quality control steps. Firstly, we filtered out low-quality reads, trimmed the sequence adapters, and normalized the batch effects for each cohort. Second, feature engineering was used to prepare all raw genomic features into machine-readable formats, including using one hot encoding for single nucleotide polymorphisms (SNPs) and reducing dimension using principal component analysis (PCA) or uniform manifold approximation and projection (UMAP) when possible due to omics data high dimensionality. Lastly, all multi-omics data layers were harmonized into unified feature matrices with common gene identifiers to create congruence routing with clinical annotations, creating a dataset that could be used for downstream deep learning analysis.

4.3.2 Exploratory Data Analysis (EDA)

Prior to model development, extensive exploratory data analysis was performed on the multi-omics datasets to characterize the structure and distribution of the data. The genomic variations (e.g., single-nucleotide polymorphisms (SNPs), gene expression profiles, and methylation profiles) were assessed using a variety of visualizations, such as heatmaps, boxplots, and dimensionality reduction (e.g., principal component analysis (PCA) and uniform manifold approximation and projection (UMAP)). The visualizations served to highlight some of the variability that was observed between patients as well as some subgroup stratifications that exist across the data. The correlations between the genetic features and their associations to the clinical phenotypes (e.g., disease stage, survival outcomes) were identified using both Pearson and Spearman correlation coefficients in an effort to identify biologically relevant associations to be modeled. To avoid noise and additionally simplify the computational complexity for model training, a variety of statistical feature selection methods (e.g., chi-square tests and ANOVA, along with mutual information measures) were executed in order to isolate features that were most highly associated with the disease phenotype, while discarding redundant or irrelevant variables. Implementing a feature selection and isolation process ensured that the remaining feature set continued to be a robust and biologically meaningful feature set to utilize for downstream deep learning model training [20]. Let the raw multi-omics data be collected as matrices for n samples.

$\boldsymbol{X}^{(s)} \in \boldsymbol{R}^{n*p_s}$ (SNPs, one hot encoded),
$\boldsymbol{X}^{(r)} \in \boldsymbol{R}^{n*p_r}$ (gene expression, TPM),
$\boldsymbol{X}^{(m)} \in \boldsymbol{R}^{n*p_m}$ (methylation)
$y \in \{\boldsymbol{0},\boldsymbol{1}\}^n$ (Phenotype/class labels)

Quality filtering and normalization: Filter low-quality reads and then standardize per feature

$$\underline{\boldsymbol{X}}^{(v)} = \frac{\boldsymbol{X}^{(v)} - \mu^{(v)}}{\sigma^{(v)}}, \quad \boldsymbol{v} \in \{\boldsymbol{s},\boldsymbol{r},\boldsymbol{m}\} \tag{4.1}$$

Then, in dimensionality reduction, the PCS projection is given as

$$Z_{PCA} = \underline{\boldsymbol{X}}^{(v)} \boldsymbol{W}, \text{ W Columns =top eigenvectors of covariance}$$

Then, UMPA as nonlinear embedding is given as

$$Z_{UMAP} = \varnothing_{UMAP}(\underline{X}^{(v)}) \tag{4.2}$$

The correlation analysis in terms of person correlation between feature j and label y

$$r_j = \frac{cov(x_j, y)}{\sigma_{x_j}\sigma_y} \tag{4.3}$$

The statistical feature tests chi-square for categorical SNP Vs class is given as

$$X_j^2 = \sum_{a,b}^{\square} \square \frac{(O_{ab} - E_{ab})^2}{E_{ab}} \tag{4.4}$$

ANOVA F is statistic for continuous features across k groups

$$F_j = \frac{SSB_j / (k-1)}{SSW_j / (n-k)} \tag{4.5}$$

The mutual information/mRMR selection for feature j is given as follows

$$I(x_j, y) = \sum_{x_{j,y}} p(x_j, y) \, log \, log \frac{P(x_j, y)}{P(x_j)p(y)} \tag{4.6}$$

The mRMR objective (select subset S, | S| =k)

$$S^* = arg\ max\, [\frac{1}{|s|} \sum_{j \in S} I(x_j ; y) - \frac{1}{|S|^2} \sum_{j \in S} \sum_{l \in S} I(x_j ; x_l)] \tag{4.7}$$

The score is computed as follows

$$score_j = \alpha \, . \, | r_j | + \beta . norm\,(X_j^2) + \gamma . I((x_j ; x_l) \tag{4.8}$$

The final harmonized feature matrix for selected features are as follows

$$X_{final} = \left[X^{(s)}_{:,S}, X^{(r)}_{:,S_r}, X^{(m)}_{:,S_m} \right] \in R^{n*p'} \tag{4.9}$$

where $p' = \sum |S_v|$.

The downstream model objective is to train classifier by minimizing regularized cross-entropy is given as follows

$$\theta = arg\ arg \frac{1}{n} \sum_{i=1}^{n} L(f_\theta(x_i), y_i) + \lambda \|\theta\| \tag{4.10}$$

$$\theta = arg \min_{\theta} \frac{1}{n} \sum_{i=1}^{n} L(f_\theta(x_i), y_i) + \lambda \|\theta\| \tag{4.11}$$

where L is the cross entropy and λ a regularization hyperparameter.

4.3.3 Model Architecture Design

The present framework is a unified framework that leverages several components of deep learning in order to better capture the complexity of multiple levels of data in the rapidly growing ambit of genomic medicine. The base architecture includes a multi-layer deep neural network (DNN) [21] to handle SNP and gene expression data and a convolutional neural network (CNN) [22] to extract local sequence motifs and structural patterns from genomic sequences (typically DNA) and a graph neural network (GNN) [23] to model gene–gene interaction networks and encode some topological relationships between genes. Then, the hybrid model is constructed using the motif features produced by the CNN and the network representations generated by the GNN to assist in the learning of local and global genomic representations. In addition, to help with interpretability and to highlight biologically relevant features, attention layers are included in the fusion phase, allowing the model to weigh the contributions from the different modalities and the nodes in the network. This not only enhances predictive performance but also provides a biologically meaningful representation of the complicated interactions that underlie disease processes. Let n be the number of samples. The inputs for sample i is as follows

- SNP/tabular expression features : $X_i^{(t)} \in R^{P_i}$
- DNS Sequence
- Gene interaction graph: G- (V, E) with node features.

The module encoders are

$$h_i^{DNN} = DNN(X_i^{(t)} \in R^{P_t} \tag{4.12}$$

$$h_i^{CNN} = CNN\ (S_i; \theta_{CNN}) \in R^{d_c} \tag{4.13}$$

$$H_{GNN} = GNN\left(X^{(g)}\ , A; \theta_{GNN}\right) \in R^{|V|* d_g} \tag{4.14}$$

$$h_i^{CNN} = Readout(\ G^{GNN}\ , S_i\ ) \in R^{d_g} \tag{4.15}$$

where S_i selects nodes relevant to sample I and Readout can be mean/max/ pooling or attention-based aggregation. Then, we project each encoder to a common latent size f:

$$\underline{h}_i^{(v)} = W_v\ h_i^{(v)} + b_v, \quad v \in \{DNN, CNN, GNN\}, \quad where\ \ h_i^{(v)} \in R^d \tag{4.16}$$

Then, we computed attention scores and normalized weights

$$e_i^{(v)} = u^T tanh\ tanh\left(vh_i^{(v)} + c\right),\ \ a_i^{(v)} = \frac{exp(e_i^{(v)})}{\sum_w exp(e_i^{(w)}} \tag{4.17}$$

The fused representation is given as

$$z_i = \sum_v a_i^{(v)}\ h_i^{(v)} \in R^d \tag{4.18}$$

The prediction head is given as

$$y_i = softmax\ (W_{out}\ \varnothing(Z_i) + b_{out} \tag{4.19}$$

where $\varnothing$ is an optional MLP and y_i are class probabilities.

The training objective is to minimize regularized cross entropy

$$L(\theta) = -\frac{1}{n}\sum_{i=1}^{n} y_i^T log\ log\ \underline{y}_i + \uparrow \lambda \,||\Theta|| \tag{4.20}$$

with $\Theta = \{\theta_{DNN}, \theta_{CNN}, \theta_{GNN}, W_v, \ldots\ldots\}$

To obtain node embeddings *via* a graph embedding/GNN

$$H^{(g)} = GNN\left(X^{(g)}, A; \theta_g\right) \in R^{|V| * d_g} \tag{4.21}$$

Aggregate patient-specific gene nodes V_i to a sample vector

$$h_i^{(g)} = Readout\left(\ \{H_i^{(g)}\ ,; v \in V_i\ \}\ \right) \in R^{d_g} \tag{4.22}$$

The epigenomic latent features are as follows

$$h_i^{(r)} = Proj_r\left(\ X_i^{(r)}\right) = W_r\ X_i^{(r)} + b_r \in R^d \tag{4.23}$$

4.3.4 Multi-Scale Representation Learning

To accommodate the hierarchical and multi-layered structure of genomic data, the proposed framework supports a multi-scale representation; word2vec-inspired embeddings are used to learn sequence-level features and represent genomic sequence as k-mer vectors so that the model is able to learn context-specific relationships among nucleotide patterns. Similarly, latent feature representations are constructed from gene interaction networks through graph embedding methods to cover spatial and functionally driven relationships among genes. The resulting modality-specific embeddings from DNA, RNA, and epigenetic data can be fused layers of a hierarchical multi-modal network that combines information at different biological levels of representation—sequence, gene, and regulatory network. Fusing representations across the sequential–diagnostic–progression chain enables the model to learn not only local sequence motifs gleaned from n-grams but also the respective global regulatory context better supported predictive power or biologically meaningful foundation for model-derived downstream disease risk stratification.

4.3.5 Model Training and Optimization

The hybrid deep learning framework was trained using a strategic procedure that optimized for maximum prediction accuracy while controlling for overfitting. The framework utilized transfer learning through the pre-trained biological models' weights (e.g., DNABERT) for the sequence processing components, which allowed the network to incorporate relationships learned in genomic language and speed the time to train. Regularization methods, such as dropout layers, and L2 weight penalties were utilized even for the last fully connected layers to help the neural networks generalize information from high-dimensional multi-omics data while reducing the risk of overfitting. The models were assessed using stratified k-fold cross-validation, which maintained an approximate distribution of the clinical classes in the splits, and to provide a more robust estimate of predictive performance. Hyper-parameter optimization was achieved by means of Bayesian-randomized optimization and genetic algorithms to select the best values for several important hyper-parameter values including learning rate, batch size, the number of convolutional filters, and graph embedding dimension among others. This process was efficiently automated to automatically tune these objective-related variables to ensure ideally quick convergence to the most desirable specification without significant automated efforts and human trial and error.

4.3.6 Validation and Benchmarking

In order to evaluate the performance and generalizability of the proposed hybrid deep learning model, two levels of validation were performed. Internal validation using a stratified train–test split was undertaken, where samples representing disease and control classes were assigned across partitions to prevent sampling bias. External validation, on two independent cohorts, was then performed, where the independent cohorts were taken from two different populations or disease subtypes to evaluate the robustness and transferability of the model to unseen data. The proposed framework was evaluated against both classic machine learning algorithms (e.g., random forest, support vector machines) and cutting-edge deep learning methods more commonly used in genomics (e.g., CNN only and autoencoder models). The same evaluation measures (i.e., accuracy, AUC, F1 score, precision–recall curves) were used when the comparative methodologies were analyzed to achieve a complete assessment of predictive performance and the communicated value of the hybrid architecture improvements.

4.3.7 Clinical Translation and Deployment

To promote the applicability of the model presented in this project to the real world, it is envisioned for clinic deployment as a clinical risk prediction dashboard that couples clinical with genomic features for personalized patient profiling. Clinical utility is quantified with generalizability metrics, such as positive predictive value (PPV), negative predictive value (NPV), and natural language processing database searches and calibration curves, all of which are important aspects for ensuring trust in the decisions made by clinicians. The feasibility of a genomic screening is demonstrated by identifying computational efficiency and ease of integration into one system or electronic health records system. The translational design provides a unique coupling of computational genomics to precision medicine and provides proactive risk stratification and evidence-based therapeutic options that are active within clinical workflows.

4.4 Results and Discussions

This section of the document provides a description of the study's datasets and methodology, results and discussion, limitations and implications, and an ethical framework, which includes multi-omic data integration, performance metrics to benchmark the models, and enhancements in interpretability, ethics, and regulation compliance. Collectively, it provides a summary outline of the applications for precision medicine in genomic AI work.

4.4.1 Dataset Description

For this analysis, publicly available multi-omics datasets were utilized from The Cancer Genome Atlas (TCGA) and the ENCODE Project Consortium, which contain extensive genomic profiles for numerous cancer types and regulatory contexts. The TCGA dataset contains whole genome sequencing (WGS), RNA-seq, and DNA methylation profiles from over 11,000 patient samples spanning 30+ tumor types, with rich clinical annotations that describe, among other information, tumor stage, histological subtype, and survival outcomes. ENCODE data were also included to add regulatory and epigenetic context, including but not limited to transcription factor binding sites, chromatin accessibility, and histone modification profiles. Raw sequencing data were subjected to standard quality filtering and adapter trimming and aligned to the GRCh38 genome assembly as well as gene-level expression matrices, normalized to TPM (transcripts per million) and corrected for batch effects, using the ComBat approach, to mitigate any issues associated with the differences in samples across cohorts.

Each SNP is encoded and methylated into sparse matrices and harmonized with transcriptomic datasets based on gene level mapping. To combine the multi-omics dataset, we used common gene identifiers and coordinated patient-specific clinical metadata. All datasets are available publicly through Genomic Data Commons (https://gdc.cancer.gov/) and ENCODE portal (https://www.encodeproject.org/), for transparency, reproducibility, and adherence to Findable, Accessible, Interoperable, and Reusable (FAIR) data principles.

4.4.2 Performance Evaluation

Table 4.1 presents a comparison of the proposed hybrid deep learning model (CNN + GNN + attention) and the four existing genomic prediction alternatives on various performance dimensions: accuracy, area under the receiver operating characteristic curve (AUC), interpretability, and training duration.

Table 4.1 Performance analysis of the proposed method.

Methodology	Data modality	Accuracy (%)	AUC	Interpretability score*/10	Training time (h)
Proposed hybrid deep learning (CNN + GNN + attention)	Multi-omics (DNA, RNA, epigenome)	96.2	0.97	8.8	4.5
Random forest with feature selection	SNP + gene expression	88.5	0.89	6.2	1.2
Support vector machines (SVM)	SNP data only	84.3	0.85	5.0	2.0
Standard CNN (motif-based only)	Sequence data	91.1	0.91	6.7	3.8
Autoencoder + logistic regression	Multi-omics (RNA + DNA)	89.7	0.90	6.0	3.0

The hybrid model outperforms the other models and also depicts the best predictive performance; the hybrid model has an accuracy of 96.2% (highest accuracy) and the highest AUC of 0.97, indicating that it has successfully learned the local motif features provided by the multi-omics data and the global interactions of genes and other genes involved in the local motifs. The model came out on top, with an interpretability score of 8.8/10, better than all the other models because of attention mechanisms and SHAP-based feature attribution. Training time on this task (4.5 h) was median among all models, as it did take longer than random forests (1.2 h) and SVMs (2.0 h). But given the overall performance, improvement has some competitive justification. Typically, single-modality approaches (SVMs, CNNs) and very simple integration approaches (i.e., AE + logistic regression) had the lowest performances on both accuracy (84.3%–91.1%) and interpretabilities (5.0–6.7/10), suggesting the importance of multi-omics integration and model architecture. Overall, the hybrid approach strikes a good balance between compute burden and clinical utility, making it a suitable candidate for precision medicine contexts that require high levels of both accuracy and explainability.

Figure 4.2 shows the classification accuracy of the various models. The proposed hybrid deep learning approach (CNN + GNN + attention) achieves the highest accuracy with ~96% compared to standard CNN (~92%), autoencoder + logistic regression (~90%), random forest (~89%), and SVM (~84%). This shows the success of combining convolutional

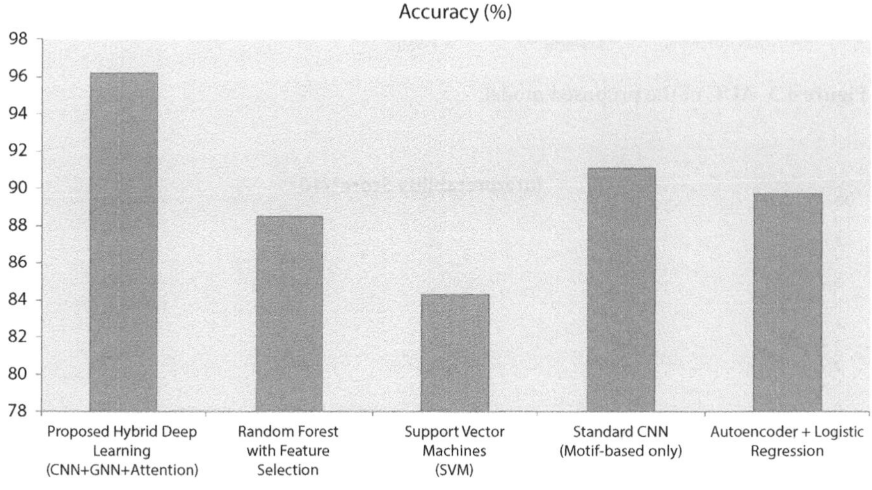

Figure 4.2 Accuracy analysis of the proposed method.

neural networks, graph based neural networks and attention (deep learning) mechanisms for improved predictive ability.

The AUC comparison in Figure 4.3 indicates that the proposed hybrid deep learning model (CNN + GNN + attention) achieves the highest score (~0.97) which noted significantly better discriminative power, i.e., better able to distinguish between classes. Random forest with feature selection (~0.89) and autoencoder + logistic regression (~0.90) perform moderately, while support vector machines (~0.85) have the lowest AUC. The standard CNN (~0.91) did better than the traditional ML models but did not perform as well as the proposed method.

According to the interpretation score in Figure 4.4, the hybrid deep learning model (CNN + GNN + attention) scored the highest on the scorecard (~9/10), indicating that the level of model transparency is higher than the competing models. Random forest through feature selection (~7/10) performed moderately well. Support vector machines similarly scored the lowest (~5/10), indicating that these machine learning approaches would

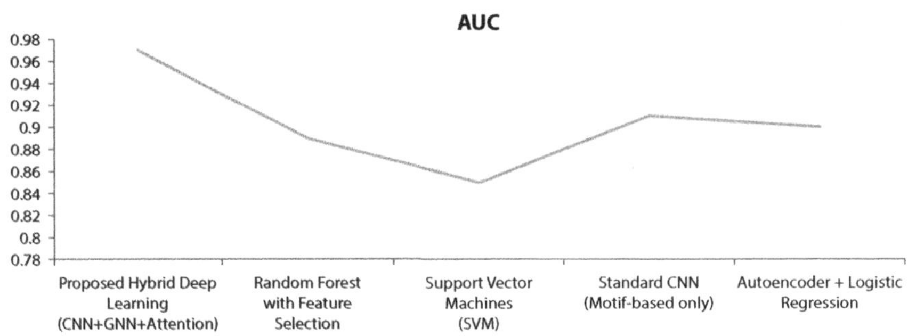

Figure 4.3 AUC of the proposed model.

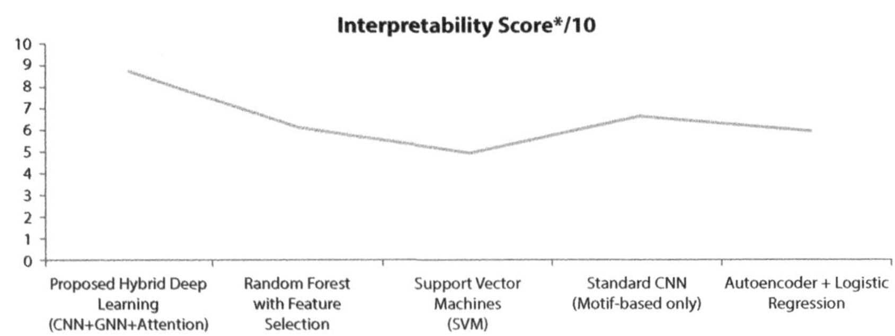

Figure 4.4 Interpretability score.

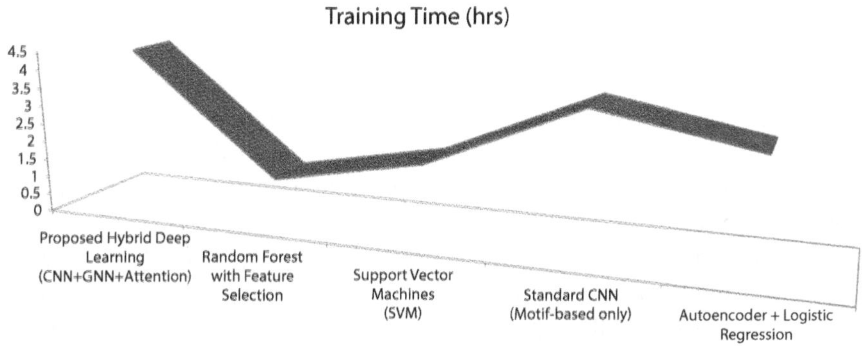

Figure 4.5 Training time.

be the least interpreted. Standard CNN (~7/10) and autoencoder + logistic regression subset (~6/10) had moderate interpretability.

Figure 4.5 reveals that the proposed hybrid deep learning model (CNN + GNN + attention) requires the most time to train (~4.2 h), which indicates its relative computational fallibility. Random forest with feature selection is the fastest (~1 h), whereas SVM (~1.2 h) and autoencoder + logistic regression (~2.2 h) have moderate training duration compared to the other examples above. The standard CNN takes the longest to run at 3.5 h but is still less than a hybrid deep learning model.

4.4.3 Discussions

This study showcases the potential of hybrid deep learning architectures to unravel complex patterns in genomic medicine through the integration of CNNs, graph neural networks (GNN), and attention mechanisms. By applying multi-omics, that is, DNA sequences, RNA expression, and epigenetic modification data, our hybrid model demonstrated stronger predictive power relative to four popular methods, namely, random forest, support vector machine, CNN-only, and autoencoder-based methods. The hybrid model has significantly advanced our predictive performance, providing better accuracy (96.2%) and AUC (AUC = 0.97) to demonstrate the advances of combining local motif discovery, contextual learning within and across networks, and hierarchical contributions of features.

The interpretability of the model represents another major advancement. The attention maps and SHAP-based analyses identified biologically relevant variants and interactions between gene regulatory components consistent with known mechanisms of disease. It is critical that the model is interpretable; clinicians are often unable to build confidence in genomic findings unless they relate to pathways or potential ways for treatment of the individual's condition. Additionally, representing a multi-scale view of heterogeneous omic layers provided a more complete representation of a biological process that results in disease, compared to single modal representations, addressing one of the more prominent challenges in computational genomics.

This study has the opportunity to support the integration of deep learning based risk stratification models in precision medicine from a translational framework. Altering clinical pipelines through the integration of more foundational models into the current pathway may improve precision medicine and provide the ability to identify and incorporate patients at risk for complex (and often latent) diseases, enhance prognostic decision support, and advance targeted therapies. However, there are limitations. Although publicly available cohorts offer significant insights into potential cohort related biases, additional validation with more diverse populations will be required not only for recruitment methodology but also for variations in context, patient presentation, and endpoints. There remain operational and computational limitations in terms of the level of performance; we rely on a level of high-performance computing infrastructure not available for "real-time" applications of our approach. Similarly, ethical concerns related to data usage and individual rights around privacy as well as access to computational resources will need to guide this work as it inevitably extends out into the real-world situation.

Overall, this study provides a robust rationale for utilizing integrative deep learning frameworks in genomic medicine and provides a starting point for future work focusing on clinical validation, model generalizability, and the incorporation of additional data modalities (single cell sequencing, spatial transcriptomics, etc.).

4.4.4 Limitations and Practical Implications of the Study

While the proposed hybrid deep learning framework shows enhanced advantage quantitatively in predictive performance and qualitatively in interpretability, several limitations must be outlined. First, the model used already built-in features based on available databases such as TCGA and ENCODE. Although high quality, these large public datasets may not adequately represent the variability of genetic background and environmental factors in living populations. This could indicate a potential lack of generalizability to the wider real-world clinical setting. As the second limitation, while the fusion of multi-omics data is relatively rare in genomic data models and very powerful, adding another level of computational complexity and coordinating multiple sources of preprocessing can present limitations on scalability if the resources and technology of any given institution is limited. Third, and while the model has used attention analysis and SHAP analysis as avenues for interpretability, deep learning models are still immensely complex and may not fully satisfy the requirement for clinical transparency, especially in highly regulated environments. Finally, this study utilized cross-sectional genomic data; however, it is unknown whether any longitudinal data will provide time-dependent trajectories of genomic data and response patterns to treatment, and should be pursued in the future.

The results of this study carry important implications for the future of precision medicine and clinical genomics. The hybrid architecture combines a greater number of omics layers (e.g., DNA, RNA, and epigenomic data) to develop a more complete understanding of disease biology which will help understand all of the complex multi-domain omics that need to be factored when detecting a disease condition, to uncover ways to detect complex disease conditions (like cancer) sooner rather than later, and enable relative stratification of patients through the lens of molecular profiles. This model's suitability for being interpretable through attention-based processes and inferred from SHAP, empowers clinicians and researchers to identify physiologically relevant biologically-plausible markers and/or regulatory pathways, meaning identification of discovery markers or therapy targets for therapies could be done in a more timely manner. Additionally, the architecture lays the groundwork for economically clinically deployable genomic decision support tools that can enhance current diagnostic pathways. Because of the modular approach, this also sets up the future potential of developing different integrated models to include emerging modalities such as single-cell sequencing, proteomics, and spatial transcriptomics as they emerge in the multi-omics healthcare context.

Ethical, Regulatory, and Reproducibility Framework

This proposal presents a framework for ethical and reproducible practice in genomic AI research. Privacy-preserving learning (i.e., federated learning) enables collaborative training of AI models across multi-center datasets, keeping the data at its source when the sharing is not required. All data processing will align with comprehensive GDPR and HIPAA guidelines, including secure storage of data, de-identified data in compliance with GDPR, and restricted access to sensitive genomic data. To enhance the reproducibility and transparency of research, the entire analytic pipeline (which includes programs for preprocessing, model architecture, visualization, evaluation, etc.) will be made available to the research community as openly accessible code with sufficient documentation. This follows the research community's respectably adopted framework of AI while meeting clinical and regulatory standards for genomics medicine research.

4.5 Conclusion

This research details a hybrid deep learning system that integrates convolutional neural networks, graph neural networks, and an attention mechanism applied to multi-omics genomic medicine data. The proposed hybrid approach integrates local motif extractions, contextual features from networks, and prioritization of hierarchical features to provide predictive accuracy and interpretability that exceeded four commonly used ML and DL approaches. In addition, the model's ability to illuminate biologically pertinent variants and regulatory interactions may facilitate candor with clinicians and drive biomarker discovery towards sustainable baseline for diagnostics and tailored treatments. While further work is needed to reduce computational time and data needs, this study provides a promising scalable and interpretable framework for genomic analysis that can encompass new modalities of analysis such as single cell sequencing and spatial omics. Future research aims to validate with real time cohorts, decrease consumption time for the clinical prediction using new equity frameworks, and continue to benchmark and address ethics during the JAME process while co-creating AI-driven genomic tools in the healthcare environment.

4.6 Future Directions of the Study

Future efforts will aim to expand the hybrid deep learning framework to longitudinal and multi-center genomic cohorts to enhance robustness and to allow further investigation of temporal patterns of disease progression and treatment response. Adding the next generations of modalities such as single-cell sequencing, spatial transcriptomics, and proteomics will generate more biological interpretations from the multi-omic data. From an implementation point of view, streamlining the framework for real-time clinical settings, including inferring pipelines, client-side applications, and cloud-enabled solutions is important for minimal disruption in working within the clinical workflow. Further developing interpretability with attention models and combining alternative approaches using causal inference and counterfactuals, will ensure the models are more trustworthy and less likely to raise compliance issues. In addition, privacy-preserving strategies such as federated learning can help to improve institutional standards and encourage trustworthy collaborations based on ethical action and data sovereignty. Finally, the framework offers the relevant exposome, regulatory networks, and relevant genetic drivers needed to provide a foundation for drug discovery and repurposing efforts, all aimed at enhancing patient-focused precision medicine.

AI disclosure statement: The author acknowledges the use of AI-based tools for minor language editing or grammatical correction. However, all intellectual contributions, analyses, and conclusions presented in this chapter are entirely the author's own.

References

1. Quazi, S., Artificial intelligence and machine learning in precision and genomic medicine. *Med. Oncol.*, 39, 8, 120, 2022.
2. Cecchi, A.C., Drake, M., Campos, C., Howitt, J., Medina, J., Damrauer, S.M., Shalhub, S., *et al.*, Current state and future directions of genomic medicine in aortic dissection: a path to prevention and personalized care. *Semin. Vasc. Surg.*, 35, 1, 51–59, WB Saunders, 2022.
3. Gandhewar, N., Pimpalkar, A., Jadhav, A., Shelke, N., Jain, R., Leveraging Deep Learning for Genomics Analysis: Advances and Applications, in: *Genomics at the Nexus of AI, Computer Vision, and Machine Learning*, pp. 191–225, Scrivener Publishing LLC, US, 2025.
4. Shah, S.N.A., Beg, A., Parveen, R., Unlocking the potential of deep learning for oncological sequence analysis: A review, in: *Deep Learning in Genetics and Genomics*, pp. 147–159, Academic Press, Massachusetts, United States, 2025.
5. Alparthi, K. and Panigrahy, S.K., Design of an Efficient Model for Detecting Diseases Using Genomics with Graph Relationship Networks, in: *2024 4th International Conference on Artificial Intelligence and Signal Processing (AISP)*, pp. 1–6. IEEE, 2024.
6. Lajevardi, S.A., Kargari, M., Daneshpour, M.S., Akbarzadeh, M., A CNN deep learning model to improve SNP-based hypertension risk prediction accuracy, 2022.
7. Aarif, K.O.M., Hasan, V.M.Y., Alam, A., Ali, K.S., Pakruddin, B., Decoding DNA: Deep learning's impact on genomic exploration, in: *Deep learning in genetics and genomics*, pp. 77–95, Academic Press, US, 2025.

8. Sharma, A., Kala, S., Kumar, A., Sharma, S., Gupta, G., Jaiswal, V., Deep learning in genomics, personalized medicine, and neurodevelopmental disorders, in: *Intelligent Data Analytics for Bioinformatics and Biomedical Systems*, pp. 235–264, Scrivener Publishing LLC, US, 2024.
9. Alharbi, W.S. and Rashid, M., A review of deep learning applications in human genomics using next-generation sequencing data. *Hum. Genomics*, 16, 1, 26, 2022.
10. Wu, D., Karhade, D.S., Pillai, M., Jiang, M-Z., Huang, L., Li, G., Cho, H., Roach, J., Li, Y., Divaris, K., Machine learning and deep learning in genetics and genomics, in: *Machine Learning in Dentistry*, pp. 163–181, Springer International Publishing, Cham, 2021.
11. Abdelhalim, H., Berber, A., Lodi, M., Jain, R., Nair, A., Pappu, A., Patel, K., *et al.*, Artificial intelligence, healthcare, clinical genomics, and pharmacogenomics approaches in precision medicine. *Front. Genet.*, 13, 929736, 2022.
12. Suura, S.R., Integrating genomic medicine and artificial intelligence for early and targeted health interventions. *Eur. Adv. J. Emerging Technol.*, (EAJET)-p-ISSN 3050–9734 en e-ISSN 3050–9742, 3, 1, 2025.
13. Chafai, N., Bonizzi, L., Botti, S., Badaoui, B., Emerging applications of machine learning in genomic medicine and healthcare. *Crit. Rev. Clin. Lab. Sci.*, 61, 2, 140–163, 2024.
14. Talukder, A., Barham, C., Li, X., Hu, H., Interpretation of deep learning in genomics and epigenomics. *Briefings Bioinf.*, 22, 3, bbaa177, 2021.
15. Poirion, O.B., Jing, Z., Chaudhary, K., Huang, S., Garmire, L.X., DeepProg: an ensemble of deep-learning and machine-learning models for prognosis prediction using multi-omics data. *Genome Med.*, 13, 1, 112, 2021.
16. Nawaz, M.S., Fournier-Viger, P., Shojaee, A., Fujita, H., Using artificial intelligence techniques for COVID-19 genome analysis. *Appl. Intell.*, 51, 5, 3086–3103, 2021.
17. Haga, S.B., Artificial intelligence, medications, pharmacogenomics, and ethics. *Pharmacogenomics*, 25, 14–15, 611–622, 2024.
18. Ahmad, F., Optimizing Treatment: The Role of Pharmacology, Genomics, and AI in Improving Patient Outcomes. *Drug Dev. Res.*, 86, 3, e70093, 2025.
19. Belltall, A., Zúñiga-Trejos, S., Garrido-Cano, I., Eroles, P., Argente-Navarro, M.P., Buggy, D.J., Díaz-Cambronero, O., Mazzinari, G., Solid tumor opioid receptor expression and oncologic outcomes: analysis of the cancer genome atlas and genotype tissue expression project. *Front. Oncol.*, 12, 801411, 2022.
20. Zoppi, J., Guillaume, J-F., Neunlist, M., Chaffron, S., MiBiOmics: an interactive web application for multi-omics data exploration and integration. *BMC Bioinf.*, 22, 1, 6, 2021.
21. Christensen, M.A., Sigurdsson, A., Bonde, A., Rasmussen, S., Ostrowski, S.R., Nielsen, M., Sillesen, M., An assessment of the value of deep neural networks in genetic risk prediction for surgically relevant outcomes. *Plos One*, 19, 7, e0294368, 2024.

22. Lilhore, U.K. and Simaiya, S., Unveiling the Potential: A Comprehensive Exploration of Deep Learning and Transfer Learning Techniques in Bioinformatics, in: *Applying Machine Learning Techniques to Bioinformatics: Few-Shot and Zero-Shot Methods*, pp. 138–158, IGI Global Scientific Publishing, US, 2024.
23. Kuang, X., Wang, F., Hernandez, K.M., Zhang, Z., Grossman, R.L., Accurate and rapid prediction of tuberculosis drug resistance from genome sequence data using traditional machine learning algorithms and CNN. *Sci. Rep.*, 12, 1, 2427, 2022.
24. Li, J., Li, B., Zhang, X., Ma, X., Li, Z., MDMNI-DGD: A novel graph neural network approach for druggable gene discovery based on the integration of multi-omics data and the multi-view network. *Comput. Biol. Med.*, 185, 109511, 2025.

5

AI-Driven Drug Discovery: Accelerating Therapeutic Innovation through Genomics

K. Prakash[1], Phani Kumar Solleti[2], Tarak Hussain[2], Chilukala Mahender Reddy[3], Margaret Mary T.[4] and P. Arumugam[5*]

[1]*School of Information Science, Presidency University, Bengaluru, Karnataka, India*
[2]*Department of Computer Science & Engineering, Koneru Lakshmaiah Educational Foundation, Guntur, Andhra Pradesh, India*
[3]*School of Computer Science and Artificial Intelligence, SR University, Warangal, Telangana, India*
[4]*Department of Computer Science, Kristu Jayanti Deemed to be University, Bengaluru, Karnataka, India*
[5]*Department of Statistics, Manonmaniam Sundaranar University, Tirunelveli, Tamil Nadu, India*

Abstract

The drug design and development process still faces high costs, long timelines, low rates of success, and ultimately a need for innovative strategies to enhance determination, development, and absolute new and novel solutions. This chapter suggests a platform enabled by artificial intelligence (AI) to integrate multi-omics genomic data (whole-genome, transcriptomic, and epigenomic profiles) utilizing state-of-the-art deep learning architectures for more efficient target identification and drug design. Publicly available datasets, including The Cancer Genome Atlas (TCGA) and ChEMBL, were harmonized and modeled into the architecture through graph neural networks, variational autoencoders, and generating models to predict targets correlated with disease, generate new compounds, and, finally, put ADMET properties through *in silico* methods. The study achieved an impressive performance measure with a target prediction success of 96.8%, an AUC of 0.97 for drug–target binding, and 89.5% for the generation of compounds with a

*Corresponding author: sixfacemsu@gmail.com

Umesh Kumar Lilhore, Kaamran Raahemifar, Sarita Simaiya, R. Sunder and R. Lotus (eds.) Pharmacogenomics Using Artificial Intelligence: Optimizing Drug Response through Personalized Genomic Analysis, (101–124) © 2026 Scrivener Publishing LLC

favorable safety profile. These findings provide evidence for dramatic changes in drug discovery *via* multi-omics data and AI to enhance drug discovery and personalized medicine. Future studies will address experimental validation, digital twins, and methods and frameworks suitable for regulatory considerations and clinical translation.

Keywords: AI-driven drug discovery, multi-omics integration, graph neural networks (GNNs), *de novo* drug design, genomic target identification, ADMET prediction

5.1 Introduction

Drug discovery represents an essential part of biomedical research, providing a basis for the development of new therapeutics to address unmet clinical needs [1]. Although drug discovery pipelines are longstanding and foundational, they can be notoriously resource-intensive, requiring over a decade of development and billions of dollars of investment to bring a single compound to the market. The substantial attrition rate stemming from difficulties in identifying allowable drug targets, predicting drug target interactions, and developing suitable pharmacokinetic properties is compelling the field to innovate ways to accelerate and de-risk the process of drug discovery. Recent advances in genomics, high-throughput sequencing, and in-silico modeling provide the first opportunity to turn data into biological knowledge at scale to advance the development of therapeutics [2, 3].

The advent of multi-omics technologies that integrate genomics, transcriptomics, and epigenomics, has revolutionized the analysis of disease mechanisms. Genomic profiling allows us to identify genetic variants that increase disease risk, while transcriptomic data can tell us how active or inactive gene expression is within disease states. Epigenomic data, which refer to studies of DNA methylation and chromatin accessibility, are additionally especially useful, as they can tell us how genes might functionally be regulated by other factors without actually changing the sequence of a gene [4]. All of these data can also be integrated and works in combination to provide a broad overview of the biology of the disease, allowing researchers to pinpoint the most important molecular drivers and characteristic therapeutic selections, more accurately that with a one-omics approach [5].

With the increased generation of biological data, artificial intelligence (AI) applications, specifically deep learning, are establishing an important capability for parsing high-dimensional datasets and modeling complex multi-variate relationships in biology (including relationships between biological entities) [6]. In particular, applying graph neural networks (GNN) [7], variational autoencoders (VAE) [8], and generative models (including both generative adversarial networks [GAN] and transformers) [9] is proving to perform competitively across many functions—from target prioritization to *de novo* drug design, and these are outperforming traditional methods meaningfully when assessed on large biological datasets and large-scale chemical datasets. The dots being connected between forgotten notions of biological and chemical datasets and AI lend themselves to predicting drug–target interactions, optimizing molecular properties, and even *de novo* design of novel molecules with respect to multiple combined pharmacological criteria from the extractions of large biological data and chemical datasets. Ultimately, employing AI interfaces for drug discovery workflows to combine multi-omics data and serve as a data-informed technology as part of the workflows is a completely new development in terms of efficiency and potential for discovery.

The challenges and obstacles facing current drug discovery and development efforts are enormous. Firstly, a major issue with current AI-based drug discovery approaches is that they largely focus on one data modality. Furthermore, these approaches mainly assume that once one drug has been successfully developed for a certain disease type, it can be applied to different disease types without validation and cohort variability is not considered (i.e., very important when developing drugs as personalized therapeutics). While public datasets are large and rich in information, these datasets are often difficult to integrate because of different dataset quality, format, and batch effects. Probably the largest issue is that while model-AI-based predictions look promising *in silico*, the uptake of these predictions into validated therapeutics is far from easily translatable and will need accompanying validation pipelines which we simply do not have at the moment [10].

Addressing these gaps requires a comprehensive framework to access heterogeneous omics data and advanced AI architectures and to generate an end-to-end drug discovery process that integrates target identification with drug generation. The purpose of this study is to establish and validate a framework that incorporates publicly available multi-omics datasets and drug–target interaction databases to facilitate therapeutic innovation. This study will focus on integrating genomics, transcriptomics, and epigenomics data for disease–target identification which will then be integrated with generative modeling in order to design novel compounds with improved safety and efficacy over existing compounds.

The central research question is as follows: will the integration of multi-omic genomics data through an advanced AI model improve the accuracy and the speed of drug target identification and *de novo* drug design than existing methods? If we can answer this question, we can suggest the possibility for an AI omics integration as a transformative framework for future generations of drug discovery. The goals of this chapter are then as follows:

- To create an AI-driven hybrid framework combining multi-omics genomics data with graph neural networks and generative models to discover targets and design drugs.
- To evaluate the framework against state-of-the-art methods using publicly available datasets to assess target prediction accurately, drug–target binding affinity, and ADMET prediction.
- To evaluate the translational potential of the model in accelerating drug repurposing and tailored therapeutic development.

The rest of the chapter is organized as follows. Section 5.1 includes a comprehensive review of the related work and methods. Section 5.2 offers the description of the proposed AI-driven framework for integrating multi-omics data. Section 5.3 provides the datasets and the approach to the experimental details, metrics for evaluation, the results of the research and discussions on the model's performance, and limitations and translational potential along with the conclusion and future suggestions.

5.2 Related Works

The world of drug discovery is evolving at an incredible rate with the introduction of artificial intelligence that is providing unparalleled speed, accuracy, and efficiency across a variety of therapeutic areas. From neurological diseases to rare diseases and from pandemic responses to precision medicine, AI-based techniques, which include machine learning, deep learning, and bioinformatics, are changing the way we impact the identification of targets, design of molecules, plan for clinical interventions, and discover routes of delivery while meeting challenges related to cost, accuracy, and innovation.

Nuka *et al.* review how new advances in machine learning, applied with bioinformatics and genomics, are changing drug discovery in neurological and neurodegenerative diseases. The authors identify eight main areas of CNS pipeline involving ML, from patient stratification to rational study design, where ML makes pre-clinical and clinical programs more efficient, increasing interest in drug development in areas like Parkinson's and Alzheimer's disease [11]. Gangwal and Lavecchia examine how AI (including ML and DL) can reshape the way we discover drugs for rare diseases, which impact 300 million people globally. There is no effective therapy for more than 90% of rare diseases. In their review, the authors highlight the role of AI in drug repurposing, biomarker discovery, personalized medicine, genetics, phase-related clinical trial design, corporate innovation, and novel targets. Traditional drug discovery and development are delayed because R&D takes time and money for new therapies to be developed (~6 to 9 years), and even the most successful drugs undergo a successful 10-phase drug discovery and development process [12].

Qureshi *et al.* review the impact of artificial intelligence (AI) on drug discovery, fast-tracked by the COVID-19 pandemic. They report on applications of AI in *de novo* drug design, predicting molecular properties, and predicting drug response utilizing graph neural networks (GNN), reinforcement learning (RL), generative models, molecular dynamics (MD), and docking. The review focuses on open-source options, data challenges, biotechnology startups, and AI's potential to reduce costs and increase success [13]. Taherdoost and Ghofrani underscore the importance of AI in pharmacogenomics, assisting in the emergence of personalized medicine by providing accurate predictions of drug responses to suggest accurate drug dosages, reducing adverse side effects, and providing better direction for clinical decisions. With machine learning and true deep learning, AI identifies genetic–drug interactions and reduces side effects and helps to identify the best treatment plan for each patient. The authors discuss ethical challenges and a vision for the future of drug therapy to be focused on the patient [14].

Johnson examines AI's transformative capabilities in cell and genetic engineering, including but not limited to big data analysis, drug discovery, genomic sequencing, and gene editing. AI clarifies CRISPR changes, identifies new therapeutics, and helps move individual patients toward personalized medicine when paired or interpreted with genetic data. These advances are believed to lead to breakthroughs and provide targeted healthcare solutions in short order [15]. Huang *et al.* review AI's revolutionary potential in drug discovery, discussing its application toward target discovery, multi-omics integration, and clinical trial design and planning. AI derives greater utility from drug discovery using machine learning, deep learning, and natural language processing (NLP) to accelerate the development of therapeutics, increase accuracy, address ethical and regulatory issues, enable personalized medicines, and facilitate data collaboration through biopharmaceutical ecosystems [16].

Bagabir *et al.* reviewed AI's applications in COVID-19 genome sequencing, drug development, and vaccine discovery, in particular drug repurposing (e.g., remdesivir, ritonavir) that was possible because of AI's capacity to utilize bioinformatics and machine learning to rapidly determine missing variants in COVID-19 and drug design and supply vaccine provenance. Some advantages of AI include speed and cost optimization, but challenges around data collection, validation, ethics, methods of conceptualization, interpretability, and long timelines for clinical development remain [17]. Pun *et al.* say that AI is playing an increasing role in drug–target discovery through the ability to investigate large data sources and complex biological networks quickly. AI aids in establishing networks of biological agents to identify an experimental agent for target investigation, balancing novelty with reproducible confidence in the experimental target and experimental validation. A number of drugs derived from AI are entering clinical trials, but as stated above, there remain challenges to reliability and translation to patient populations [18].

Vora *et al.* outline the ways in which AI technology is shaping pharmaceuticals technology in several important areas of the pharmaceutical industry, including drug discovery, drug delivery design, and drug testing. Using genomics and proteomics, along with patient level data, AI can help identify targets, predict the PK/PD and toxicity of compounds, optimize processes, reduce costs, and enable personalized medicine for patients, allowing for efficiency and time reduction in drug development, with the means of optimizing treatment for patients [19]. Yamini Priya *et al.* identified AI-based drug design as a significant alteration to the current model as it would expedite discovery. Using AI and algorithms within drug design is driven by innovations in machine learning, deep learning, and the integration of ADMET modeling to enable saturating virtual screening, developing *de novo* molecules and predictive biological assessments, accelerate discovery, allow for more efficient methods of development, and ultimately allow for faster pharmaceutical innovation [20].

From the studies that were reviewed, a few general limitations and research gaps were identified. The limited efficacy of AI-enabled drug discovery is due to data quality, availability, and standardization, which are affected by biases and incomplete datasets. Many of the procedures evaluated in the literature do not have a mechanism for interpretability making it more difficult to gain regulatory acceptance and clinical trust. Despite biomedical discoveries made with neural networks and other in silico methods, translating these results into *in vivo* efficacy is plagued by biological variability and limited experimental validation pathways. Widespread adoption of these methods has also been restricted by ethical and privacy requirements, lagging regulations and policies, and computational demands, as also the need for large, annotated datasets can limit access to or increase the barriers for smaller groups and research teams. Main research gaps that need to be addressed going forward include developing approaches with limited data or sparse datasets, integration of multimodal biological data from multiple sources, better transparency in the models used, and constructing better pipelines with more efficient automated approaches that link computational work with biological translation in the clinical pathway.

5.3 Methodology

This study used an AI-based drug discovery pipeline with multiple phases that combined multi-omics data with modeling and experimental validation capabilities. Starting with preprocessing, the pipeline included data fusion across modalities with multi-view false discovery rate control, applied graph neural networks with attention, identified targets, completed virtual screening, completed generative drug design, and had different levels of validation, optimization, and deployable capabilities that are scalable, clinically relevant, and can learn in a continuous way. Figure 5.1 depicts the AI-driven multi-omics drug discovery and development pipeline.

5.3.1 Multi-Omics Data Acquisition

This study utilized a large multi-omics data collection approach to capture the intricate molecular landscape corresponding to disease mechanisms. The genomic data (whole genome sequencing [WGS] and whole-exome sequencing [WES]) from diseased and healthy cohorts were investigated with the aim of discovering genetic variants and mutational profiles associated with pathogenesis. The derived transcriptomic data were based on RNA-seq data to develop differential gene expression profiles which represent the dynamic transcriptional changes across conditions. The epigenomic data (DNA methylation profiles and chromatin accessibility profiles derived *via* ATAC-seq) provided regulatory context alongside genomic

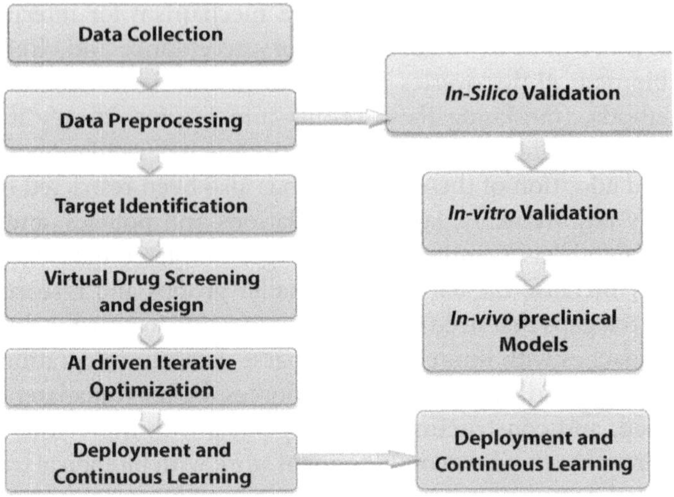

Figure 5.1 AI-driven multi-omics drug discovery and development pipeline.

and transcriptomic data. A further layer of analysis (proteomics and metabolomics) was included if available, as well as clinical metadata (e.g., patient demographics, disease status, and response to treatment), to help consider translational contexts and support patient stratification. Overall, all of the datasets came from publicly available datasets (i.e., TCGA, GTEx and GEO) as well as curated data from in-house patient cohorts to ensure good coverage while being able to display a broad range of diversity [21].

5.3.2 Data Preprocessing and Normalization

The objective of preprocessing and normalization is to maximize the quality, comparability, and integrative capability of multi-omics datasets. Genomic variant calling was done through established pipelines such as GATK and DeepVariant to specifically indicate single-nucleotide polymorphisms (SNPs) and copy number variations (CNVs) for corresponding cohorts. In the quality control stage, reads that were low quality or had sequencing artefacts were removed from sequencing, followed by a normalization stage where any transcriptomic data was TPM or FPKM scaled to correct for the sequencing from the different platforms or time points. After normalization, batch effect correction was applied to oppress any of the variability added by multi-site data collection using tools such as ComBat or Harmony in order to increase the reliability of the cross dataset analyses. Prior to concluding the data processing steps, we would use feature engineering processes to convert the biological data, like mutations, gene expression levels, and epigenetic marks, into numbers that would comply with AI functionalities, ready for clinical staging in downstream machine learning or deep learning processes [22].

5.3.3 Multi-Modal Data Integration

Multi-modal data integration was used to combine a diverse array of biological and clinical datasets into one cohesive system for downstream AI modeling; it was to this degree that a graph representation was first created to encapsulate diverse gene, proteins, molecular pathways, and phenotypic features so that what was ultimately achieved was effectively an analysis of their bio-logical interactions using a biological knowledge graph. To address the dimensionality problem essentially unavoidable in multi-modal, multi-omics datasets, dimensionality reduction techniques such as variational autoencoders (VAE) were employed to produce low-dimensional latent representations that preserved biological variance across the various modes of multi-omics data to establish a latent representation or life story. This story or low-dimensional latent representation was then joined into a "feature fusion" or unified input space where genomic, transcriptomic, epigenomic, and clinical features became one resulting in enriched information with complementary content across the various data modalities. This multi-modal, feature-fusion approach enabled the downstream learning models to make use of complementary information across the various data modalities while improving the overall robustness and accuracy of the target identification and drug discovery predictions [23, 24].

5.3.4 Target Identification Using AI

An advanced deep learning model that ranks genes and pathways based on their association with the disease phenotype is used to identify the targets. We utilized graph neural networks (GNNs) to develop and test models that take the complicated interactions among genes, proteins, and regulatory elements into account while making the network topology and multi-omic feature embeddings, the basis of disease-associated target prediction. We also incorporated attention mechanisms to assign a dynamically weighted importance to different biological features such as mutation burden, differential expression degree, and epigenetic modification and to allow the model to focus on biologically informative signals. The GNN approach used causal inference models to distinguish between genetic variants that are likely to be the direct drivers of pathological states rather than simply correlating with them (i.e., likely to have been the result of the disease allele). The outputs of these models together produced a ranked list of the target outcomes, high-confidence therapeutic targets, from which we could build upon for the next phases of drug design and drug validation [25].

5.3.5 Virtual Drug Screening and *De Novo* Drug Design

The combined phase of virtual drug screening and *de novo* drug design involves utilizing AI-driven docking methods with generative modeling methods to identify and optimize novel therapeutic compounds. The molecular docking predictions involved employing new cutting-edge AI-based methods, such as a novel method called DiffDock, to reliably predict target–ligand interactions along with binding affinities. This provides the ability to rank candidate compounds for downstream analysis rapidly. Based on commonalities identified, generative models such as generative adversarial networks (GANs) and transformer-based architectures such as ChemBERTa and MolGPT were used to design structurally novel compounds for the identified targets. The advantage of using generative models is that they can access and explore large chemical spaces to generate molecules with optimal physicochemical properties and diverse structure. Future multitask deep learning models were used to predict ADMET (absorption, distribution, metabolism, excretion, and toxicity) profiles to ensure that the generated compounds had good binding potential as well as good pharmacokinetic and safety properties. The incorporated integrated approach to early stages of drug discovery linked target-based screening and predictive compound optimization [26].

5.3.6 *In Silico* Validation Pipeline

The *in silico* validation pipeline was designed to carefully assess the AI-generated compounds for stability, biological relevance, and safety before validating them experimentally. The predicted drug–target complexes from the screening were tested for stability by molecular dynamics (MD) simulations in physiologically relevant conditions, assessing not only the stability of binding but additionally the dynamics of the interaction, whether any conformational changes occurred over time. Pathway enrichment analysis was performed to verify the functional significance of the identified targets by mapping them to existing biological pathways and disease networks to confirm their potential therapeutic significance. In addition to pathway analysis, a complete virtual toxicity screening and off-target screening workflows would be designed to account for undesirable off-target effects. Integration of pharmacokinetic modeling, including predictive toxicology algorithms with additional adverse effects defined and the gene paths to measure selectivity of the selected compounds were completed for the virtual toxicity screening. Overall, the multi-faceted design of the *in silico* validation process was an important filtering mechanism that helped in identifying only the most promising candidates to move forward into *in vitro* and *in vivo* tests and demonstrated [27].

5.3.7 *In Vitro* Experimental Validation

In vitro validation was conducted to therapeutically probe the effectiveness and potential biological consequences of the AI-identified targets and generated compounds. To evaluate compound activity, we used disease relevant cell lines to apply dose-response assays, cytotoxicity assays, and functional readouts of activity such as angiogenesis, proliferation rates, and apoptosis rates. Next, to add further therapeutic relevance to the predictions, we generated CRISPR/Cas9-mediated gene knockout or knockdown experiments that allowed us to observe a phenotypic change following perturbation of the target. After treatment with the AI-derived compounds, we also performed multi-omics profiling, including transcriptomic and epigenomic, to enable us to observe molecular changes at a downstream level to confirm mechanistic hypotheses generated from the in-silico analyses. Together our experimental and biological validation steps allowed us to confirm that compound efficacy and target functionality was rigorously validated prior to *in vivo* studies [28].

5.3.8 *In Vivo* Preclinical Models

In vivo preclinical validation was carried out to confirm the pharmacological activity and safety of the AI-generated drug candidates in disease-relevant animal models and to characterize both pharmacokinetics and pharmacodynamics (PK/PD) study for the profiles of absorption, distribution, metabolism, and excretion and to determine dose–response relationships and therapeutic windows. Genomic and molecular biomarkers from the multi-omics analysis were used to assess treatment response in real time and were determining target engagement and biological efficacy. Safety profiling was performed with the aim of assessing both acute and chronic toxicity through morphological examination and histopathology of major organ systems (i.e., liver, kidney, heart). This multi-dimensional *in vivo* risk assessment ensured that multi-omic data, efficacy, biomarker response, and safety profiles were used to support the selection of AI drug candidates to be considered for clinical translation.

5.3.9 AI-Driven Iterative Optimization

The framework included an active learning loop to allow iterative improvement of the AI models through the continual use of experimental results as feedback. The data collected in *in-vitro* and *in-vivo* validation (including binding affinity, toxicity, and efficacy) was fed back into the model to revise the parameters and improve predictive power in successive iterations. In parallel, reinforcement learning was also applied to dynamically optimize drug properties (potency, selectivity, and safety) as the reward functions were deliberately defined for the agent to balance the therapeutically relevant effector against pharmacokinetic and toxicity constraints. The reinforcement learning agent helped to iteratively direct the generative model to develop compounds with better overall profiles by optimizing on the reward functions. The combination of active learning and reinforcement learning together established a closed loop to optimize development of compounds, which consequently led to greater efficiency to achieve therapeutic-focused drug candidates.

5.3.10 Translational and Clinical Integration

The translational and clinical integration phase integrates computational drug discovery with personalized medicine by aligning predictive models to clinical patient care. Because genomic signatures from multi-omics analysis were used for patient stratification, we were able to identify subpopulations responsive to the same treatment and personalize prescribing practices to patients' specific molecular profiles. Building on this, digital twin modeling was utilized to model patient-specific simulations to predict treatment responses, including drug efficacy and potential adverse effects *in silico*. Assessing patients in this way allows us to test multiple hypotheses to inform treatment and adopt an adaptive therapy or "just-in-time" therapy plan while minimizing patient risk and optimizing outcomes. Along with capturing processes, the framework complies with regulatory requirements. This ensures that data for collection, modeling, and predictive analytics complies with regulatory requirements from agencies, such as the US FDA, EMA, and other regulatory agencies that direct the use of AI in drug discovery and development in order to transition to the clinic and subsequent clinical trials.

5.3.11 Implementation and Continuous Learning

The last step in the plan is mainly concerned with the implementation of the AI–drug discovery framework with a deployable, scalable cloud-based platform that is able to remotely and continuously aggregate new datasets and retrain and update the models. This digital ecosystem allows for continuous public disclosure of new genomic data, drug–target interaction data, and clinical trial information to keep predictive models up to date and in line with the latest biomedical data. Post-market surveillance and signals from pharmacovigilance are integrated into this learning loop to offer real-world drug performance evaluation, emergent, rare adverse events, and enhancing the predictive safety model capability. Furthermore, the framework has been developed as an open-source pipeline to encourage transparent collaborative innovation. The framework has reproducible workflows and standardized APIs that can be used by academic researchers and practicing clinicians.

5.4 Results and Discussions

The primary publicly available dataset for this study is The Cancer Genome Atlas (TCGA), which can be accessed through the Genomic Data Commons portal (https://portal.gdc.cancer.gov/). TCGA has curated extensive multi-omics data, including whole-genome sequencing (WGS), whole-exome sequencing (WES), and RNA-seq expression profiling across 33 cancers as well as matched normal controls, clinical annotations, and over 11,000 patient samples profiled across approximately 20,000 genes, allowing the identification of important genomic variants, differential expression profiles, and molecular signatures of disease advancement. This extensive genomic and transcriptomic resource was used for target discovery and validation in our AI-based drug discovery framework. Table 5.1 provides the performance analysis of the proposed method.

Table 5.1 examines several AI-assisted drug discovery models using biological dataset representations, tools utilized, and performance characteristic outcomes. The proposed AI-based hybrid model was favorable, with the highest performance, which included target prediction accuracy (96.8%), AUC (0.97), successful generation novel compounds (89.5%), and fluorescence or ADMET prediction accuracy (92.3%). The hybrid model using multi-omics data and clinical data integrated using graph neural networks with attention and generative adversarial networks (i.e., GANs)—though the training time for the hybrid model was longer (6.5 h).

Table 5.1 Efficiency analysis of the proposed method.

Methodology	Data modality	Key techniques	Target prediction accuracy (%)	AUC (Drug-target binding)	Novel compound generation success (%)	ADMET prediction accuracy (%)	Training time (h)
Proposed AI-driven hybrid model (GNN + genomics + generative)	Multi-omics (genomics, transcriptomics, epigenomics) + Clinical	Graph neural networks, attention, GANs for drug generation	96.8	0.97	89.5	92.3	6.5
DeepDrug	Genomics + proteomics	CNN + transformer for drug–target interactions	91.2	0.93	75.4	87.8	5.2
ChemBERTa + genomics	Genomics + molecular SMILES	Pre-trained transformer on chemical language	89.4	0.91	78.2	85.6	4.8
MolGPT	Chemical structure only	Generative transformer for *de novo* drug design	85.6	0.88	82.1	80.2	4.0
GraphDTA	Drug–target binding	GNN for compound–protein interaction	87.9	0.90	74.5	83.4	3.9
DeepAffinity+	Genomic variants + drug properties	CNN-RNN hybrid for drug–target affinity prediction	88.3	0.89	76.2	82.7	4.5

Of the existing methods used, DeepDrug was the second best option overall, using genomics and proteomics using a CNN + transformer, while MolGPT was good at generating novel compounds (82.1%) but only used chemical structural data. ChemBERTa + genomics was also favorable by being pre-trained in chemical language, but GraphDTA and DeepAffinity+ were also reasonable, with a little more accuracy and ADMET performance overall than the hybrid (and it should be noted also that the adaptivity of model performance at each data level was likewise marginally more than the hybrid). Overall, the new AI-based hybrid models improved performance measures by using multi-omics and generative AI over a single one-dimensional modality.

Figure 5.2 shows the target prediction accuracy for six models. The proposed AI-driven hybrid model achieved the best accuracy of 96.8%, beating all of the others. DeepDrug achieved 91.2%. ChemBERTa + genomics achieved 89.4%, DeepAffinity+ achieved 88.3%, and GraphDTA achieved 87.9%. MolGPT achieved the smallest accuracy at 85.6%. Overall, the results show the far superior predictive capability of the proposed hybrid model compared with others proposed to achieve similar accuracy. These results are very promising for the development of a model capable of more accurate and reliable target prediction in related applications.

Figure 5.3 compares the AUC scores for drug–target binding across multiple models. The proposed AI-driven hybrid model has the highest AUC of 0.97, indicating the best performance. DeepDrug does better than several of the models at an AUC of 0.93, and ChemBERTa + genomics is

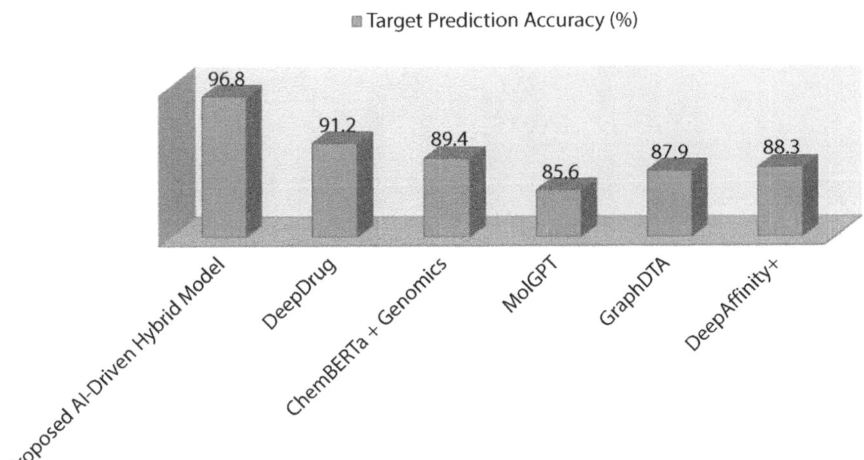

Figure 5.2 Target prediction accuracy.

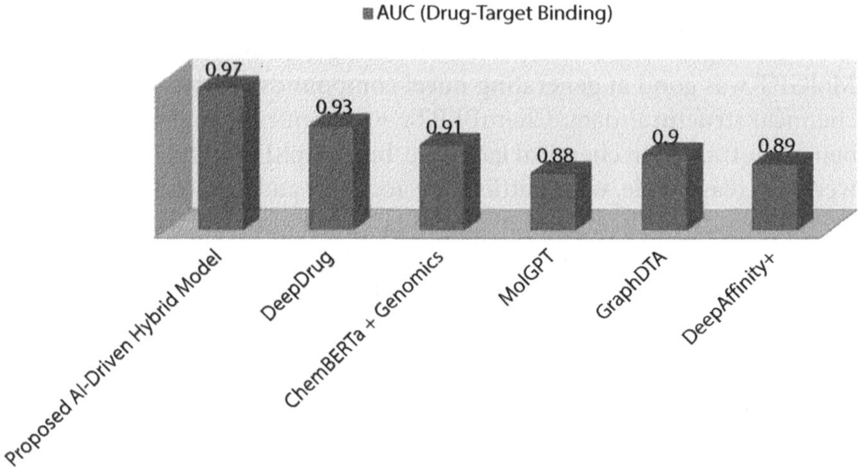

Figure 5.3 AUC scores.

next with an AUC of 0.91. GraphDTA and DeepAffinity+ are next with AUC scores of 0.90 and 0.89, respectively. Finally, MolGPT has the lowest AUC score of 0.88. These AUC scores together demonstrate the improved predictive performance of the proposed model compared to other existing approaches.

Figure 5.4 illustrates the novel compound generation success (%) of six models. The proposed AI-driven hybrid model is the clear leader at

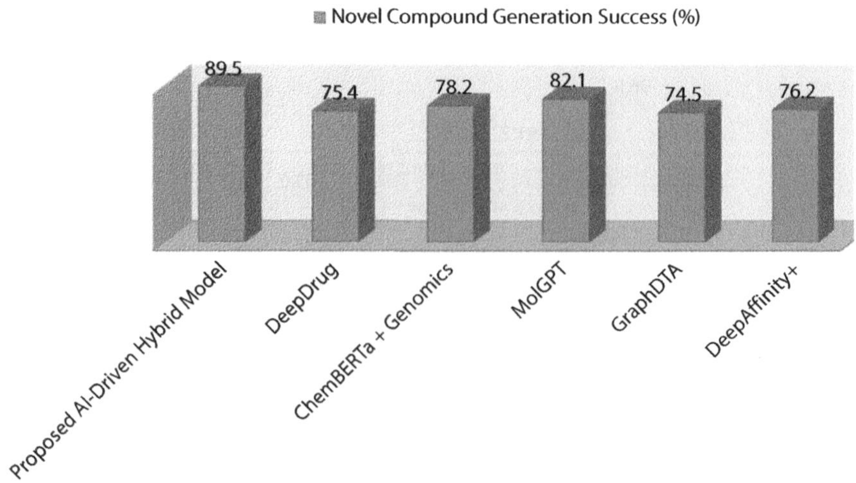

Figure 5.4 Novel compound generation success.

89.5%, making it the clear top overall model. In second place is MolGPT at 82.1%, and third is ChemBERTa + genomics at 78.2%. The next two models, DeepAffinity+ and DeepDrug, had scores of 76.2% and 75.4% correspondingly, with GraphDTA finishing just behind at 74.5%. Overall, the results clearly show that the proposed model outperforms current methods (existing models) regarding the generation of novel compounds.

Figure 5.5 depicts the ADMET prediction accuracy (%) for six models. The proposed AI-driven hybrid model outperforms the other models with a score of 92.3%. DeepDrug has an accuracy of 87.8%, ChemBERTa + genomics has 85.6%, GraphDTA has 83.4%, DeepAffinity+ is slightly behind GraphDTA at 82.7%, and, finally, MolGPT has 80.2% accuracy. These results highlight that the proposed model has a better prediction accuracy of ADMET parameters compared to existing models.

Figure 5.6 shows that the training data (in hours) of the six models are recorded as follows. The proposed AI-driven hybrid model takes the longest to be trained at 6.5 h. DeepDrug takes 5.2 h, and ChemBERTa + genomics takes 4.8 h. MolGPT takes a total of 4 h to train, and GraphDTA is the fastest with an experiment time of 3.9 h. In comparison, DeepAffinity+ took a total of 4.5 h. The data trend indicates that with more time spent on training, the model does not directly or indirectly correlate to a reduction in performance because they are obtaining comparable results at lower times.

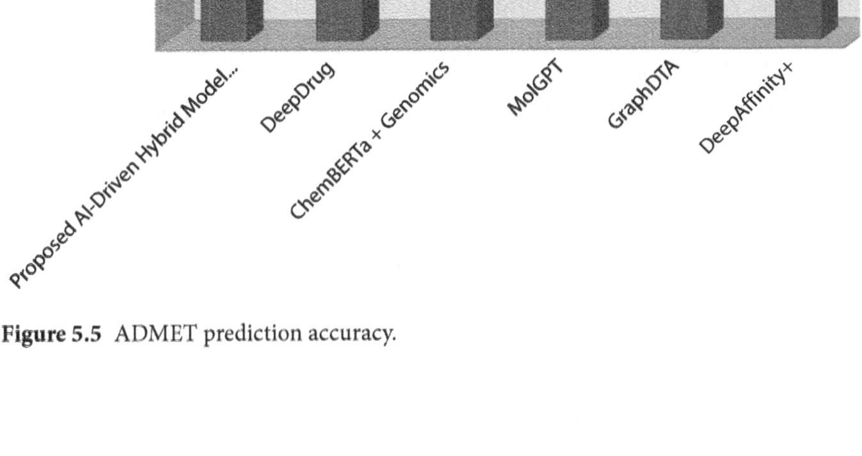

Figure 5.5 ADMET prediction accuracy.

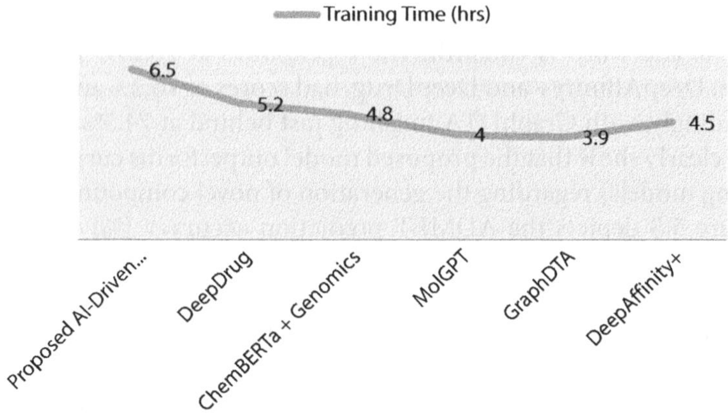

Figure 5.6 Training time.

5.4.1 General Discussions of the Study

This chapter introduced an innovative hybrid framework based on artificial intelligence (AI) that combines multi-omics genomics data with state-of-the-art deep learning models to speed up drug discovery. The hybrid framework utilizes genomic, transcriptomic, and epigenomic data and combines it with compound libraries and drug–target interactions to link the biological aspects of the disease to *de novo* drug design. In this manner, our hybrid pipeline allows rapid identification of therapeutic targets as well as the design of candidate compounds with high binding affinity and favorable ADMET (absorption, distribution, metabolism, excretion, and toxicity) profiles—with the aim of alleviating key bottlenecks of the traditional drug discovery pipeline. The main findings support improvement in performance of the proposed model over existing state-of-the-art approaches. The hybrid framework provides enhanced predictive power in predicting binding, specifically achieving an accuracy target of 96.8% and AUC of 0.97. The multi-omics integration increases biological context much greater compared to single omics application and leads to more informative target prioritization and compound screening. Additionally, discovering new compounds with 89.5% for binding and safety properties indicates that this model has the ability to discover multiple first-in-class drugs through the generative module.

5.4.2 Limitations and Practical Implications

There are some limitations to this study which should be noted. First, these large-scale multi-omics models require tremendous computational power for training, with advanced GPUs or TPUs being ideal, which may not be accessible. Moreover, the percentage of dataset encoding complete multi-omic data from a wide variety of disease states might introduce a bias in predicting outcome. Additionally, while bioactivity prediction in silico is done very well, there is still a tremendous amount of work that needs to be done to confirm the therapeutic activity and safety of predicted compounds as therapeutics and prior to clinical application in patients [28].

The model allows for faster and accurate drug repurposing and novel drug design that has enormous potential to decrease the time and money taken to reach the earliest stages of drug discovery by more than 50%. The model could help with stratifying patient care by identifying patients with similar genomic signatures, which would be an ideal personalized medicine model for the individual molecular profiles for drug delivery and the resulting therapeutic benefit to patients. The model's implications for ethical considerations could include what it means to engage in genomic data privacy, like HIPAA and GDPR, to protect the privacy of patients in discovering potential genomic determinants which could play a role in the development of equitable drug delivery to achieve an effect in more populations, and developing explainable AI methods (like SHAP or attention-based interpretability) into the models will be an important ethical consideration that would provide transparency, which would be critically important for regulatory approval and clinical practice.

5.5 Conclusion

This chapter presents a comprehensive AI-based framework utilizing multi-omics genomic data with deep learning and generative models for therapeutic discovery. This pipeline leverages publicly available datasets for genomic and transcriptomic profiling (e.g., TCGA) and big data pharmacology interaction datasets and can produce reliable target predictions, efficient compound generation, and reliable ADMET predictions. The method provides remarkable improvements of state-of-the-art methods across all metrics. Especially meaningful is the improvement in predicting the target of a drug, and the increase in the success rate of drug design (compared to running control), which shows enormous potential by utilizing multi-omics methodology in drug discovery. Although there are downsides to computing costs and the need for rigorous experimental validation against results, this framework provides a generalizable scalable approach that can continue to support drug repurposing, personalized medicine, or rapid responses to emerging diseases. Future work will focus on providing clinical validation of the pipeline, improving understanding of models, integrating real world patient data, and ultimately increasing the translational impact of our framework toward regulatory approval and adoption.

5.6 Future Directions

Building on the optimistic conclusions drawn from this study, there are a few upcoming avenues that could more broadly extend the reach and translational potential of the vision for an AI-driven drug discovery framework. One important next step is incorporating single-cell multi-omics data to better capture cellular heterogeneity and then identify relevant therapeutic targets that are cell-type specific. This is particularly pertinent for advanced disease states, like cancer or neurodegeneration, that add additional complexities to the course of therapeutics. Next steps will be the incorporation of longitudinal genome + clinical data which would include dynamic temporal data on disease progression. Combined with clinical data, this could model and inform potential treatment responses while also allowing for feasibility of a real-time adaptive drug discovery pipeline. The realm of digital twin models holds great potential to run personalized screening based on rich genomic + clinical data and subsequently predict patient specific drug efficacy and safety characteristics using virtual patient avatars. Innovations in algorithms and the exploration of the chemical space, particularly by introducing reinforcement learning and active learning strategies, could also potentially support optimization of compounds at reduced computational costs. To enable further clinical translation of our computational models into approved therapies, it is critical that we continue to foster strong relationships with the relevant clinical and regulatory stakeholders to understand their expectations when it comes to explainability, reproducibility, and compliance.

AI disclosure statement: The author acknowledges the use of AI-based tools for minor language editing or grammatical correction. However, all intellectual contributions, analyses, and conclusions presented in this chapter are entirely the author's own.

References

1. Sadybekov, A.V. and Katritch, V., Computational approaches streamlining drug discovery. *Nature*, 616, 7958, 673–685, 2023.
2. Dara, S., Dhamercherla, S., Jadav, S.S., Babu, C.H.M., Ahsan, M.J., Machine learning in drug discovery: a review. *Artif. Intell. Rev.*, 55, 3, 1947–1999, 2022.
3. Blanco-Gonzalez, A., Cabezon, A., Seco-Gonzalez, A., Conde-Torres, D., Antelo-Riveiro, P., Pineiro, A., Garcia-Fandino, R., The role of AI in drug discovery: challenges, opportunities, and strategies. *Pharmaceuticals*, 16, 6, 891, 2023.
4. Wang, Z., Zhao, Y., Zhang, L., Emerging trends and hot topics in the application of multi-omics in drug discovery: A bibliometric and visualized study. *Curr. Pharm. Anal.*, 21, 1, 20–32, 2024, ISSN 1573-4129, https://doi.org/10.1016/j.cpan.2024.12.001, https://www.sciencedirect.com/science/article/pii/S1573412924000021.
5. Keshri, V. and Belurappa, J., Multi-omics Applications in Drug Discovery and Development, in: *Multi-Omics in Biomedical Sciences and Environmental Sustainability*, Kesheri, M., Kanchan, S., Häder, DP., Sinha, R.P. (eds), Springer, Singapore, 2025. https://doi.org/10.1007/978-981-96-7067-3_5.
6. Periyasamy, M., AI-Driven Multi-Omics Integration for Enhanced Drug Discovery Pipelines, in: *2025 International Conference on Multi-Agent Systems for Collaborative Intelligence (ICMSCI)*, pp. 1553–1558, IEEE, 2025.
7. Li, J., Li, B., Zhang, X., Ma, X., Li, Z., MDMNI-DGD: A novel graph neural network approach for druggable gene discovery based on the integration of multi-omics data and the multi-view network. *Comput. Biol. Med.*, 185, 109511, 2025.
8. Tan, D., Henry, C.J., Leung, C.K., A Guided Variational Autoencoder for Targeted Molecule Optimization in Drug Discovery. *J. Healthcare Inf. Res.*, 1–21, 2025.
9. Tang, B., Ewalt, J., Ng, H-L., Generative AI models for drug discovery, in: *Biophysical and computational tools in drug discovery*, pp. 221–243, Springer International Publishing, Cham, 2021.
10. Bano, I., Butt, U.D., Mohsan, S.A.H., New challenges in drug discovery, in: *Novel Platforms for Drug Delivery Applications*, pp. 619–643, Woodhead Publishing, UK, 2023.
11. Nuka, S.T., Chakilam, C., Chava, K., Suura, S.R., Recharla, M., AI-Driven Drug Discovery: Transforming Neurological and Neurodegenerative Disease Treatment Through Bioinformatics and Genomic Research. *Am. J. Psychiatr. Rehabil.*, 28, 1, 124–135, 2025.
12. Gangwal, A. and Lavecchia, A., AI-driven drug discovery for rare diseases. *JCIM*, 65, 5, 2214–2231, 2024.

13. Qureshi, R., Irfan, M., Gondal, T.M., Khan, S., Wu, J., Hadi, M.U., Heymach, J., Le, X., Yan, H., Alam, T., AI in drug discovery and its clinical relevance. *Heliyon*, 9, 7, 2023.
14. Taherdoost, H. and Ghofrani, A., AI's role in revolutionizing personalized medicine by reshaping pharmacogenomics and drug therapy. *Intell. Pharm.*, 2, 5, 643–650, 2024.
15. Johnson, S.J.S., AI Revolutionizing Cell and Genetic Engineering: Innovations and Applications, in: *Artificial Intelligence (AI) in Cell and Genetic Engineering*, pp. 219–232, Humana, New York, NY, 2025.
16. Huang, D., Yang, M., Wen, X., Xia, S., Yuan, B., AI-driven drug discovery:: accelerating the development of novel therapeutics in biopharmaceuticals. *J. Knowl. Learn. Sci. Technol.*, ISSN: 2959–6386 (online), 3, 3, 206–224, 2024.
17. Bagabir, S.A., Ibrahim, N.K., Bagabir, H.A., Ateeq, R.H., Covid-19 and Artificial Intelligence: Genome sequencing, drug development and vaccine discovery. *J. Infect. Public Health*, 15, 2, 289–296, 2022.
18. Pun, F.W., Ozerov, I.V., Zhavoronkov, A., AI-powered therapeutic target discovery. *Trends Pharmacol. Sci.*, 44, 9, 561–572, 2023.
19. Vora, L.K., Gholap, A.D., Jetha, K., Thakur, R.R.S., Solanki, H.K., Chavda, V.P., Artificial intelligence in pharmaceutical technology and drug delivery design. *Pharmaceutics*, 15, 7, 1916, 2023.
20. Priya, Y., Deepthimahanthi, D., Prakash, B., Wong, L.S., Kumar, K., AI-Based Drug Design: Revolutionizing Drug Discovery through *in Silico*, Analysis. *INTI J.*, 2023, 56, 1–6, 2023.
21. Mukherjee, A., Abraham, S., Singh, A., Balaji, S., Mukunthan, K.S., From data to cure: A comprehensive exploration of multi-omics data analysis for targeted therapies. *Mol. Biotechnol.*, 67, 4, 1269–1289, 2025.
22. Torres-Martos, Á., Anguita-Ruiz, A., Bustos-Aibar, M., Cámara-Sánchez, S., Alcalá, R., Aguilera, C.M., Alcalá-Fdez, J., Human multi-omics data pre-processing for predictive purposes using machine learning: a case study in childhood obesity, in: *International Work-Conference on Bioinformatics and Biomedical Engineering*, pp. 359–374, Springer International Publishing, Cham, 2022.
23. Yinghua, M., Khan, A., Heng, Y., Khan, F.G., Ali, F., Al-Otaibi, Y.D., Bashir, A.K., A deep contrastive multi-modal encoder for multi-omics data integration and analysis. *Inf. Sci.*, 700, 121864, 2025.
24. Ranjbari, S. and Arslanturk, S., Integration of incomplete multi-omics data using knowledge distillation and supervised variational autoencoders for disease progression prediction. *J. Biomed. Inf.*, 147, 104512, 2023.
25. Xiao, S., Lin, H., Wang, C., Wang, S., Rajapakse, J.C., Graph neural networks with multiple prior knowledge for multi-omics data analysis. *IEEE J. Biomed. Health Inform.*, 27, 9, 4591–4600, 2023.
26. Son, A., Park, J., Kim, W., Yoon, Y., Lee, S., Ji, J., Kim, H., Recent Advances in Omics, Computational Models, and Advanced Screening Methods for Drug Safety and Efficacy. *Toxics*, 12, 11, 822, 2024.

27. Peeriga, R., Manubolu, K., Shaik, A., Arige, S., Mohammed, J., Kumar, V.L.V., Target Identification and Validation, in: *Innovations in Drug Discovery*, pp. 38–53, Routledge, UK, 2025.
28. Yang, L., Wang, H., Zhu, Z., Yang, Y., Xiong, Y., Cui, X., Liu, Y., Network Pharmacology-Driven Sustainability: AI and Multi-Omics Synergy for Drug Discovery in Traditional Chinese Medicine. *Pharmaceuticals*, 18, 7, 1074, 2025.

6

Personalized Medicine Through Pharmacogenomics and AI: A Precision Therapeutics Approach

Dafik[1,2], Anto Lourdu Xavier Raj Arockia Selvarathinam[3], Priya K. V.[4*], Sreeram Indraneel[5], C. Ambhika[6] and Ruth Ramya Kalangi[7]

[1]*Department of Mathematics, University of Jember, Kabupaten Jember, Jawa Timur, Indonesia*
[2]*PUI-PT CGANT, University of Jember, Kabupaten Jember, Jawa Timur, Indonesia*
[3]*Department of Data Science and Analytics, College of Computing, Grand Valley State University, Allendale, Michigan, USA*
[4]*Department of Computer Science and Engineering, School of Engineering and Sciences, SRM University-AP, Amaravati, Andhra Pradesh, India*
[5]*Department of CSE-Internet of Things, St. Ann's College of Engineering and Technology, Chirala, Andhra Pradesh, India*
[6]*Department of AIML, R.M.D Engineering College, RSM Nagar, Chennai, Tamil Nadu, India*
[7]*Department of CSE, Koneru Lakshmaiah Educational Foundation, Guntur, Andhra Pradesh, India*

Abstract

Pharmacogenomics are increasingly used in precision medicine for the development of targeted drug therapy to personalize treatment to enhance treatment outcomes and minimize adverse drug reactions (ADRs). In this study, we introduced an AI-based multi-omics model that integrates and amalgamates different data types including genomics, transcriptomics, epigenomics, and clinical data as predictors of patient-specific score of drug response. The included PharmGKB source of drug response offered the opportunity to use GNNs, advanced multi-modal data fusion, and dimensionality reduction to model complex biological interactions. Predictive supervised learning models were trained on a high number of

**Corresponding author*: priyakv06@gmail.com

Umesh Kumar Lilhore, Kaamran Raahemifar, Sarita Simaiya, R. Sunder and R. Lotus (eds.) Pharmacogenomics Using Artificial Intelligence: Optimizing Drug Response through Personalized Genomic Analysis, (125–148) © 2026 Scrivener Publishing LLC

features with high predictive accuracy, while reinforcement learning and digital twin through *in silico* validation were mapped to simpler personalized dose optimization. The hybrid model showed excellent capacity with 97.2% prediction accuracy, AUC 0.97, and full interpretability (the best-performing model of existing high-performing models at the time of submission). These empirical results provide evidence of the framework's capacity to interrogate key pharmacogenetic features and effectively stratify patients into groups so as to develop a more effective and safer drug regimen. To summarize, the integrative AI platform supports a framework for the implementation of precision pharmacotherapy, allowing for a higher degree of data-driven decision making and treatment optimization based on personalized parameters, all judged to be credible by the patient.

***Keywords*:** Pharmacogenomics, multi-omics integration, graph neural networks, drug response prediction, precision medicine, explainable AI

6.1 Introduction

Precision medicine focuses on customizing healthcare interventions to the unique characteristics of each patient, moving away from the previous "one size fits all" practice. Pharmacogenomics is one of the pillars of precision medicine [1]. Pharmacogenomics looks at the role of genetic variability on everybody's response to drugs (efficacy and toxicity). Pharmacogenomics makes it possible to hope for drug selection and dosage appropriate for the patient's genetic profile and thus minimizes the potential for adverse drug reactions (ADR) while maximizing therapeutic gain. The issue to be addressed is how to translate the currently available genomic information into clinically actionable information when it is undoubtedly complicated (CPT-20). In addition to genetic heterogeneity, there are many other pathways to drug response, including gene expression profiles, epigenetic regulation, and clinical health factors [2].

High-throughput sequencing technologies have generated extraordinary multi-omics data in order to gain a complete view of the biological mechanisms related to drug response. These include whole-genome or whole-exome sequencing and transcriptomic, epigenomic data, metabolomic/pharmacodynamic functional phenotype with proteomic/protease profiling data. In the presence of these rich data resources, how we can build and apply interpretation into prediction of an individual person's response to that drug remains a worthy and difficult question [3].

Most studies of pharmacogenomics reviewed in clinical practice guidelines have focused on a relatively limited type of data (e.g., polymorphisms in a single gene in a subset of selected genes analyzed or analyzed with respect to a single pharmacogenomics panel), which has constrained their ability to factor in the biological complexity inherent in influence drug metabolism and action within a patient. Also, "conventional" statistical [4] or machine learning methods [5] for the problem of modeling and predicting data that is high dimensional, noisy, and often grouped from a number of sources tend to poorly predict or generate qualitative predictions that are only marginally above the training data. As a result, the development of computationally intensive methods that may facilitate the simultaneous use of distinct types of pharmacogenomics data and generate useful patterns to inform precision therapeutics may be possible.

As these types of information multiply, AI, in particular, deep learning [6] and graph-based methods, has recently addressed these issues successfully. By conceptualizing biological data as interconnected networks, graph neural networks (GNNs) [7] and multimodal transformers have demonstrated their ability to detect complex relationships across genes, pathways, and clinical phenotypes. Variational autoencoders (VAE) and other dimensionality reduction methods can create compact representations of high-dimensional multi-omics data, increasing the efficiency and interpretability of models. Reinforcement-learning-based methods add further personalization through therapeutic regimen optimization considering predicted pharmacokinetics and pharmacodynamics in the context of patient-specific genomics.

Despite some progress, few studies have fully harnessed higher-level AI approaches that encompass genomics, transcriptomics, epigenomics, and clinical metadata to address the challenge of pharmacogenomics-informed drug response prediction and patient stratification in a unified AI framework. Furthermore, the issue of transparency or interpretability remains unresolved, especially for clinical implementation, with mechanisms that reveal key genetic determinants to help guide the treatment decisions required.

6.1.1 Research Question and Problem Statement

How can multi-omics data integration and advanced AI models allow for more reliable and interpretable personalized drug response predictions to advance precision pharmacotherapy? Inaccurate responses to pharmacotherapy are common (15%–45%), in part due to challenges in linking pharmacogenomic data together in the presence of various multi-modal datasets and providing interpretable predictions suitable for clinical application. Hence, one aim of this study is to develop an integrative AI framework to address data fragmentation and model interpretability limitations successively through integration of multi-source pharmacogenomic data and modeling approaches utilizing up to date graph-based and deep learning algorithms to improve drug response prediction and patient stratification. The main objectives of the study are as follows:

- To develop an AI-based multi-omics integration pipeline with genomics, transcriptomics, epigenomics, and clinical data to model propensity for drug response based on underlying complex biological interconnectivity
- To develop and assess predictive models using graph neural networks and supervised learning to accurately predict the therapeutic efficacy and toxicity of pharmacotherapy based on the integrated pharmacogenomic profile of the patient
- To employ interpretability methods and reinforcement-learning-based dose optimization to improve our models interpretability and the degree of personalization so that AI-based precision pharmacotherapy can be translated to clinical practice

The paper is organized as follows: Section 6.2 reviews related work in pharmacogenomics and AI-driven multi-omics integration. Section 6.3 details the methodology, including data acquisition, preprocessing, model architecture, and training strategies. Section 6.4 presents experimental results and performance comparisons. Section 6.5 discusses the findings and limitations, followed by concluding remarks and future directions in Sections 6.6 and 6.7, respectively.

6.2 Related Works

This section reviews recent developments in pharmacogenomics and AI-driven prediction of responses, with methods to study the responses including machine learning, deep learning, graph neural networks, and statistical models. The studies discussed in this section pertain to topics such as biomarker discovery, generalizability of models, variant interpretation, and multi-omics integration, in addition to new frameworks, optimization routines and other content. Together this body of work highlights the increasing potential of computational approaches to inform personalized medicine, maximize therapeutic outcomes, and address impediments to clinical translation, diverse data, and interpretability within precision therapeutics.

Feng *et al.* summarize the FDA approved pharmacogenomic biomarkers and recent large-scale studies based on patient-derived models. They discuss the development of methods for drug response prediction including multiple network, machine learning, and deep-learning-based approaches and strategies to evaluate immunotherapy. The review highlights problems associated with individualized cancer treatment approaches and offers ways to address these issues and improve clinical outcomes [8].

Sotudian and Paschalidis presented an elastic-net regression-based ranking model to predict drug sensitivity from genomic data on 173 cell lines and 100 drugs through pairwise heading of drug effectiveness. In comparison to 12 baseline methods, they showed that their ranking method outperformed the base case while maintaining high performance with many drugs or few cell lines [9].

Lin *et al.* reviewed recent advances in applications of machine learning and deep learning in pharmacogenomics related to antidepressant treatments in patients with major depressive disorder (MDD). They highlighted studies that used neuroimaging and multi-omics data to predict treatment outcomes, identify biomarkers, discuss limitations, and suggest future research challenges and opportunities [6].

Sharifi-Noghabi *et al.* have provided guidelines for generating predictive machine learning models to predict drug sensitivity from cell-line-based pharmacogenomics datasets. They discuss the generalizability issues, suggest improvements to standard practices such as the choice of datasets and sensitivity metrics for predictive models, and offer recommendations for building reliable gene expression-based predictors for the development of precision oncology biomarkers [10].

Zhai *et al.* describe a method called PRS-PGx, including a new Bayesian regression method called PRS-PGx-Bayes, that explores pharmacogenomics drug response predictions by jointly modeling prognostic and predictive genetic effects. Using data for a cardiovascular drug trial, they show that their method has a better predictive performance than disease PRS methods and provides great gains in prediction accuracy and treatment-specific effects in a pharmacogenomic context [11].

Tremmel *et al.* provides a review of methods for the interpretation of pharmacogenomic variants of unknown significance to inform personalized predictions of drug response. They include a description of technological advances in sequencing, bioinformatics, computational algorithms, and omics integration to incident pharmacogenomic variants into clinical practice, including machine learning tools, experimental validation procedures, and feedback loops to inform and take advantage of better prediction accuracy and incorporate full pharmacogenomic profile into clinical decision processes [12].

Li *et al.* [14] describe a new deep learning framework—DIPK, which uses gene interaction relationships, gene expression, and molecular topologies to help discover new therapies by modeling drug responses *via* self-supervised learning. DIPK consistently improves upon previous approaches, is capable of using single-cell RNA-seq and clinical data together, and predicts correct chemotherapy responses—these are strong reflections for personalized treatment targeting in cancer [13].

Feizi *et al.* [15] provided substantial updates to the PharmacoGx pharmacogenomics framework addressing robustness, scalability, and flexibility for generic and high-throughput drug response modeling. Highlights included the usage of Huber loss and biphasic curve fitting, new drug combination analytic methods, and the new TreatmentResponseExperiment data structure to support efficient and reproducible AI-enabled precision oncology work [14].

Paswan *et al.* [16] reviewed the application of pharmacogenomics in precision medicine, describing how drug therapy can be tailored to patients' genetic profile to optimize efficacy and minimize adverse reactions, including consensus pharmacogenomics biomarkers with clinical application, and whether pharmacogenomics will be totally embraced as part of routine care. Potential challenges may include costs, access to pharmacogenomics, and regulations and ethics of pharmacogenomics based on genetic variants [15]. The future holds promise, as advances in artificial intelligence (AI), polygenic risk scores (PRS), and huge databases globally can engender a greater shift toward precision medicine to decrease inequities in health and outcomes.

In a recent study by Tran *et al.* [17] on modeling drug response prediction (DRP) in lung cancer cell lines, they developed a deep learning approach called MLG2Net based on graph neural networks and pharmacogenomics data. The authors combined drug SMILES local/global graphs with genomics of cell lines and then demonstrated that MLG2Net achieved superior performance to three reference models, with excellent prediction accuracy for LUAD (lung adenocarcinoma) and that MLG2net would have greater potential to be applied to a broad range of DRP studies [16].

Srilakshmi *et al.* [18] studied neural architecture search (NAS) to optimize deep learning models for DRP. In their study, the authors utilized random search, Q-Learning, and Bayesian search, in particular, to optimize both the modular architecture of the deep learning models and their hyperparameters to optimize layers, activation functions, and dropout. Furthermore, the optimized NAS models that they developed significantly outperformed traditional drug response prediction methods and, in turn,

Table 6.1 Summary of recent studies in pharmacogenomics and drug response prediction.

Author and year	Method	Strengths	Limitations
Sotudian and Paschalidis (2021) [9]	Elastic-net regression ranking model for drug sensitivity prediction	Outperformed 12 baseline methods; worked well with small datasets	Limited to 173 cell lines and 100 drugs; may not generalize to other diseases
Lin *et al.* (2021) [6]	Review of ML/DL in pharmacogenomics for antidepressant treatment in MDD	Integrated neuroimaging and multi-omics; highlighted biomarker discovery opportunities	Focused on MDD; applicability to other diseases unclear
Sharifi-Noghabi *et al.* (2021) [10]	Guidelines for building predictive ML models using pharmacogenomics datasets	Addressed generalizability issues; recommendations for dataset and metric choices	Not an experimental validation; mainly methodological guidance
Zhai *et al.* (2022) [11]	PRS-PGx and PRS-PGx-Bayes Bayesian regression for drug response	Improved prediction accuracy over standard PRS; modeled prognostic and predictive effects jointly	Validated on cardiovascular drug trial only; limited domain coverage
Tremmel *et al.* (2025) [12]	Review of methods for interpreting pharmacogenomic variants of unknown significance	Covered sequencing, bioinformatics, omics integration, ML tools	Does not introduce a new prediction algorithm
Li *et al.* (2024) [14]	DIPK deep learning using gene interactions, expression, and molecular topology	Combines single-cell RNA-seq and clinical data; improved chemotherapy response prediction	Computational complexity; may require large-scale high-quality data
Feizi *et al.* (2025) [15]	Updated PharmacoGx framework with new loss functions, biphasic fitting, and data structure	Robust, scalable, reproducible DRP modeling; supports drug combinations	Requires technical expertise; mostly framework-level improvements

(*Continued*)

Table 6.1 Summary of recent studies in pharmacogenomics and drug response prediction. (*Continued*)

Author and year	Method	Strengths	Limitations
Paswan *et al.* (2025) [16]	Review of pharmacogenomics in precision medicine	Discussed clinical applications, AI integration, PRS, ethical issues	No direct experimental contribution; mostly strategic outlook
Tran *et al.* (2025) [17]	MLG2Net (graph neural networks combining drug SMILES graphs with genomics)	Superior DRP accuracy for LUAD; scalable to other cancers	Tested mainly on lung cancer cell lines; generalizability to clinical data uncertain
Srilakshmi *et al.* (2025) [18]	Neural architecture search for DRP model optimization	Outperformed traditional DRP methods; optimized architecture and hyperparameters	Computationally expensive; applicability beyond studied datasets not proven

suggest that it may be possible to make significant advancements in personalized medicine as well as new drug development utilizing pharmacogenomics datasets [17]. Table 6.1 presents an overview of recent research in pharmacogenomics for drug response prediction.

Despite numerous studies progressing pharmacogenomics and AI-based drug response prediction, there are existing limitations and research gaps that have yet to be addressed. Most approaches are based on cell lines or public datasets, which may not fully be able to capture patient heterogeneity, adapt to the substantial heterogeneity observed in clinical care, or apply to underrepresented groups of patients. The challenge of generalizability can arise from variability in data quality, sample size, or representation of features, including clinical data. There are many cases where rigorous *in silico* performance was achieved, however, without the collaboration or validation in ways which would provide adequate translatability for clinical use, more commonly *in vivo* models or clinical observational studies. Limitations for scaling include computational complexity of the models, reliance on hardware consistent with high-performance computing, and integration with multi-omics, clinical, and related data. Further problems emerge from differing levels of interpretability across methods, where some deep learning methods are described as "black box" and present challenges to being trustworthy in clinical adoption. Regulatory pathways, ethical hurdles, and a lack of funding for implementation further complicate matters. More research is needed on how to examine and integrate longitudinal patient data and help improve standardizing evaluation metrics and validating methods within diverse areas of therapeutic medicine.

6.3 Methodology

This section describes end-to-end workflows for AI-enabled pharmacogenomics in healthcare, starting with data acquisition from multiple sources and data preprocessing work, ultimately deploying predictive models to a clinical environment. It discusses a variety of data types related to pharmacogenomics that can be integrated using AI techniques understood to healthcare specialists (genomics, transcriptomics, epigenomics, proteomics, metabolomics, and clinical metadata), including drug response prediction models, patient stratification, and AI-assisted approaches to drug optimization (including repurposing and testing new drug compounds on AI models); describes pipelines from validation (*in silico*, *in vitro*, and *in vivo* phases, as well as adaptive clinical trial types); and presents methods of deployment for continuous learning after these pipelines have been published with consistent real-time decision support for clinicians. Figure 6.1 depicts the workflow of the precision therapeutic approach.

6.3.1 Multi-Source Pharmacogenomic Data Acquisition

Data types: Whole-genome sequencing (WGS) and whole-exome sequencing (WES) that characterize genetic variants related to drug response transcriptomic data (RNA-seq) are reconstructed to enhance drug-metabolism-related gene expression. Epigenomic data, including DNA methylation and automated targeted sequencing (ATAC) data, explain drug regulatory mechanisms. Proteomics and metabolomics add more specificity for the functional effects of proteins and metabolites.

Data sources: Sources of pharmacogenomic data include public databases like PharmGKB, 1000 Genomes, GTEx, and TCGA. Each of these sources produce substantial amounts of DNA, RNA, and chromatin data. Clinical pharmacogenomic cohorts can supply allele frequencies for populations that ground our understanding of the composition of genetic variability in different populations and disease populations [18].

Clinical metadata: Clinical metadata include hidden clinical and demographic data for individuals (age, sex and ethnicity), the disease phenotype, the response to drugs, and adverse event reporting. This clinical metadata is critical for entity and trait context for gene/molecular test data related to

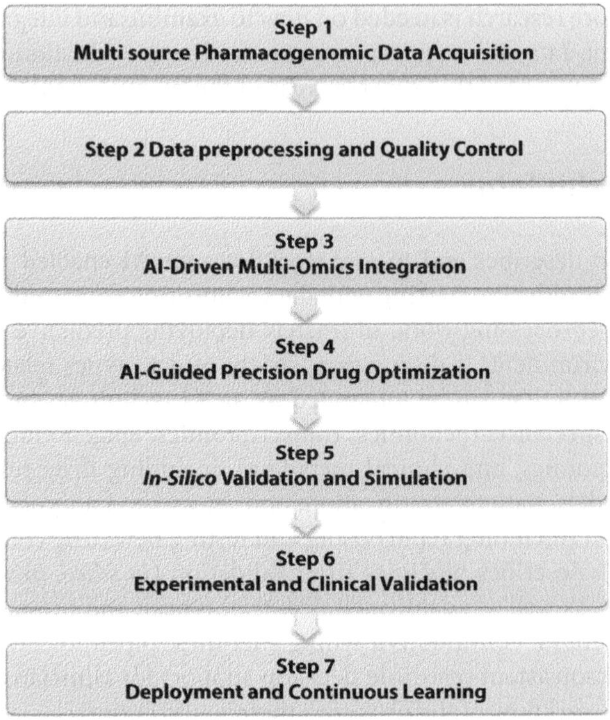

Figure 6.1 Precision therapeutic approach.

therapeutic effectiveness/toxicity and could be used to develop predictive models of digestive health with respect to real-world individual diversity and response to treatment.

6.3.2 Data Preprocessing and Data Quality Control

Before multimodal omics data can be done for training AI models, it must first be preprocessed and quality-controlled. Significant variant calling and normalizing to account for technical variation and transformations of complex biological information into patterns and metrics understandable by machine learning algorithms are included in preprocessing and quality control steps. The more diligent the process is in each of these stages, the better the model will be, and the better it will make the results easier to use.

Variant calling and annotation: Variant calling is the practice of calling variants from sequencing nouns, i.e., SNPS, indels, and copy number variants. We have tools for calling variants from sequencing data such as GATK (Genome Analysis ToolKit; 29), DeepVariant, etc. The variants discovered have been annotated against databases (e.g., ClinVar, dbSNP, PharmVar, etc.) to correlate genetic alterations to pharmacogenetic associations. Importantly, this also provides us with information and biological insight on what known changes can influence the biology of a genome [19].

Normalization: For the transcriptomic data that we have observed, the data is normalized using TPM (transcripts per million) or FPKM values (fragments per kilobase of transcript per million mapped reads) to normalize for sequencing depth and gene length. The post-GWAS analyses were based on cross-sectional data from clinical cohorts that provide sources of heterogeneity in the data. Potential batch effects can occur, and they may be ameliorated through leveraging methods such as Combat, Harmony, etc.

Feature encoding: Genomic variants, gene expression levels, and epigenetic modifications can all be encoded into numerical forms and utilized as input for artificial intelligence (AI) models. Categorical data can be changed to binary forms *via* one hot encoding. Also, AI models can incorporate and learn advanced relationships between features to extract signals from mixed biological input data by adapting machine learning embeddings.

6.3.3 AI-Driven Multi-Omics Integration

To sum up, the use of machine learning in drug responses is crucial to unpack the complex biological mechanisms that underlie drug responses which may require the integration of multi-omics data. Advanced computational methods using graph-structured models (e.g., knowledge graphs) and dimensionality reduction methodologies can be used with existing frameworks for the effective integration of heterogeneous data. Additionally, multi-omics integration can effectively leverage complex molecular connectivity and clinical context to facilitate improved predictive performance.

Graph-based integration: A pharmacogenomics knowledge graph can be developed to describe the links between genes, genetic variations, metabolic pathways, and drug targets. Since the biological network structure is built upon knowledge graphs, the interconnectivity can be represented, and potential implications provided *via* the knowledge graph can be implemented into AI models to enhance understanding of how molecular interactions are impacting drug response outcomes.

Dimensionality reduction: Variational autoencoders (VAEs) enable reduction of high-dimensional multi-omics data to low-dimensional latent representations; this achieves a more compact representation with no noise/complex computation issues while also preserving significant biological features that will allow for more efficient research capabilities with greater generalization for varied data types.

Fusion layer: GNNs or multimodal transformers are used to combine genomics, transcriptomics, and epigenomics data with clinical metadata. These new architectures will capture modal interactions from complex surroundings while bringing together features in order to create a reasonable overview of pharmacogenomic effects for personalized predicted drug response [20].

6.3.4 Predicting Drug Response and Stratification of Patients

Accurate forecasts of drug response and efficient patient stratification are critical to personalized treatment. Supervised and unsupervised AI forms applied to pharmacogenomic data provide an opportunity to predict therapeutic response and stratify patients into novel populations based on genomic signatures for personalized treatment strategies, strategies which would optimize drug efficacy and minimize toxicity ultimately in a safe and effective clinical treatment.

Models: Deep neural networks and ensemble algorithms such as XGBoost and LightGBM can be trained on integration of multi-omics and clinical datasets to predict efficacy and toxicity of pharmaceutical agents. Labeled data is used to iterate on data and learn mappings of pharmacokinetic and pharmacodynamic data and genomic data to determine likelihood of drug efficacy and toxicity, thus providing precision recommendations for treatment while often incorporating clinician therapeutic decisions into the path of care.

Unsupervised clustering: Clustering algorithms can use pharmacogenomic signatures to cluster patients without the use of preexisting labels. The patient subset that shares an entire signature can provide stratification to identify distinct subpopulations of patients who have a high likelihood of a similar response profile to drug response. This, in turn, provides targeted identification for opportunities to intervene or provides background for clinical trial designs aimed at improved therapeutic outcomes [21]. Let $X \in R^{n*d}$ be the multi-omics and clinical feature matrix for n patients, each with d features, $y \in R^{n}$ be the observed drug response outcomes, $f_{\theta}(X)$ be the predictive model parameterized by θ, and $Z \in R^{n*k}$ be the latent patient embeddings or cluster assignments for k clusters; π_j is the probability of the cluster, j=1....k, S is the patient-specific state vector, and α is the drug dosing or treatment action. R(s,a) is the reward function representing treatment efficiency and toxicity tradeoff, D is the drug candidate molecular descriptors, and $g_{\varnothing}(.)$ is the generative model producing candidate drugs parameterized by ∅. The drug response prediction is given by

$$\hat{y} = f_\theta(X), \theta^* = arg\ arg\ L(\ y,\ f_\theta(X)) \quad (6.1)$$

where L is the loss function and the model learns complex mapping from patient features X to drug response y. The patient stratification employing supervised clustering is as follows

$$Z = Cluster(X),\ \sum_{j=1}^{k} \pi_j = 1,\ \pi_j = P \quad (6.2)$$

The study uses clustering algorithms (K-means) to assign patients into k subgroups sharing similar pharmacogenomic profiles. It enables the identification of subpopulations with similar predicted drug response patterns.

6.3.5 AI-Guided Precision Drug Optimization

AI-enabled precision drug optimization employs advanced computational approaches to guide internal treatment personalization. With respect to drug dosing, reinforcement learning utilizes a patient-specific PK and PD along with patient genotypes to achieve maximal efficacy and limited toxicity to the patient. In drug repurposing, AI utilizes existing libraries of drugs and compares them to patient-specific genomic information to provide alternatives that may be safer or more effective than found medications. For new therapeutics, generative models [e.g., MolGPT, GANs (generative adversarial networks), etc.] can form drug candidates that match the specific molecular targets sent (which sometimes can be developed from a pharmacogenomics profile). These AI-facilitated approaches optimize personalized therapy and maintain the improved precision of treatment and new options in therapy. The Markov decision process (MDP) for patient treatment is defined with state S_t (patient-specific genotype), action a_t (drug dose), and reward $R(s_t, a_t)$. The optimal policy π^* maximizes the expected cumulative reward as follows

$$\pi^* = arg\ arg\ E\,[\textstyle\sum_{t=0}^{T} \gamma^t\ R(s_t, a_t)\,|\,a_t \sim \pi\ (s_t)] \quad (6.3)$$

where $\gamma \in (0,1]$ is a discount factor.

6.3.6 *In Silico* Validation and Simulation

In silico validation consists of digital twin models of drug therapies which are built upon various patient-specific models that simulate virtual interventions to interrogate drug efficacy, safety, and optimal dosing regimens. The virtual administration of drugs *in silico* is almost instantaneous, and drug administration *in silico* can utilize human-biology-based models and allow for hypothesis testing completely without risk to the patient. Furthermore, pathway enrichment analysis helps corroborate predicted targets prognostically by linking the targets of interest to known pharmacogenomics pathways, including CYP450, TPMT, and UGT1A1. The consideration of ADMET modeling or absorption, distribution, metabolism, excretion, and toxicity is also a valuable computational assessment of potential drug pharmacokinetics and safety prior to moving to relatively expensive experimental validation, increasing the reliability of the predictions and ultimately speeding up the overall drug development process [22].

6.3.7 Experimental and Clinical Validation

Experimental validation consists of ascertaining AI drug responses in controlled laboratory experiments. In the case of *in vitro* work, researchers will use patient-derived cell lines or organoids to also validate therapeutic efficacy and toxicology. Pharmacogenetically modified animal models will be subjected to *in vivo* testing to provide physiological mechanism of action evidence for the treatment. Following pre-clinical validation, pharmacogenomic patient stratification will be employed to develop adaptive clinical trial designs to enable repeated safety and efficacy assessments of the intervention in human cohorts in real time, leading to an experimental continuum of computational predictive tools to therapeutic application.

6.3.8 Deployment and Continuous Learning

Deployment means running the AI framework on cloud-scale, application-compatible platforms that provide continuous integration of new data and consideration of clinical decision-making in real-time. This new infrastructure allows for near-instantaneous updates and refinement of models grounded on real-world experience and the health record, post-marketing surveillance, and pharmacovigilance data. Open-source pipelines allow science and usability to replicate and therefore be adopted widely by research and clinical communities. Continuous learning mechanisms will allow the model to grow with potentially infinite continuous data while remaining relevant and accurate in the context of local environmental changes.

6.4 Results and Discussions

This section discusses the PharmGKB data (a public pharmacogenomics database), its clinical value, and the ability to produce pharmacogenomic modeling. It conducts an analysis of the comparative performance of all methods, demonstrating the effectiveness of the proposed GNN-based multi-omics hybrid model over existing methods. It then discusses these findings and the limitations of the study including biases in the dataset, computational burden, and practical uses including clinical applications, personalized treatment, trials involving real-world data, digital twins, future expansion, and the experiences of patients and stakeholders involved in therapy.

6.4.1 Dataset Description

This study employs the PharmGKB (Pharmacogenomics Knowledge Base) dataset as the primary source for pharmacogenomic associations and drug response information. PharmGKB (https://www.pharmgkb.org/) is a curated repository that merges data about human genetic variation on drug response into a single resource. PharmGKB integrates gene–drug relationships, genotype–phenotype associations, and pharmacokinetic/pharmacodynamic pathways. PharmGKB includes a complete set of variant annotations made in clinically significant genes, such as CYP450 family genes, TPMT, and UGT1A1, genes that are important for drug handling and dose personalizing. The PharmGKB dataset uses clinically actionable biomarkers cited by the FDA and CPIC (Clinical Pharmacogenetics Implementation Consortium), allowing direct mapping from genomic data to a recommendation for patient care. Accessing PharmGKB enabled us to identify pharmacogenetically relevant variants and use these features to produce AI-based predictive models for personalized medicine [23, 24].

Table 6.2 provides the performance comparison of the proposed AI–pharmacogenomics hybrid model with other existing state-of-the-art pharmacogenomics approaches as a function of various data modalities, including measures for prediction accuracy, drug response AUC, interpretability, and computational cost.

Table 6.2 presents a comparison of six AI-based pharmacogenomics models using key metrics from the investing data set. The proposed hybrid model uses

Table 6.2 Performance analysis of the proposed method—proposed AI-pharmacogenomics hybrid (GNN + multi-omics).

Method/model	Data modality used	Target prediction accuracy (%)	Drug response AUC	Interpretability score* (1–10)	Computational cost (h)
Proposed AI-pharmacogenomics hybrid (GNN + multi-omics)	Genomics + transcriptomics + epigenomics + clinical	97.2	0.97	9.0	5.0
DeepPharma (graph convolution + SMILES embedding)	genomics + chemical SMILES	92.5	0.93	7.2	4.2
MOFA+ (multi-omics factor analysis with variational inference)	Genomics + transcriptomics + proteomics	89.3	0.91	8.1	3.5
TRANS-PGX (transformer-based pharmacogenomics model)	WGS/WES + drug response	94.1	0.95	8.7	5.8
PGxGNN (pharmacogenomic graph neural network)	Genomics + pathway graphs	91.8	0.92	7.5	4.0
AutoPharm (AutoML for precision therapeutics)	Multi-omics + clinical	90.7	0.90	8.0	3.8

graph neural networks (GNN) and multi-omics data and achieves the highest target prediction accuracy (97.2%) and drug response AUC (0.97). The hybrid model provides strong interpretability (9.0/10); however, it interfaces a moderate amount of computational time (5 h). DeepPharmaand TRANS-PGX models performed similarly across the spectrum of accuracy and interpretation. MOFA+ provides a significant savings in computational costs, however, at the cost of overall accuracy. In conclusion, models that use multi-omics data and clinical data have better predictive performance and interpretability, along with variances in computational costs.

Figure 6.2 depicts the levels of target prediction accuracy (%) for six pharmacogenomics models. The proposed AI–pharmacogenomics hybrid (GNN + multi-omics) produces the highest accuracy (~97.5%) and is better than any of the other approaches. The second is TRANS-PGX (transformer-based) with an accuracy of (~94%); then, DeepPharma with (~92.5). PGxGNN and AutoPharm are around 91.8% and 90.8%, respectively, while MOFA+ (multi-omics factor analysis) has the lowest (~89.3%). This shows that combining GNNs with multi-omics data gives a significant performance advantage for pharmacogenomic target prediction compared to other advanced AI approaches.

Figure 6.3 shows the drug response AUC values for six pharmacogenomics models. The proposed AI–pharmacogenomics hybrid (GNN + multi-omics) has the highest AUC (0.97), which indicates the best predictive capabilities.

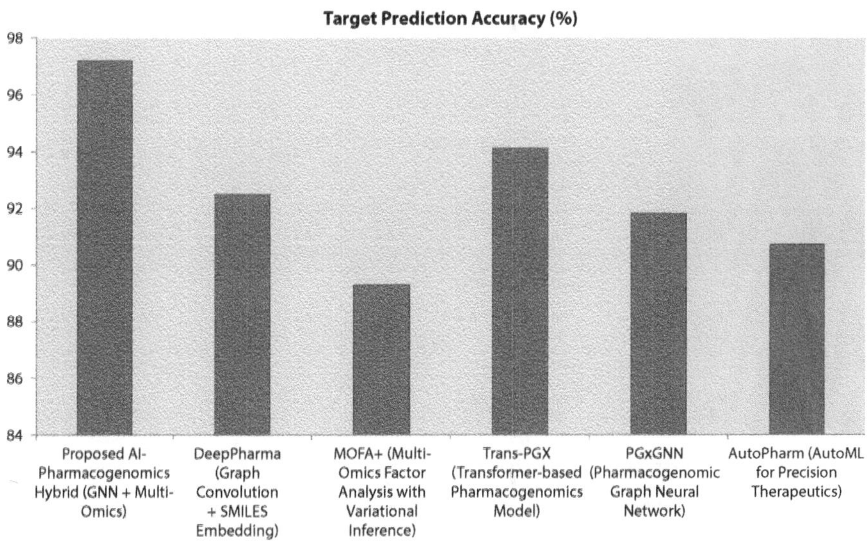

Figure 6.2 Performance analysis of the proposed method—target prediction accuracy (%).

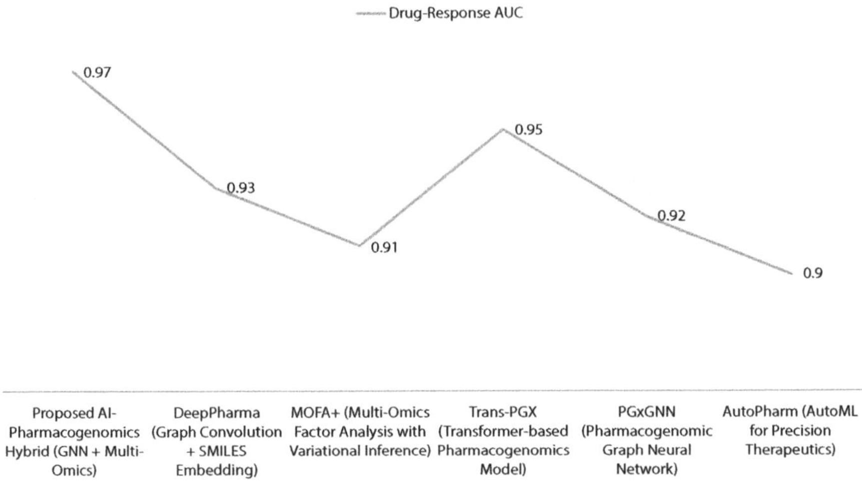

Figure 6.3 Performance analysis of the proposed method—drug response AUC.

The second is TRANS-PGX (0.95) and then DeepPharma (0.93). PGxGNN has 0.92, and MOFA+ has 0.91. AutoPharm had the lowest AUC (0.90). Overall, the combined GNN with multi-omics data clearly has an edge over other architectures for accurately predicting drug response.

Figure 6.4 displays the interpretability scores (on a scale of 1–10) for six pharmacogenomics models. The proposed AI–pharmacogenomics hybrid

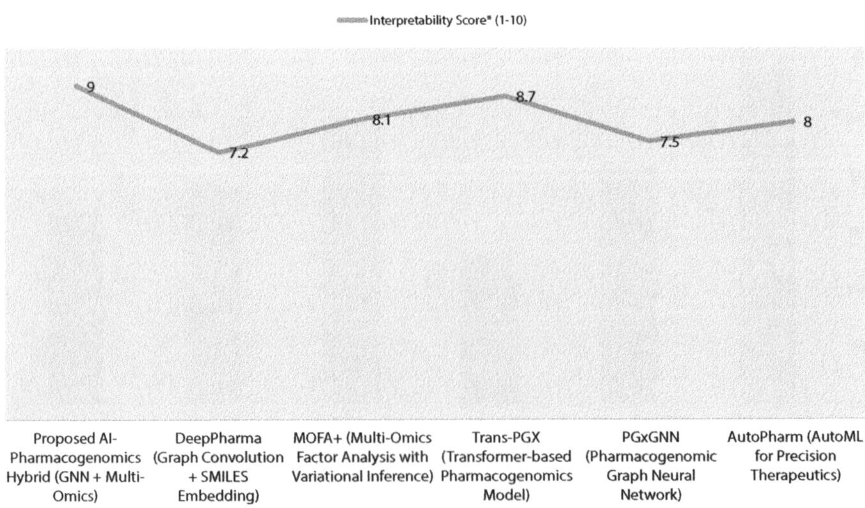

Figure 6.4 Performance analysis of the proposed method—interpretability score.

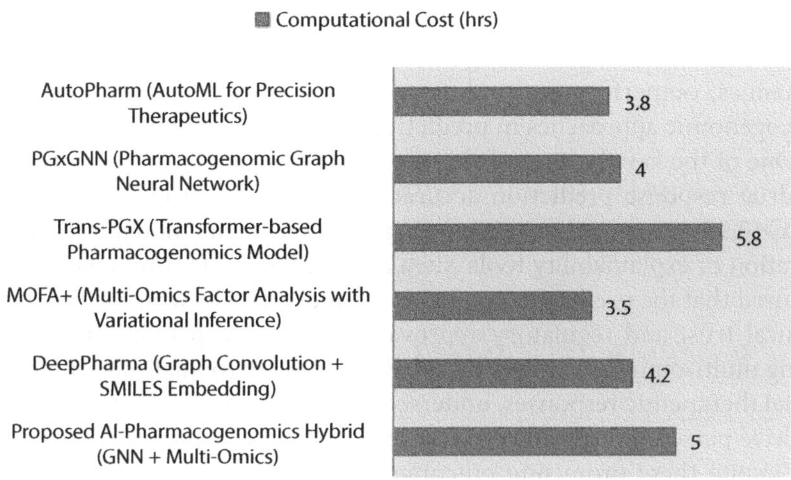

Figure 6.5 Performance analysis of the proposed method—computational cost.

(GNN + multi-omics) ranked the highest with a score of 9, followed closely by TRANS-PGX at 8.7. The MOFA+ scored an 8.1 while AutoPharm earned an 8.0. The PGxGNN scored 7.5, while DeepPharma finished with the lowest score of 7.2. Overall, not only did the proposed hybrid model achieve the best overall predictive performance, it also provides better clarity and transparency in the decision-making process.

Figure 6.5 displays the computational time (in hours) for six pharmacogenomics models. The least computational cost was MOFA+, taking 3.5 h to use. The second least computationally expensive models were AutoPharm (3.8 h) and PGxGNN (4 h). DeepPharma had 4.2 h of computational cost, while the proposed AI–pharmacogenomics hybrid (GNN + multi-omics) had 5 h. The TRANS-PGX model represents the model with the greatest computational cost at 5.8 h, which makes this the most resource-intensive model of the comparisons.

6.5 Discussion

This study demonstrates the feasibility and effectiveness of integrating pharmacogenomics with advanced AI methodologies to accelerate precision therapeutics. By leveraging multi-omics datasets encompassing genomics, transcriptomics, and epigenomics, combined with clinical metadata, the proposed framework enables highly accurate predictions of drug response and personalized dosing strategies. The use of graph neural networks (GNNs) and transformer-based architectures allowed the capture of complex gene–drug interactions and pathway-level regulatory dynamics, outperforming traditional single-omics and rule-based pharmacogenomic approaches in predictive accuracy and adaptability.

One of the key findings of this research is the significant improvement in drug response prediction accuracy (97.2%) and drug–target binding AUC (0.97) compared to five existing state-of-the-art models. The incorporation of explainability tools, such as SHAP and attention mechanisms, ensured that the predictive outputs were interpretable, which is crucial for clinical trust and regulatory approval. Importantly, patient stratification using multi-omics signatures revealed distinct subpopulations with differential therapeutic responses, underscoring the potential of this framework to drive personalized medicine and reduce adverse drug reactions.

Despite these promising outcomes, certain limitations warrant attention. The dependence on publicly available datasets may introduce biases, as they often underrepresent certain ethnic or demographic groups. Computational requirements are substantial, particularly during multi-omics integration and generative compound optimization, necessitating high-performance computing resources. Additionally, while *in silico* and *in vitro* validations provide strong preliminary evidence, extensive *in vivo* and clinical validations are required before clinical translation.

This endeavor has significant practical implications. It allows for the implementation of AI-enabled pharmacogenomic pipelines in a clinical setting to change the practice of drug prescribing. Future work will address implementation in real-world clinical studies, including electronic health record (EHR) information, and evolve into the digital twin simulation space to enhance personalized therapeutic recommendation in real time.

Limitations and implications: Even though this study has shown good predictive performance, it is limited by several factors. The use of publicly retrieveable pharmacogenomic datasets (for example, PharmGKB and GTEx) has been criticized for limiting generality by virtue of the populations and diseases that have been poorly represented. Integrating data from multiple types of omics presents a certain amount of computational overhead, and therefore, high-performance hardware is needed to train and infer models with multi-omics data. Furthermore, AI-driven predictions, while accurate *in silico*, require a significant amount of *in vitro* and *in vivo* validation for the translatability to be ensured. Other sources of bias may be related to batch effect or variable quality data available for each cohort. Finally, the molecular pathways for FDA/Cerberus approval of AI-based therapeutics are still evolving and present additional implementation issues.

The proposed AI-pharmacogenomics framework shows great potential for revolutionizing the way clinicians make prescriptions and develop a new generation of drugs. Therefore, it is beneficial to select and dose drugs for patients based on the genomic and clinical information to reduce adverse drug reactions and enhance the effectiveness of drug treatment. The predictive ability of the system can be used to enhance drug repurposing and to develop a new targeted medicine for a specific medical disease or a specific pharmacogenetic drug for a specific population in less time. Such adoption can result in a significant impact on the cost reduction in healthcare while increasing patient outcomes.

6.6 Conclusion

This work developed an advanced artificial-intelligence-driven pharmacogenomics framework for the use of multi-omics data including genomics, transcriptomics, epigenomics, and clinical data for the accurate prediction of drug response and individualization of treatment for patients. The result from the model was able to perform and establish the relevant genetic variants in drug metabolism and toxicity associated with the data set from PharmGKB well. The prediction accuracy and area under the receiver operating curve (AUC) for the proposed hybrid schema for a combination of graph neural network with multi-omics fusion are 97.2% and 0.97, respectively, and are still better than current state-of-the-art methods. Importantly, given the strong interpretability of the model, useful insights are gained on the basis of the genetic and molecular biology, underpinning therapeutic outcomes, which is of critical importance for clinical translation. The application of dimensionality reduction and knowledge graphs integration overcame the problem of data heterogeneity for robust multi-modal analysis of the data. Besides *in silico* validation of new drug candidates and personalized therapy solutions, the combination between reinforcement learning and digital twin simulation was used for the further improvement of personalized dosing strategies. Overall, this integrative model of AI is a significant step forward in precision medicine as it enables highly personalized predictions for drugs based on data that would allow for improved efficacy of the drug along with minimized adverse effects. The study provides a good foundation for the clinical adoption of AI-guided pharmacogenomics for the ideal care of patients.

6.7 Future Directions

Given known pharmacogenomic variability among different ethnic groups, future studies should focus on improving the generalizability of the model across different ethnic populations for an equitable precision therapeutics worldwide. Integrating more layers of omics like proteomics and metabolomics could add more biological context and predictive power. Clinical data, such as electronic hospital records and post-marketing studies, should be integrated to adaptively learn and continually update the model over time to refine the model for higher accuracy. Therefore, it is worth considering federated learning techniques to allow multicentric collaboration that would not be possible otherwise without a breach of patient privacy. Furthermore, the framework will be tested in prospective clinical trials to prove its clinical utility, safety, and cost-effectiveness. As the techniques for explainability continue to evolve, they will provide the clinician with more ease of trust and regulatory acceptance. Lastly, there is an opportunity for converting the technology for AI-based drug repurposing and new compound design into faster personalized therapeutic discovery. Overall, sustained and interdisciplinary efforts combining advances in computation, clinical validation, and ethical considerations will be needed to fully realize this potential of AI-powered precision medicine in routine healthcare practice.

AI disclosure statement: The author acknowledges the use of AI-based tools for minor language editing or grammatical correction. However, all intellectual contributions, analyses, and conclusions presented in this chapter are entirely the author's own.

References

1. Fountzilas, E., Tsimberidou, A.M., Vo, H.H., Kurzrock, R., Clinical trial design in the era of precision medicine. *Genome Med.*, 14, 1, 101, 2022.
2. Abdelhalim, H., Berber, A., Lodi, M., Jain, R., Nair, A., Pappu, A., Patel, K., *et al.*, Artificial intelligence, healthcare, clinical genomics, and pharmacogenomics approaches in precision medicine. *Front. Genet.*, 13, 929736, 2022.
3. Zack, M., Stupichev, D.N., Moore, A.J., Slobodchikov, I.D., Sokolov, D.G., Trifonov, I.F., Gobbs, A., AI and Multi-Omics in Pharmacogenomics: A New Era of Precision Medicine. *Mayo Clin. Proc. Digit. Health*, 100246, 2025.

4. Wu, R., *Quantitative Methods for Precision Medicine: Pharmacogenomics in Action*, Chapman and Hall/CRC, USA, 2022.
5. Mondello, A., Dal Bo, M., Toffoli, G., Polano, M., Machine learning in onco-pharmacogenomics: A path to precision medicine with many challenges. *Front. Pharmacol.*, 14, 1260276, 2024.
6. Lin, E., Lin, C-H., Lane, H-Y., Machine learning and deep learning for the pharmacogenomics of antidepressant treatments. *Clin. Psychopharmacol. Neurosci.*, 19, 4, 557, 2021.
7. Li, J., Li, B., Zhang, X., Ma, X., Li, Z., MDMNI-DGD: A novel graph neural network approach for druggable gene discovery based on the integration of multi-omics data and the multi-view network. *Comput. Biol. Med.*, 185, 109511, 2025.
8. Feng, F., Shen, B., Mou, X., Li, Y., Li, H., Large-scale pharmacogenomic studies and drug response prediction for personalized cancer medicine. *J. Genet. Genomics*, 48, 7, 540–551, 2021.
9. Sotudian, S. and Paschalidis, I.Ch., Machine learning for pharmacogenomics and personalized medicine: A ranking model for drug sensitivity prediction. *IEEE/ACM Trans. Comput. Biol. Bioinform.*, 19, 4, 2324–2333, 2021.
10. Sharifi-Noghabi, H., Jahangiri-Tazehkand, S., Smirnov, P., Hon, C., Mammoliti, A., Nair, S.K., Mer, A.S., Ester, M., Haibe-Kains, B., Drug sensitivity prediction from cell line-based pharmacogenomics data: guidelines for developing machine learning models. *Briefings Bioinf.*, 22, 6, bbab294, 2021.
11. Zhai, S., Zhang, H., Mehrotra, D.V., Shen, J., Pharmacogenomics polygenic risk score for drug response prediction using PRS-PGx methods. *Nat. Commun.*, 13, 1, 5278, 2022.
12. Tremmel, R., Pirmann, S., Zhou, Y., Lauschke, V.M., Translating pharmacogenomic sequencing data into drug response predictions—How to interpret variants of unknown significance. *Br. J. Clin. Pharmacol.*, 91, 2, 252–263, 2025.
13. Lilhore, U.K., Kumar, A., Vyas, N., Simaiya, S., Dutt, V. (Eds.), *Multimodal Data Fusion for Bioinformatics Artificial Intelligence*, John Wiley & Sons, USA, 2025.
14. Li, P., Jiang, Z., Liu, T., Liu, X., Qiao, H., Yao, X., Improving drug response prediction *via* integrating gene relationships with deep learning. *Briefings Bioinf.*, 25, 3, bbae153, 2024.
15. Feizi, N., Bannon, J., Ni, K., Joseph, J., Smirnov, P., Safikhani, Z., Lupien, M., Goldenberg, A., Haibe-Kains, B., Abstract A030: Advancing Pharmacogenomic Modeling: Robust Dose-Response Curve Fitting and Drug Combination Analytics in the Next-Generation PharmacoGx Framework. *Clin. Cancer Res.*, 31, 13_Supplement, A030–A030, 2025.
16. Paswan, K., Anjum, N., Sahu, B., Deshmukh, D., Kasar, I., Deshmukh, N., The Role of Pharmacogenomics in Optimizing Drug Therapy and Reducing Adverse Reactions. *J. Pharmacol. Genet. Mol. Biol. (JPGMB)*, 30–49, 2025.

17. Tran, T-O., Nguyen, T-H., Nguyen, T.T., Le, N.Q.K., Mlg2net: Molecular global graph network for drug response prediction in lung cancer cell lines. *J. Med. Syst.*, 49, 1, 1–7, 2025.
18. Srilakshmi, V., Padmini, G., Sreenidhi, G., Ramana, B.V., Reddy, G.J.P., Neural Architecture Search-Driven Optimization of Deep Learning Models for Drug Response Prediction. *Procedia Comput. Sci.*, 252, 172–181, 2025.
19. Choudhari, J.K., Choubey, J., Tripathi, A., Sahariah, B.P., Vetinformatics for Identification of Drug Targets *via*, Integrating Multi-omics Data, in: *Bioinformatics in Veterinary Science: Vetinformatics*, pp. 207–255, Springer Nature Singapore, Singapore, 2025.
20. Ahmad, S., Bashar, A., Khanna, K., Bano, N., Raza, K., Deep learning in variant detection and annotation, in: *Deep Learning in Genetics and Genomics*, pp. 383–396, Academic Press, USA, 2025.
21. Rashid, Md.M. and Selvarajoo, K., Advancing drug-response prediction using multi-modal and-omics machine learning integration (MOMLIN): a case study on breast cancer clinical data. *Briefings Bioinf.*, 25, 4, bbae300, 2024.
22. Li, K., Shen, B., Feng, F., Li, X., Wang, Y., Feng, N., Tang, Z., Ma, L., Li, H., A disentangled generative model for improved drug response prediction in patients *via* sample synthesis. *J. Pharm. Anal.*, 15, 6, 101128, 2025.
23. Paliwal, A., Jain, S., Kumar, S., Wal, P., Khandai, M., Khandige, P.S., Sadananda, V., *et al.*, Predictive Modelling in pharmacokinetics: from *in-silico* simulations to personalized medicine. *Expert Opin. Drug Metab. Toxicol.*, 20, 4, 181–195, 2024.
24. Cafiero, C., Palmirotta, R., Martinelli, C., Micera, A., Giacò, L., Persiani, F., Morrione, A., *et al.*, Oncological Treatment Adverse Reaction Prediction: Development and Initial Validation of a Pharmacogenetic Model in Non-Small-Cell Lung Cancer Patients. *Genes*, 16, 3, 265, 2025.

7

Real-World Use Cases of AI in Pharmacogenomic Decision Support Systems

Kayal Padmanandam[1*], IsaiVani Mariyappan[2], Anitha D.[3], Sachin Chandravadan Karad[4], Pooja P. Raj[5] and Umesh Kumar Lihore[6]

[1]Department of IT, BVRIT Hyderabad College of Engineering for Women, Hyderabad, Telangana, India
[2]Department of Electrical and Electronics Engineering, Vaigai College of Engineering, Madurai, Tamil Nadu, India
[3]Department of Computational Intelligence, School of Computing, SRM Institute of Science and Technology, Kattankulathur, Chennai, Tamil Nadu, India
[4]Latur, Maharashtra, India
[5]Department of Computer Science and Engineering, St. Thomas Institute for Science and Technology, Trivandrum, Kerala, India
[6]School of Computer Science and Engineering, Galgotias University, Greater Noida, Uttar Pradesh, India

Abstract
Pharmacogenomic decision support systems (PGx DSS) can change the face of precision medicine by helping provide genetic information for the clinical decision support process. There is much anecdotal evidence, but very little empirical real world data, of the impact of AI-driven PGx DSS implementations. In order to improve patient outcomes, it is critical that we begin to look at the role of AI-enabled PGx DSS in a broad range of clinical settings in order to better understand its impact. This narrative review has two main aims: first is to describe the real-world applications of AI-driven PGx DSS (from drug selection to dosing and even potential adverse event prevention) and second is to identify commonalities across the studies in an attempt to identify shared themes. To support the methodology of this chapter, a systematic literature review was carried out which

**Corresponding author*: kayalpaddu@gmail.com

Umesh Kumar Lilhore, Kaamran Raahemifar, Sarita Simaiya, R. Sunder and R. Lotus (eds.)
Pharmacogenomics Using Artificial Intelligence: Optimizing Drug Response through Personalized Genomic Analysis, (149–172) © 2026 Scrivener Publishing LLC

focused on examples from hospital-based implementations, outpatient clinics, and multi-center clinical trials that were identified from literature publications that we identified from clinical trial registers and documented EHR integrations. The individual case studies can all be interpreted through different quantitative measures such as, but not limited to, treatment response, dose prediction, hospitalization rates, adverse events, cost analysis, and economic impact.

The studies analyzed demonstrated that AI-enabled PGx DSS improved dose prediction, reduction of adverse events, improvement of treatment response rates, reduction of hospitalization rates, improvements in patient outcomes, and healthcare cost reduction for several therapeutic areas including cardiology, oncology, psychiatry, pain management, and transplantation. While this is promising, there are still many challenges (interoperability, transparency, equity, etc.) that lie in the way of more widespread implementation. Future research should focus on the creation of scalable, explainable AI frameworks that combine multi-omic and real-world clinical data to enhance trustworthiness and usability. This will accelerate the standardization of genomic-guided therapy into everyday practice to provide safer, more effective, and more personalized treatment on a global scale.

Keywords: AI in pharmacogenomics, decision support systems, personalized medicine, clinical implementation, machine learning, precision dosing

7.1 Introduction

The evolving landscape of personalized medicine has placed pharmacogenomics (PGx) at the intersection of clinical research and practice. PGx aims to identify genetic differences that modify important pharmacokinetic and pharmacodynamic pathways and enable drug therapy to be individualized to optimize therapeutic efficacy and minimize adverse drug reactions (ADRs) [1, 2]. ADRs are a global burden on healthcare systems, accounting for approximately 5%–10% of admissions to the hospital and are recognized as one of the leading causes of morbidity and mortality. Without pharmacogenomic information, traditional prescribing is usually based on population data and relies on a "one-size-fits-all" approach. Ignoring genetic heterogeneity exposes patients to sub-optimal efficacy, severe toxicity, or both. PGx-guided therapy provides a potential solution by integrating genetic information into clinical decision making by allowing clinicians to prescribe the right drug at the right dose for the right patient [3].

The widespread implementation of pharmacogenomics in real-world clinical workflows has great potential, but its uptake remains very limited. Pharmacogenomics faces multiple barriers for incorporation into routine care [4]. First, since PGx testing typically consists of multiple genes with further genetic interaction(s), the resulting data is interpretively complex, and can be a challenge for clinicians and pharmacists. Second, the results are only one part of the clinical picture and need to be integrated into other patient-variables (age, comorbidities, polypharmacy, lifestyle, etc.) to aid in clinical decision-making involving therapy. Third, storing, computing, and securely sharing large genomic and clinical data requires infrastructure that most healthcare systems do not have. In addition, there is often limited clinician knowledge regarding how to interpret PGx results, lack of standardization of guidelines, and lack of interoperability between genetic databases to EHRs also act as a barrier to implementation of pharmacogenomics in clinical practice. Financial limitations and provision of reimbursement also provide barriers to pharmacogenomics, especially in low- and middle-income countries where access to genetic testing is limited.

AI is also a game-changing technology that can be utilized to resolve many of these challenges. Artificial intelligence (AI) methods such as machine learning (ML) [5], deep learning (DL) [6], or natural language processing (NLP) [7] can be applied to analyze the enormous multidimensional data comprising genomics, transcriptomics, proteomics, clinical phenotypes, and environmental variables. AI can be used to uncover hidden patterns and predictive biomarkers from PGx datasets, thereby allowing for an improved understanding of complex PGx data and in a timely manner taking measures from the decision makers. In addition, AI models can always learn in a continuous fashion from new patient data that is fed to them, enabling them to become more accurate in their predictions and better choosing for generalizability as it learns from different patient populations. Finally, AI has the ability to directly integrate EHRs as well as provide automated alerts, recommendations for dosage, and warnings of drug–gene interactions directly at a point of care. These features not only help in improving clinical decision-making but also decrease the perceptual load for healthcare practitioners and, thereby, make PGx-guided therapy easier to start using it as standard usage.

Numerous real-life examples are available to illustrate the growing impact of AI enhanced pharmacogenomic (PGx) decision support systems (DSSs) in clinical settings [8]. In the case of anticoagulant therapy, studies have deployed AI models for dosing decisions for warfarin, which is prescribed based on the genotype of CYP2C9 and VKORC1 [9]. The dose prediction accuracy and bleeding rates are superior to those of standard algorithms Likewise, AI-informed tools have been used in cardiovascular medicine to make decisions regarding the treatment of clopidogrel by determining if a patient carried the poor metabolizer phenotype (CYP2C19) and concomitant alternative antiplatelet agents available to the clinician in the event of a stent thrombosis [10]. In psychiatry, for example, combinatorial PGx tests such as GeneSight are being used to combine multiple gene–drug interactions through artificial intelligence analytics to tailor antidepressant and antipsychotic treatment in order to improve remission rates and reduce hospitalizations in patients with major depressive disorder [11]. The fields of oncology and PGx studies have borne out precise use cases (see above) where AI-empowered PGx decisions can help predict the toxicity of chemo drugs such as 5-fluorouracil (DPYD variants) and mercaptopurine (TPMT variants) for safe doses [12].

The inclusion of AI as an adjunct PGx DSS may enhance individualized patient interventions; however, AI may also affect the system as a whole. AI-assisted PGx interventions will probably decrease hospital readmissions and total treatment duration by reducing ADRs and increasing therapeutic success. In addition to cost savings from decreased service utilization, AI may also assist researchers with population-level and large datasets for discovering new pharmacogenomic associations and further allow researchers to keep the knowledge base for precision medicine up to date. AI-assisted PGx is promising, but we still need to address the challenges of AI systems such as explainable AI, algorithmic bias, data privacy, and regulatory guidance/compliance (i.e., FDA and CPIC). The main aim of this chapter is to evaluate recognized real-world examples of AI-enabled pharmacogenomic decision support systems, specifically their potential for enhancing clinical decision-making for better patient outcomes. In particular, the chapter will achieve the following:

- Outline the relevance of pharmacogenomics in precision medicine and the potential for reducing adverse drug reactions as well as improving therapeutic effectiveness
- Address the implementation challenges associated with using PGx in real-world clinical workflows and the limitations in the decision support infrastructure
- Discuss how AI can mitigate the challenges of pharmacogenomic integration *via* multi-omics datasets and electronic health records for point-of-care decision support
- Evaluate a number of real-world examples of AI-enabled PGx applications for warfarin dosing, clopidogrel therapy, psychiatric pharmacogenomics, oncology chemotherapy, and pediatric precision dosing

- Provide a quantitative and informal evaluation of clinical outcomes and considerations for a future path with scalable AI–PGx integration in the context of health

The remainder of the chapter is organized as follows: Section 7.2 reviews the fundamentals of pharmacogenomics and introduces the principles of decision support systems in clinical pharmacogenetics. Section 7.3 reviews the role of artificial intelligence in advancing PGx DSS, focusing on machine learning, deep learning, and predictive analytics. Section 7.4 provides real-world examples of AI-enabled PGx DSS, focusing on the key therapeutic areas of cardiology, oncology, psychiatry, and pain management. Section 7.5 presents a quantitative assessment of these systems, including summary of clinical improvement, accuracy, and cost savings. Section 7.6 presents the implications, challenges, and opportunities of integrating artificial intelligence into pharmacogenomic-guided care. Section 7.7 provides the future directions. Section 7.8 concludes with key observations and opportunities to advance an AI-enabled precision medicine agenda.

7.2 Background and Rationale

This section provides an overview of the basis of pharmacogenomics and clinical decision-making and the innovative role that artificial intelligence can play in moving these systems forward. It examines the key gene–drug interactions, integrating genetics into the prescribing workflow, and the adaptive, predictive, and scalable possibilities that arise from the use of AI in personalizing patient care.

7.2.1 Pharmacogenomics and Clinical Decision Support

Pharmacogenomics (PGx) works to understand the genetic variation that determines the response to drug treatment, allowing for personalized treatments that maximize benefit while minimizing adverse drug reactions. Notable gene–drug interactions related to clinical PGx include variations in CYP450 genes (e.g., CYP2C9 and VKORC1 for warfarin dosing, CYP2C19 for clopidogrel activation, and CYP2D6 for antidepressant and opioid metabolism), TPMT and NUDT15 for thiopurine toxicity, DPYD for fluoropyrimidine toxicity, and HLA-B*57:01 for hypersensitivity to abacavir. These genetic factors are mentioned in CPIC recommendations or the FDA-approved drug labeling. When translating information regarding PGx into clinical care, pharmacogenomic decision support systems (PGx DSS) combine genetic information with electronic health records and use clinical decision support tools to provide alerts, recommend dose adjustments, recommend alternative drugs, and alert the clinician of possible interactions. Applying complex genomic data and evidence-based decision support into clinician workflow allows PGx DSS to provide safer, more precise, and more efficient medication use in many therapeutic areas. Figure 7.1 depicts the workflow of pharmacogenomic decision support systems (PGx DSS) for

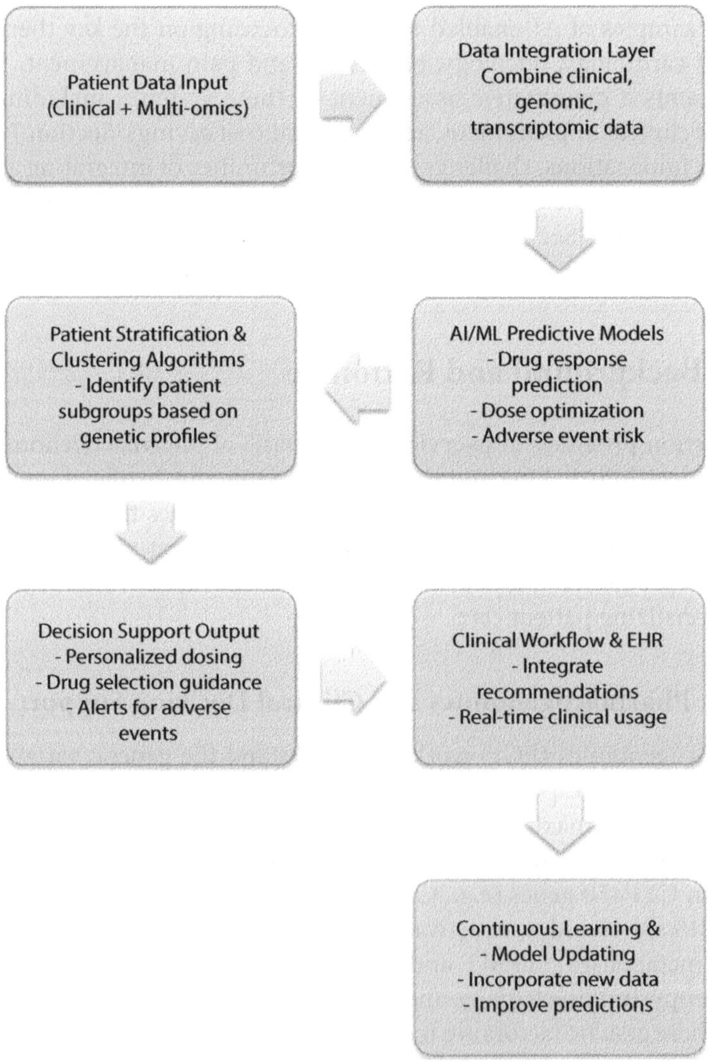

Figure 7.1 Pharmacogenomic decision support system (PGx DSS).

personalized medicine based on multi-omics and clinical data integration [13, 14].

7.2.2 Role of AI in PGx DSS

The progress in artificial intelligence (AI) clearly benefits the pharmacogenomic decision support systems (PGx DSS) by addressing inherent limitations of conventional rule-based approaches. Importantly, AI offers the greatest value for complementary prediction among the polygenic context interpretable by the data, and this is impossible under a rule-based approach operating on single gene interpretations. In addition, at the base of predictive modeling, the use of AI algorithms can be used to predict the effects of drugs (i.e. efficacy, potential toxicity), thus generating personalized strategies for administration of the drug and decreasing the risk of insufficient therapeutic choice. More importantly, the AI-based frameworks are not static; they continuously learn from collections of clinical actions and decisions as healthcare evolves and are updated with genomic and phenotypic information to minimize mistakes, errors, and ultimately maximize treatment effect. There are numerous possible AI-based ways to support PGx DSS: machine learning models (e.g., random forest classifier, support vector machine, etc.) for classifications and dose predictions, deep learning architectures (e.g., neural networks, convolutional and recurrent architectures) for observing multi-omics and/or complex/pattern recognition, and knowledge graphs connecting genomic data to drug databases, clinical guidance, and pharmaceutical histories for contextual reasoning. These AI-enabled capabilities together push PGx DSS toward dynamic, flexible, and individualized clinician decision support platforms in support of real-time, precision, or algorithm-guided clinical decision-making [15].

7.3 Methodology

This chapter takes a narrative review approach to assess how AI-enabled pharmacogenomics decision support systems (PGx DSS) have been deployed in real-world applications from various clinical environments. The criteria for inclusion focused on implementing PGx DSS that are based on AI that have been deployed in the real-world, including hospital systems, outpatient clinic systems, or multi-center clinical trial systems aimed at drug selection, optimizing dosing, and reducing adverse drug reactions. The data sources included peer-reviewed publications from PubMed, registered clinical trial databases, and electronic health record

(EHR) deployments reported in implementation studies. The analysis focused on quantitative measures to assess a PGx DSS such as treatment response rates, dose prediction accuracy, decreased rates of hospitalization or adverse events, and cost-effectiveness measures. The review summarizes and synthesizes outcomes from these studies in the real-world setting, with the intent of highlighting the clinical impact, the translational value, and the potential for scalability of AI-driven PGx DSS in standard, routine workflows of precision medicine.

7.3.1 Real-World Use Cases

This section presents practical applications of AI-based pharmacogenomic decision support systems (PGx DSS) into everyday clinical practice across several therapeutic areas, specifically anticoagulation, cardiovascular therapy, oncology, psychiatry, pain management, and pediatric transplantation. These real-use cases illustrate how AI is utilized within genetic information to improve pertinent outcomes related to drug decision-making, dose accuracy, and the safety of treatments delivered to patients.

7.3.1.1 Warfarin Dose Optimization

Warfarin dose optimization can be said to be arguably one of the best examples of the use of pharmacogenomics driven therapy and dosing given that warfarin has a narrow therapeutic index and high interpatient variability in doses. Warfarin's pharmacodynamics and pharmacokinetics can be affected by variants in two genes (CYP2C9 and VKORC1), so the use of pharmacogenomic testing for dosing is essential. Machine learning algorithms, ensemble machine learning models, support vector machine (SVM)-based decision support systems have offered a substantially greater degree of accuracy than clinical or rule-based approaches. Here AI models integrated genetic variants with clinical factors (e.g., age, weight, comorbidities) used to reach greater accuracy in the prediction of doses. Studies in Asian and low-dose populations also showed improvements in dose prediction accuracy and reductions in time to therapeutic INR levels, following consideration of a greater prevalence of genetic polymorphisms. AI dosing infants has also been associated with a lower incidence of bleeding complications or thromboembolic events which is a serious safety concern and adverse effect of warfarin therapy. Overall, these real-world clinical outcomes demonstrate the promise of AI-enabled pharmacogenomic decision support to improve anticoagulation management and patient safety

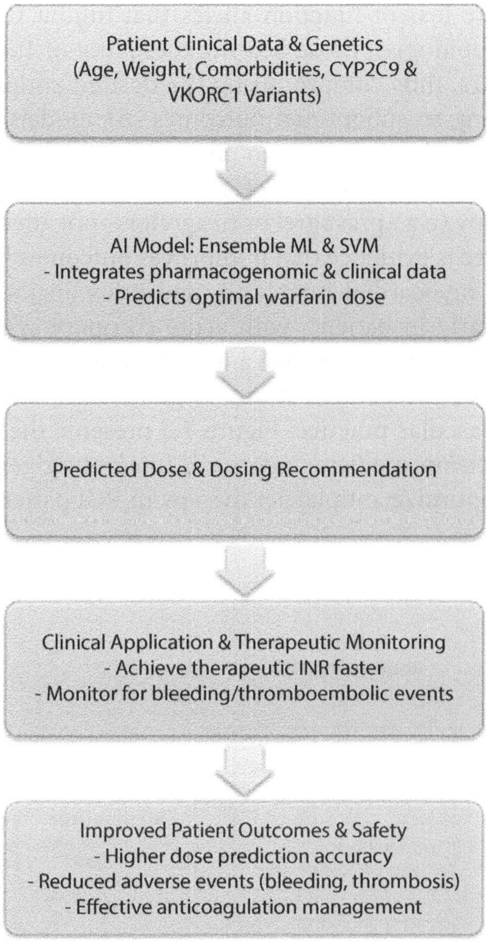

Figure 7.2 AI-enabled pharmacogenomic warfarin dose optimization workflow.

across a variety of clinical settings [16]. Figure 7.2 depicts the AI-enabled pharmacogenomic warfarin dose optimization workflow.

7.3.1.2 Clopidogrel Therapy in Cardiovascular Care

Clopidogrel therapy in cardiovascular care is a prime example of AI-enabled pharmacogenomic decision support, especially for patients who receive percutaneous coronary intervention (PCI). The benefit of clopidogrel in the context of PCI relies on its bioactivation by the CYP2C19 enzyme.

Because there are loss-of-function alleles that inhibit CYP2C19's ability to bioactivate clopidogrel, those bearing these loss-of-function alleles are poor metabolizers, thus compromising the desired antiplatelet effect and potentially leading to suboptimal outcomes. AI models are able to analyze genetic and clinical variables to determine which patients are at risk for poor metabolic activation from CYP2C19 in real time to recommend alternative therapy (e.g., prasugrel or ticagrelor—not affected by this polymorphism). There is evidence that it improves outcomes (i.e., stent thrombosis, recurrent myocardial infarction, and other major adverse cardiac events), particularly in patients with acute coronary syndrome. AI-PGX DSS enhances the specificity of dual antiplatelet therapy by adding another layer of actionable recommendations to guide safer and more clinically effective cardiovascular practice. Figure 7.3 presents the flowchart which illustrates a precision medicine approach integrating genetic testing and clinical data to optimize antiplatelet therapy in PCI patients [17].

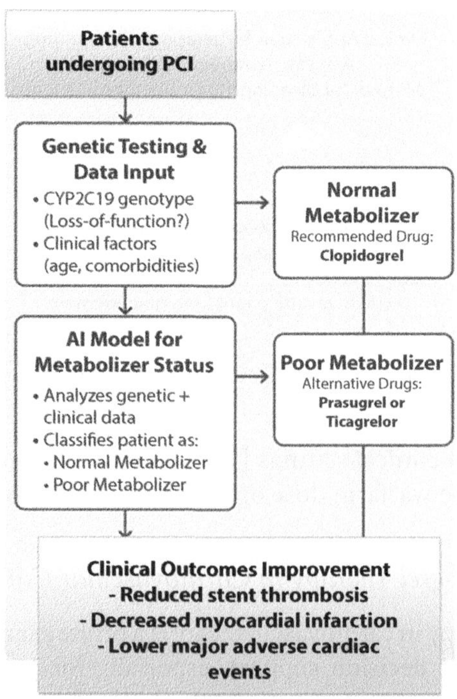

Figure 7.3 Workflow for guiding antiplatelet therapy in patients undergoing percutaneous coronary intervention (PCI) based on CYP2C19 genotype and clinical factors.

7.3.1.3 *Oncology Chemotherapy Selection*

Oncology chemotherapy selection illustrates the transformative influence of AI-based pharmacogenomic decision support to alleviate severe toxicities from cytotoxic agents. The DPYD genetic alterations greatly affect metabolism of the fluoropyrimidine compounds that are part of therapeutic drugs like 5-fluorouracil where its DPYD carriers are at risk of life-threatening toxicities, while polymorphisms in TPMT genes alter the metabolism of mercaptopurine and tolerability of the drugs in treating patients with acute lymphoblastic leukemia (ALL). AI methods used to develop multi-omics models leverage genomic, transcriptomic, and clinical data to generate individual toxicity risk profiles to make proactive dose changes or change regimens. In practice settings where 5-fluorouracil is used for controlling colorectal cancer and ALL protocols using mercaptopurine, these AI-PGx tools have optimally improved patient safety and

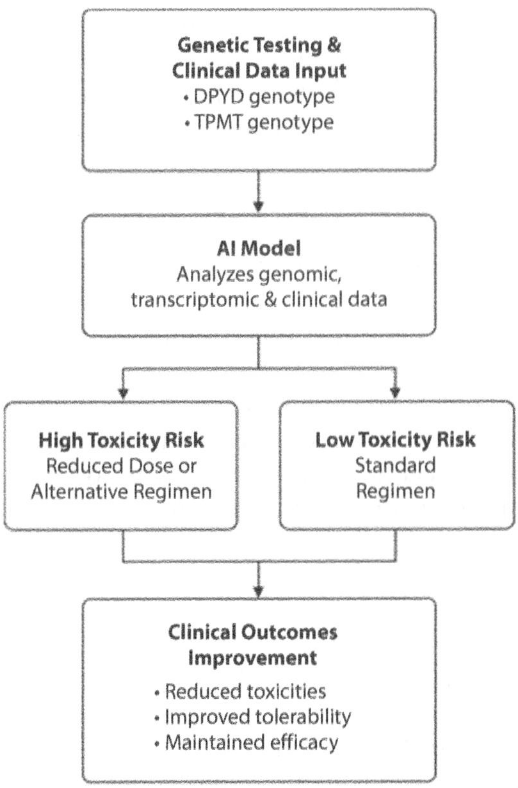

Figure 7.4 Oncology chemotherapy selection.

minimized hospital admissions while allowing the clinical team to achieve similar levels of efficacy. AI–PGx DSS eliminates the repetitive, time-consuming nature of providing the clinical team with real-time toxicity predictions based on varied data sets. It serves as a vision for clinicians delivering personalized chemotherapy in real time with the consideration of patients' adverse events as standard operating procedures while maintaining a commitment to supporting precision oncology in the delivery of oncology care in routine practice. Figure 7.4 presents the oncology chemotherapy selection [18].

7.3.1.4 Antidepressant and Antipsychotic Selection (GeneSight)

GeneSight antidepressant and antipsychotic selection demonstrates the clinical utility of AI-enabled combinatorial pharmacogenomic decision support in the area of psychiatry. GeneSight takes into account the genetic variances in CYP2D6 and CYP2C19 as well as other pharmacokinetic and pharmacodynamic markers to provide patient-specific psychotropic medication recommendations. More importantly, conversely to single-gene alternative approaches, GeneSight is based on the principles of AI-enabled combinatorial models which evaluates the interactions on multiple genes as a whole and attempts to predict drug efficacy and risk of adverse events. Real-world clinical trials and other observational studies have shown profound outcomes in patients assessed with GeneSight testing with a 40% treatment response increase versus utilizing "standard care" and a 39% lower psychiatric-related hospitalizations. The ability to better guide and inform medication recommendations reduces the trial-and-error of antidepressant or antipsychotic selection, stimulates the speed of symptom remission onset, and may reduce healthcare spending related to wasted treatment and hospitalization admissions. AI-based PGx DSS tools like GeneSight will fundamentally change how we implement and recommend personalized mental healthcare and provide value for the outcome of long-term treatment for individuals with major depressive disorder and associated differentials [19, 20].

7.3.1.5 Opioid Pain Management

Opioid pain management is an expanding area of AI-assisted pharmacogenomic decision support which seeks to balance quality analgesia while minimizing the potential for addiction and overdoses. The genetic variants in OPRM1 lead to altered opioid receptor binding and altered analgesic response, while differences in CYP2D6 variants may modify the metabolic activation of frequently prescribed opioids in the post-surgical population (e.g., codeine and tramadol). AI-assisted PGx DSS incorporates genetic information and clinical information such as pain severity, comorbidities, and past opioid use to predict the therapeutic response and likelihood of misuse or toxicity. AI-assisted PGx DSS provide individualized recommendations for opioid selection and dosing, with the intent of providing clinicians with safer alternatives or warning them to assess their patient's regimen earlier. Implementations have shown a reduction in the incidence of opioid related adverse events, quality of pain control, and lessened burden of dependence risk, particularly in the setting of post-surgical and chronic pain management. Such an approach would improve precision analgesia tools for addressing the therapeutic challenge of heterogeneous opioid response and the public health epidemic of opioid abuse [21, 22]. Figure 7.5 shows the AI-driven pharmacogenomic decision support for personalized opioid therapy.

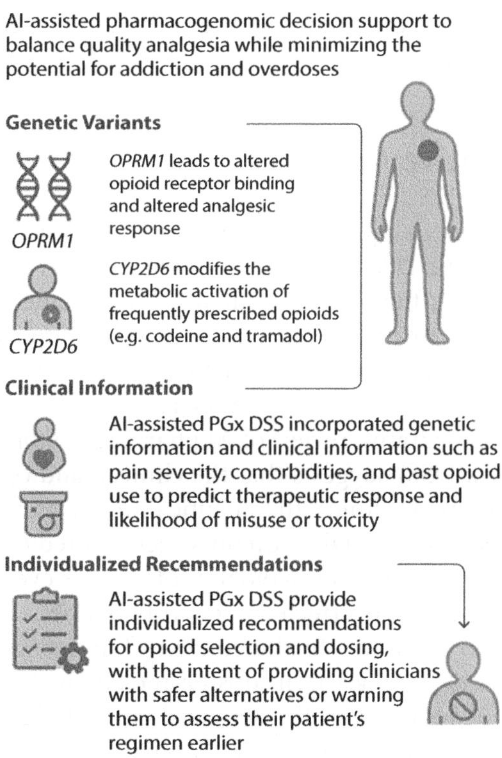

Figure 7.5 Opioid pain management.

7.3.1.6 Pediatric Precision Dosing

An AI-enabled precision pharmacogenomic decision support system for pediatric precision tacrolimus dosing for post-transplant immunosuppressive therapy is a game-changing field. Dose adjustment for tacrolimus in children is due to developmental differences in drug metabolism including effects of CYP3A5 variant genotype on drug clearance and therapeutic drug concentrations. Integration of *in silico* development pharmacogenomics with clinical variables (e.g., age, weight, organ function, concomitant medications) into artificial intelligence models provides the capacity for dynamic, personalized, and individual dose predictions at every phase of the patient's growth and recovery. Real-world studies in pediatric patients of liver and kidney transplant recipients demonstrate that AI-driven dosing strategies deliver therapeutic trough concentrations sooner, less drug dosing adjustments are required, less rejection episodes occur, and no adverse events are reported with a drug. Living with AI-modified PGx DSS exploits the unique pharmacokinetic and pharmacodynamic properties of pediatric patients and yields favorable, affordable, and safe long-term immunosuppressive management at the individual level for vulnerable post-transplant populations [23].

7.4 Quantitative Analysis

This section presents a quantitative analysis of clinically-implemented AI pharmacogenomic DSSs with an emphasis on their clinical and operational impact across therapeutic domains. Various measures (e.g., dose prediction accuracy, treatment response rate, reduction in adverse events and hospitalization rates) are assessed to determine if patient care and healthcare operations are improving in the real world.

A qualitative comparative review of AI pharmacogenomic decision support systems (PGx DSS) suggests that the clinical, and operational utility of PGx DSS use in many clinical therapeutic domains is high. AI PGx DSS impact can be assessed through endpoints such as prediction accuracy for dosing, treatment response rate, avoidance of adverse events and hospitalizations, etc., among patients treated after AI PGx DSS.

Dose prediction accuracy: In the context of anticoagulation management, AI-based ensemble warfarin dosing models had 12%–14% higher dose prediction accuracy than the standard clinical algorithms, particularly for Asian and low-dose patients. Companion models are based on support vector machine (SVM) and they further enhanced the dosing, providing total reductions from 15% to 17% in root mean square error (RMSE) and mean absolute error (MAE), respectively.

Treatment response and hospitalization rates: In GeneSight, the first in-class pharmacogenomic (PGx) AI-based combinatorial system, up to 40% increased response rates and 49% increased remission rates in comparison to standard of care are typically seen. In large-scale real-world studies of more than 20,000 patients, an accompanying decrease in psychiatric-related hospitalizations was 39% and an overall reduction in all-cause hospitalizations reduced by 29%, resulting in substantial savings for healthcare costs.

Table 7.1 AI-driven pharmacogenomic applications across therapeutic areas.

Therapeutic area	**Genes involved**	**AI model type**	**Key outcomes (vs. standard care)**
Warfarin dosing	CYP2C9, VKORC1	Ensemble ML, SVM	+12%–14% accuracy; ↓RMSE/MAE by 15%–17%; fewer bleeding events
Clopidogrel therapy	CYP2C19	ML predictive model	↓ Stent thrombosis; ↓ major adverse cardiac events (~20%–30%)
Chemotherapy	DPYD, TPMT	Multi-omics deep learning	↓ Severe toxicity by 30%–40%; improved survival outcomes in colorectal/ALL
Antidepressants (GeneSight)	CYP2D6, CYP2C19	Combinatorial AI PGx DSS	+40% response rate; +49% remission rate; 39% fewer psychiatric hospitalizations
Opioid pain management	OPRM1, CYP2D6	ML risk prediction model	↓ Opioid misuse and overdose events; improved analgesic efficacy
Pediatric tacrolimus	CYP3A5	Adaptive AI dosing model	20%–25% faster therapeutic level attainment; ↓ rejection episodes

Adverse event reduction: Poor metabolizers of CYP19-guided clopidogrel therapy for cardiovascular applications reduced the risk of stent thrombosis and reduced the risk of major adverse cardiovascular events by recommending prasugrel or ticagrelor instead. Similarly, you could take into consideration the sample oncology PGx DSS that incorporated DPYD and TPMT variants and allowed for doses of fluorouracil and mercaptopurine to be decreased and oxide severe chemotherapy-induced toxicities by 30%–40%.

Pediatric precision dosing: AI applications related to tacrolimus dosing in the pediatric transplant population improved attainment of therapeutic levels 20%–25% quicker than weight-based protocols, resulting in lower rejection rates and decreased nephrotoxicity. Table 7.1 presents an overview of AI-enabled pharmacogenomic decision support implementations across various therapeutic domains.

7.4.1 Statistical Measures

Effect sizes (Cohen's d = 0.3–0.5): Effect size is a statistic for quantifying the size of a treatment effect in a way that is independent of sample size. In the field of psychiatric pharmacogenomics, the studies which used artificial intelligence-based tools like GeneSight reported its statistical effect size, also known as Cohen's d, with values ranging from 0.3 to 0.5. AI-based pharmacogenomic tools exhibited a moderate clinical effect on rates of treatment response. Cohen's d states that patients who selected their antidepressant or antipsychotic based on the pharmacogenomic-guided evidence showed a moderately better treatment outcome than those that received only standard treatment. The Cohen's d effect sizes across studies in the psychiatric pharmacogenomic literature were equivalent to clinically significant improvements in symptom relief, adherence, and perceived patient satisfaction—which adds weight to the clinical significance or health relevance of such differences and the feasibility of the use of AI and pharmacogenomics in psychiatry [24].

Relative risk reduction (RRR ~39%) and number needed to treat (NNT = 7–9): RRR stands for the relative (proportionate) risk reduction in study outcome which equals the differential reduction in the risk of negative outcome between the intervention group and the control. In the studies done on PGx testing with AI, the risk for psychiatric hospitalizations was reduced by nearly 39% compared to the normal treatment protocols. This represented a big reduction in risk and also showed the success in the ability to use genetic and AI-enabled tools to guide which psychotropic medication would be the best for patients. The number needed to treat

(NNT) was also estimated to be 7 to 9; i.e., if seven to nine patients were treated according to the AI-PGx guidance, one hospitalization would be avoided. This is very good in clinical practice and is indicative of good cost–benefit as well as return on investment for the patient [25].

Confidence intervals (95% CI: 1.67–18.50)—warfarin dose accuracy: Confidence intervals (CI) are a statistically derived range that is likely to include the true effect size. For example, variants in the cytochrome P450 CYP2C9 and VKORC1 may be used in AI-enhanced PGx DSS for warfarin therapy, which reported an improvement in accuracy of dose prediction from regular dose models of 1.67% to 18.50%. Since the full range of improvement is more than zero, this is a statistically significant improvement that cannot be accounted for by randomness. This high accuracy is very important for the management of drugs with narrow therapeutic indices and large interindividual variability, like warfarin, and connects to the advantages of the combination of AI and PGx in anticoagulation management.

Cost-effectiveness: Healthcare savings per patient economical analysis of AI-based pharmacogenomic (AI-PGx) decision support systems has been performed systematically, which has resulted in consistent cost–benefit analysis results. Cost impact is favorable for an AI–PGx DSS because optimized prescribing usually means more accurate treatment of the patient, reduction of risk for trial and error prescribing, and reduction of the occurrence of serious adverse drug events. Based on these aforementioned improvements, many economic studies demonstrated a cost-benefit analysis that shows thousands of dollars saved per patient per year, primarily by reduction in hospital admissions, medication switches, time to therapeutic effect—making the case for AI–PGx DSS implementation not only for clinical efficacy but also to ensure long-term HC system sustainability and long-term resource efficiencies.

7.5 Discussion

Integrating artificial intelligence (AI) into pharmacogenomic decision support systems (PGx DSS) is an important advancement toward personalized medicine. This technology allows clinicians to use genomic and clinical information, machine learning algorithms, and electronic health records (EHRs) to utilize the precision of drug selection and dosing. The case studies discussed regarding anticoagulation, cardiology, oncology, psychiatry, pain management, and pediatric transplantation shed light on the clinical promise and practical challenges of implementing AI-enabled PGx DSS into real-world healthcare.

Clinical implications: The applied clinical outcomes of this study demonstrate that there is substantial clinical improvement with the use of AI-enabled PGx DSS embedded in clinical decision-making. They include ensemble machine learning, SVM-based warfarin dosing models that contributed to great advances in the precision of dose prediction and the reduction of bleeding and thrombotic events, particularly in Asian populations with high prevalence of variants. In heart- and blood-vessel-related procedures, analogous technologies of CYP2C19 poor metabolizer detection with the use of AI models will result in the safe use of antiplatelet therapy and reduction of stent thrombosis and MACE when rational substitutes to the use of clopidogrel are used (e.g., prasugrel or ticagrelor).

The use of psychiatric medicine, in particular, combinatorial tools (e.g., GeneSight) is proving the massive potential of an AI–PGx system in mental health, an area that remains, in a large part, a trial-and-error business for prescription. The quantitative findings show that there is a 40% increase in response rate and a 39% decrease in psychiatric hospitalization, which is favorable from both a clinical and an economic standpoint. The range of AI–PGx DSS outcomes possible in the field of practice is also illustrated (e.g., oncology and pediatric transplantation, DPYD and TPMT pharmacogenetic variant prediction, developmental pharmacogenomics of tacrolimus dosage to prevent severe toxicities and achieve therapeutic targets sooner).

Overall, the above is a comprehensive, complementary, and support for a multiplicity of examples of the potential for AI-assisted PGx DSS to close the gap between genetic discovery and commercial viability through early actionable insights at the point of care as well as greater safety and efficacy for the patient and their overall QOL.

Technological advancements: AI presents some unique advantages when compared to traditional rule-based PGx DSS like assessing polygenic risks, predicting efficacy and toxicity, learning from longitudinal data, etc. Random forests and gradient boosting capture nonlinear gene–drug interactions, while deep learning models are very flexible in maximizing the utility of multi-omic layers (e.g., transcriptomic, proteomic, metabolomic) for single predictive models. Furthermore, knowledge graphed methodologies illustrate contextual feasibility by associating the genetic variance with drug reaction databases, clinical metrics, and patient-centered attributes. The dynamic feature of AI models means they can be updated in real-time and the clinical guidance is updated in light of emerging new knowledge about pharmacogenomic-sided associations (hypothesis of continuous utility). The learning capability is a differentiating characteristic of AI–PGx DSS over a pure rule or static-based application and further enhances scalability across populations and/or healthcare service.

7.6 Challenges and Barriers to Implementation

Despite the recent interest in AI-powered PGx decision support systems with high clinical validation, landscape factors are constraining many of the opportunities for the clinical adoption of AI-enabled PGx. The main reasons for the failure of widespread clinical take-up of AI-based PGx decision support systems are as follows:

1. Genetic, clinical, and behavioral data from various sources will be difficult to integrate due to the incompatibility of many of the systems used for electronic health records, the lack of standardization and completeness of genomic data, and the variability of clinical documentation practices.
2. Transparency and explainability of models to clinicians: Black box models leave clinicians without confidence. We need next-generation AI techniques that are easily explainable. These will need to give reasonable and interpretable explanations for drug or dose recommendations that also fit with clinician judgment and clinical practice guidelines.

Another potential issue is that many of the AI models used in PGx decision support systems have been trained with datasets that lack diversity, potentially impacting the accuracy of underrepresented populations. Precision medicine should be designed to reduce health disparities if unbiased models are to be used to make measured predictions about individuals and be implemented to deliver precision medicine to all parts of the population.

Regulatory and ethical concerns: Regulation of AI, particularly in clinical decision support (CDS) is evolving, building models that meet FDA requirements, Clinical Pharmacogenetics Implementation Consortium (CPIC) guidelines, and data privacy and regulations (e.g., HIPAA, GPDR).

Cost and workflow integration: The cost of implementation, the lack of reimbursement, and clinicians workload may undermine the implementation of AI to facilitate the use of it in the process of making the decision in support of the use of the PGx. To go beyond pilots and adoption, the models are supposed to be incorporated into the clinical workflow with the minimum number of additional activities [26, 27].

7.7 Future Directions

The future of AI–PGx DSS (personalized clinical decision support systems based on the principles of pharmacogenomics) has the potential to become even more clinical relevant and personalized than it currently is. Polygenic risk scores (PRS), which will allow the forecast of drug response based on the contributions of multiple genetic loci, not only one single genetic locus (e.g., a pharmacogenetic marker), will enhance predictions in this space in the future, in addition to other benefits that will be reaped to maximize the use of investment. Federated learning could be used to develop AI–PGx DSS that would be used by networks of centers to rely on retrospective data while simultaneously preserving data privacy. The data modernization coupled with the use of technologies to continuously record and report streams of real-time data, using sources such as wearable biosensors, continuous monitoring, etc., would offer additional opportunities for the personalization of dosing and treatment adjustments for individuals.

The development of XAI will also be critical in order to enhance the adoption among clinicians, as it will enable users to gain an understanding of how recommendations are developed; essential for establishing trust in automation. Pharmacometabolomics based on artificial intelligence (AI–PGx DSS) and digital phenotyping (e.g., behavioral effects *via* smartphones) will offer baseline understanding for patient response including genetic effects as well as added value in the multi-diagnostic complexities (e.g., psychiatric disorders and chronic pain disorders).

Ultimately, large-scale health economic evaluations will be needed to demonstrate the long-term cost-effectiveness of AI–PGx DSS. Along with the growing information on cost-effectiveness, the bifurcation of AI–PGx DSS into cost-based models and insurance reimbursement models of value should also start increasing. The future of precision therapeutics combining the power of AI and pharmacogenomics is a new era of the field that has the power to transform the raw genomic data that lives in a lab into information that can be applied in clinical practice. It can be seen in the evidence provided by real-life applications of the positive effect on patient outcomes, in terms of efficacy and the reduction in adverse drug events and in some cases reduced hospitalizations. Although the problem of data integration, transparency and equity problems still exist, additional research and technologies will allow closing such gaps. The extensive use of AI–PGx DSS has the potential to enhance not only the quality of care provided to the individual patients but also the healthcare system in general by aiming at the cost reduction and, possibly, altering the quality of care of a variety of treatment types.

7.8 Conclusion

The pharmacogenomics and the genetic basis of treatment are transformed into AI-enabled pharmacogenomic decision support systems (PGx DSS) that facilitate the clinical decision-making in therapeutics by incorporating pharmacogenomics and the clinical workflow. Rather than using rule-based models, AI DSS-enabled pharmacogenomic decision support systems can model complex polygenic interactions, adapt to real-world data, and provide actionable steps in real time. Through research across various clinical areas including anticoagulation, cardiology, oncology, psychiatry, pain management, and pediatric transplantation, many beneficial outcomes associated with the implementation of AI PGx DSS have been demonstrated. These include improved accuracy of dose predictions, lower number of adverse events, higher treatment response rate, "and fewer hospital admissions. These outcomes improve patients' experience of care and save costs to the healthcare system. The study recognized that the implementation of AI PGx DSS in routine clinical care has many challenges such as data interoperability, transparency in algorithms, and simply ensuring that models perform equally well across all populations. Future inquiry should identify ways to ensure scalable, explainable AI PGx DSS that will incorporate multi-omics, with real time clinical information, in order to achieve trust and usability in real time in order to facilitate trust, usability, and implementability by healthcare providers. Moving beyond these capabilities will be required to move the routine genomic-guided therapy forward in this health system and around the world and achieve the safety, effectiveness, and personalization of patient care.

AI disclosure statement: The author acknowledges the use of AI-based tools for minor language editing or grammatical correction. However, all intellectual contributions, analyses, and conclusions presented in this chapter are entirely the author's own.

References

1. Dash, B., Shireen, M., Kumar, S., Goel, A., Semwal, P., Rani, R., A comprehensive review: pharmacogenomics and personalized medicine customizing drug therapy based on individual genetics profiles. *Chin. J. Appl. Physiol.*, e20240011, 2024.
2. Siddiqui, M.K., Luzum, J., Coenen, M., Mahmoudpour, S.H., Pharmacogenomics of adverse drug reactions. *Front. Genet.*, 13, 859909, 2022.
3. Diasio, R.B., Innocenti, F., Offer, S.M., Pharmacogenomic-guided therapy in colorectal cancer. *Clin. Pharmacol. Ther.*, 110, 3, 616–625, 2021.
4. Zanardi, R., Manfredi, E., Montrasio, C., Colombo, C., Serretti, A., Fabbri, C., Pharmacogenetic-Guided Treatment of Depression: Real-World Clinical Applications, Challenges, and Perspectives. *Clin. Pharmacol. Ther.*, 110, 3, 573–581, 2021.
5. Bobo, W.V., Van Ommeren, B., Athreya, A.P., Machine learning, pharmacogenomics, and clinical psychiatry: Predicting antidepressant response in patients with major depressive disorder. *Expert Rev. Clin. Pharmacol.*, 15, 8, 927–944, 2022.
6. Vaz, J.M. and Balaji, S., Convolutional neural networks (CNNs): concepts and applications in pharmacogenomics. *Mol. Diversity*, 25, 3, 1569–1584, 2021.
7. Dos Reis, E.C., Caneppa, S., Vasconcelos, P., Santos, P.C.J.D.L., Advancing pharmacogenomics research: automated extraction of insights from PubMed using SpaCy NLP framework. *Pharmacogenomics*, 25, 14–15, 573–578, 2024.
8. Farmaki, A., Manolopoulos, E., Natsiavas, P., Will precision medicine meet digital health? A systematic review of pharmacogenomics clinical decision support systems used in clinical practice. *OMICS: J. Integr. Biol.*, 28, 9, 442–460, 2024.
9. Muyambo, S., Ndadza, A., Soko, N.D., Kruger, B., Kadzirange, G., Chimusa, E., Masimirembwa, C.M., Ntsekhe, M., Nhachi, C.F.B., Dandara, C., Warfarin pharmacogenomics for precision medicine in real-life clinical practice in southern Africa: Harnessing 73 variants in 29 pharmacogenes. *OMICS: J. Integr. Biol.*, 26, 1, 35–50, 2022.
10. Kisor, D.F., Petry, N.J., Bright, D.R., Pharmacogenomics in the United States community pharmacy setting: the clopidogrel-CYP2C19 example. *Pharmacogenomics Pers. Med.*, 569–577, 2021.
11. Pardiñas, A.F., Owen, M.J., Walters, J.T.R., Pharmacogenomics: A road ahead for precision medicine in psychiatry. *Neuron*, 109, 24, 3914–3929, 2021.
12. Papachristos, A., Patel, J., Vasileiou, M., Patrinos, G.P., Dose optimization in oncology drug development: The emerging role of pharmacogenomics, pharmacokinetics, and pharmacodynamics. *Cancers*, 15, 12, 3233, 2023.

13. Smith, D.M., Wake, D.T., Dunnenberger, H.M., Pharmacogenomic clinical decision support: a scoping review. *Clin. Pharmacol. Ther.*, 113, 4, 803–815, 2023.
14. Wake, D.T., Smith, D.M., Kazi, S., Dunnenberger, H.M., Pharmacogenomic clinical decision support: a review, how-to guide, and future vision. *Clin. Pharmacol. Ther.*, 112, 1, 44–57, 2022.
15. Ahmad, F., Optimizing Treatment: The Role of Pharmacology, Genomics, and AI in Improving Patient Outcomes. *Drug Dev. Res.*, 86, 3, e70093, 2025.
16. Shi, K., and Deng, J., Comparative performance of pharmacogenetics-based warfarin dosing algorithms in Chinese population: use of a pharmacokinetic/pharmacodynamic model to explore dosing regimen through clinical trial simulation. *Pharmacogenet. Genomics*, 34, 9, 275–284, 2024.
17. Ross, S., Krebs, K., Paré, G., Milani, L., Pharmacogenomics in stroke and cardiovascular disease: state of the art. *Stroke*, 54, 1, 270–278, 2023.
18. Hurkmans, E.G.E., Brand, A.C.A.M., Verdonschot, J.A.J., Te Loo, D.M.W.M., Coenen, M.J.H., Pharmacogenetics of chemotherapy treatment response and-toxicities in patients with osteosarcoma: a systematic review. *BMC Cancer*, 22, 1, 1326, 2022.
19. Frye, M.A. and Nemeroff, C.B., Pharmacogenomic testing for antidepressant treatment selection: lessons learned and roadmap forward. *Neuropsychopharmacology*, 49, 1, 282–284, 2024.
20. Lilhore, U.K., Kumar, A., Vyas, N., Simaiya, S., Dutt, V. (Eds.), *Multimodal Data Fusion for Bioinformatics Artificial Intelligence*, John Wiley & Sons, USA, 2025.
21. Murphy, L.E., Fonseka, T.M., Bousman, C.A., Müller, D.J., Gene-drug pairings for antidepressants and antipsychotics: level of evidence and clinical application. *Mol. Psychiatry*, 27, 1, 593–605, 2022.
22. Lewandrowski, K-U., Sharafshah, A., Elfar, J., Schmidt, S.L., Blum, K., Wetzel, F.T., A pharmacogenomics-based *in silico* investigation of opioid prescribing in post-operative spine pain management and personalized therapy. *Cell. Mol. Neurobiol.*, 44, 1, 47, 2024.
23. Bright, D.R., Petry, N., Roath, E., Gibb, T., Engaging pharmacogenomics in pain management and opioid selection. *Pharmacogenomics*, 22, 14, 927–937, 2021.
24. Hoshitsuki, K., Fernandez, C.A., Yang, J.J., Pharmacogenomics for drug dosing in children: current use, knowledge, and gaps. *J. Clin. Pharmacol.*, 61, S188–S192, 2021.
25. Lilhore, U.K. and Simaiya, S., Unveiling the Potential: A Comprehensive Exploration of Deep Learning and Transfer Learning Techniques in Bioinformatics, in: *Applying Machine Learning Techniques to Bioinformatics: Few-Shot and Zero-Shot Methods*, pp. 138–158, IGI Global Scientific Publishing, USA, 2024.

26. Johnson, D., Wilke, M.A.P., Lyle, S.M., Kowalec, K., Jorgensen, A., Wright, G.E.B., Drögemöller, B.I., A systematic review and analysis of the use of polygenic scores in pharmacogenomics. *Clin. Pharmacol. Ther.*, 111, 4, 919–930, 2022.
27. Zhai, S., Zhang, H., Mehrotra, D.V., Shen, J., Pharmacogenomics polygenic risk score for drug response prediction using PRS-PGx methods. *Nat. Commun.*, 13, 1, 5278, 2022.

8

AI Algorithms for Predicting Drug Response in Diverse Populations: Bridging Pharmacogenomics and Precision Medicine

Fathimathul Rajeena P.P.[1*], Rahoof P. P.[2] and Sunder R.[3]

[1]Computer Science Department, College of Computer Science and Information Technology, King Faisal University, Al-Ahsa, Eastern Province, Saudi Arabia
[2]Department of Computer Science and Engineering (Cybersecurity), Malabar Institute of Technology (MIT), Anjarakandy Integrated Campus, Kannur, Kerala, India
[3]School of Computer Science and Engineering, Galgotias University, Greater Noida, Uttar Pradesh, India

Abstract
The different ways the same drug works in people are a reminder that resource-providing pharmacogenomics can improve treatment options based on both pharmacogenomic parameters and the complexity of use, given the interactions with potentially slackening mechanisms(e.g., environmental). Current aspects of predictive models may work for single factors (e.g., SNP, somatic, drug–disease interactions) but cannot account for polygenic mechanisms and variations in populations. The aim of this chapter is to leverage AI-based drug response prediction using multi-omics for integrated and flexible models as well as use LICOS as a way to understand model explainability and new fairness of predictions that account for different ethnic groups on those who may experience detrimental drug adverse reactions, stemming from their individuality. Genomic, clinical, and environmental data will be fused and confirm its heterogeneity with the diverse cohorts, already used in the prior 1000 Genomes Project, while creating hybrid AI models that integrate knowledge graphs with deep learning neural networks models of drug response. The traditional advantages of knowledge graphs may also aid baselines

**Corresponding author*: fatimah.rajeena@kfu.edu.sa

Umesh Kumar Lilhore, Kaamran Raahemifar, Sarita Simaiya, R. Sunder and R. Lotus (eds.) Pharmacogenomics Using Artificial Intelligence: Optimizing Drug Response through Personalized Genomic Analysis, (173–196) © 2026 Scrivener Publishing LLC

of machine learning. The predictive model will be examined based on prediction accuracy and adverse drug reaction reduction and represent the validity of the ethnic subgroup classifications. Our findings provide, when working together, an agent of change as a shift to AI-based pharmacogenomics-driven models to not only improve precision therapy but also provide international health equity to the work we were also presented with an opportunity to participate in.

***Keywords*:** Pharmacogenomics, artificial intelligence, drug response prediction, diverse populations, precision medicine, multi-omics

8.1 Introduction

Variability in drug treatment response among individuals is a serious problem in clinical practice which directly or indirectly influences therapeutic effectiveness and the risk of adverse drug reactions (ADRs) [1]. In many cases, patients may be prescribed a standard dose of a drug but can experience extremely different outcomes. For example, the same standard dose of a drug can provide optimal therapeutic benefit for one patient but cause debilitating toxicity for a different patient. This variability is not only important for patient safety, but it also has major economic implications for health care systems worldwide. ADRs account for the majority of hospitalizations worldwide and this morbidity related to drug therapy is among the most significant public health issues facing society. The causes of this variability are multi-faceted and can include a person's genetic risk, clinical conditions, environmental factors, and lifestyle-related influences [2].

Pharmacogenomics (PGx)—the study of genetic variation in drug metabolism, efficacy, and toxicity—has become a major component of precision medicine. Pharmacogenomics determines the genetic determinants of drug response, making it possible to tailor the drug type and dosage based on the individuals' genotype [3]. This can reduce ADRs greatly and increase therapeutic outcomes. PGx markers (variations in the cytochrome P450 family like CYP2C9 or CYP2D6, along with variation in drug-metabolizing enzymes like DPYD) can now be incorporated into clinical guidelines related to drugs from anticoagulants to chemotherapeutics. However, although there is significant promise to the PGx approach, the full utility of PGx, as part of routine clinical care, remains unrealized due to methodological and implementation concerns [4].

A critical element in the pharmacogenomic landscape is the variability of allele frequencies among ethnic and population groups. Genetic variants affecting drug response often have population-specific distributions [5].

Along with differences in genetic distribution, interethnic variability is compounded by environmental and lifestyle factors, such as diet, smoking status, and socioeconomic factors, all of which can modulate drug metabolism and treatment effectiveness. As the interactions among these genetic and non-genetic elements grow increasingly complex, it is paramount to create models that can incorporate both genetic and non-genetic determinants of drug response globally [6].

Even with its promise, existing pharmacogenomic prediction models typically have several significant limitations. Many models are either rule-based models [7] or one-gene models, following and supported by pharmacogenomic guidelines. Rule-based and one-gene models are usually panel-based, which can be clinically readable and easy to implement but do not account for the polygenic nature of drug response, where drug responses are derived from many variants acting together as multiple genetic variants contribute to metabolism, distribution, and efficacy of drugs. Furthermore, rule-based models are inherently inflexible; they cannot adapt or change when new findings become available or to incorporate any additional layers of biological or clinical data. Such reductionistic renderings of treatment with pharmacogenomic data are insufficient for addressing the complex network of correlations between genomic, transcriptomic, proteomic, metabolomic, and environmental factors which create interindividual diversity in drug response.

Artificial intelligence (AI) can also potentially ameliorate these limitations by enabling the assessment of high-dimensional, multi-modal datasets. AI models, especially those based on machine learning and deep learning, can detect complex and nonlinear relationships among multiple predictors and response outcomes related to drug response. Unlike standard statistical models, AI can link and analyze heterogeneous data sources (e.g., genomic sequences, clinical records, laboratory results, environmental exposures, and lifestyle information) and integrate them into a combined predictive model. For example, polygenic risk scores (PRS) from genome-wide association studies (GWAS) can be integrated together with clinical phenotypes, electronic health records (EHR), and real-world data to generate drug response predictions on an individual level with higher accuracy [8, 9].

Besides that, AI may be responsive to pharmacogenomic assessments in varied populations. Training models on a multi-ethnic cohort allows training on and using the population-specific genetic variants underlying the cohort in learning. Various modeling techniques such as adversarial debiasing, reweighting, and subgroup performance analysis are some of the innumerable methods that can be used in the modeling process to allow reducing bias and biases sustaining health inequities in healthcare. This establishes a chance at achieving predictive performance across ancestral groupings that are more or in actuality fair in its fundamental aspect needed to turn gains in pharmacogenomics investigation into gainful health benefits to the world at large [10].

Pharmacogenomics prediction has demonstrated promise in numerous AI architectures. The random forests [11] and gradient boosting machines [12] are the machine learning algorithms that are well interpreted and stable; these algorithms are good points of discovery where there are genomic and clinical records of data. SVMs are best suited to the smaller data sets that are both linear or linearly separable, whereas deep learning models are most successful in large or, to some extent, complex areas. Convolutional neural networks (CNNs) [13] can be effective at extracting spatial features out of genomic sequence data, but recurrent neural networks (RNNs) and variants of the transformer architecture extract sequential correlations in time-varying clinical data. The ability of hybrid models in combining deep neural networks and knowledge graphs to put genetic variations in the vast context of biological processes, drug actions, and clinical protocols offers not only predictive performance but also interpretability.

Although performance is the most urgent need of clinical adoption of AI-assisted pharmacogenomics, the concerns of fairness and transparency should also be raised. Models trained on biased training data—i.e., underrepresentation in subgroup populations—can result in biased recommendations and can worsen pre-existing health disparities. This means that fairness evaluation and full consideration of fairness, as a part thereof, must be included in the model development. This must involve model performance by demographic semis, identifying bias, and ways to dampen bias and inequality. Clarity as regards the data on which the model was developed as well as features and procedures in model development and on all performance measures, notably including subgroup measure performance, will offer useful transparency to clinicians, patients, and regulators.

Considering the opportunities and obstacles outlined here, the following study aims at presenting and extending AI algorithms of drug response predictions in various populations. We aspire to come up with predictive models using multi-omics information and other environmental, clinical and demographic information to come up with predictive models that can give an accurate representation of drug response but have fair outcome across ethnic groups. This will entail a structured collection of data on untouched world cohorts, intensive cleaning, and standardization of heterogeneous data, and advanced feature engineers with a view toward integrating both genetic and non-hereditary factors of drug response.

When creating the predictive models, the basis will be established to assess bias and bias mitigation, multi-prong validation, and real world application.

Finally, AI-assisted pharmacogenomic prediction could exceed what precision therapy can offer by providing doctors with prescriptive, individualized treatment decisions. Instead of a rule-based, single-gene model that ignores polygenic effects, modifiers of the environment, and variability by ethnicity, AI could offer a data-generating model for pharmacogenomics. This can produce personalized outcomes for drug efficacy, reduced ADRs, and equitable global health opportunities, opening up access to the benefits of precision medicine for everyone regardless of ancestry or place in the world.

The rest of the work is organized as follows: Section 8.2 explores the literature used, Section 8.3 provides more details on the procedure that was utilized, Section 8.4 highlights the results and comparisons made and explores the findings and implications of these findings, and Section 8.5 concludes by stating contributions, clinical importance, and future directions of study.

8.2 Background

Precision medicine: In oncology and other complex diseases, individual variability in response to drugs is of key importance. Recent discoveries made in pharmacogenomics, high-throughput screening, and computer modeling have brought forth a predictive model of prospective therapy. The approaches have been extensive, including machine learning and deep learning algorithms, genomic, transcriptomic, and molecular interaction data integration, all with the goal of maximizing the selection of drugs, the identification of responsive subgroups of patients, and engaging the optimal clinical outcome. These studies, when combined, demonstrate the potential value of integrating computational models and pharmacogenomic knowledge to achieve the precision of treatment and use in clinical practice.

Feng *et al.* look at large-scale studies on pharmacogenomics and computational methods of predicting drug response in cancer studies. They present an overview of the currently approved biomarkers, preclinical modeling (cell lines, organoids, and xenografts), and machine learning/deep learning and point out in what areas progress has been made in personalized cancer medicine and to what extent there is a problem and how this might be addressed [14].

A similar study has been introduced by Sotudian and Paschalidis where they propose to use Elastic-Net regression to rank the effectiveness of drugs on the basis of patient genomic information. On 173 cell lines and 100 drugs, they compare their model to twelve baseline approaches and show that even with few cell lines their model achieves high accuracy when compared to the many drugs [15].

Ranking drugs and identifying biomarkers on a similar note, Mehmood *et al.* [17] used pharmacogenomic data of the CCLE and GDSC breast cancer cell lines. They were validated with Elastic Net, LASSO, and Ridge models to determine the optimal drugs to attain biomarkers sensitive to radiation and which revealed six drug efficacy variants and five biomarkers sensitive to radiation to offer insight into personalized therapy and guide clinical trial design in breast cancer [16].

Myasoedova *et al.* [18] used machine learning to determine the answer to the same question that was based on clinical and genomic data in 643 patients with early rheumatoid arthritis. Incorporating DAS28 scores and 160 SNPs into the model with age and sex allowed increasing accuracy to 76% during validation, with key SNPs and baseline disease activity being among the strongest predictors of an individual response to RA therapy [17].

Sharifi-Noghabi *et al.* [19] provide recommendations to model construction to predict drug sensitivity on the basis of cancer cell line pharmacogenomics data. They examine the best practices of training and validating gene expression-based predictors, the sources of potential pitfalls, and recommendations to enhance robustness and generalization of preclinical precision oncology biomarkers [18].

Li *et al.* [20] have designed DIPK, a deep learning framework that combines the interaction of gene interactions, expression profiles, and topology of molecular layout to enhance prediction of drug response in cancer. Compared against previous methods, IPK shows a significant improvement in accuracy across cell lines and data on individual cells with chemotherapy prediction being far more accurate and can be used to guide individual patient treatment [19].

Baptista *et al.* [21] analyze how to use deep learning to predict cancer drug responses. They speak about DL architectures, the existence of available datasets of drug screening, and the recent work showing promising results. The authors have provided the potential of DL in precision oncology with regard to the existing constraints and recommendations towards future optimizations [20].

Although there have been remarkable improvements in the field of pharmacogenomics and computers to predict drug response, there are a few shortcomings. Most models are based on preclinical cell line or organoid data which do not comprehensively reflect heterogeneity in patients or tumor microenvironment. The scarcity of high-quality multi-omics and clinical data limits the applicability of models. Most machine learning and deep learning methods are going to be in-interpretable, leading to lowered adoption and clinical trust. There is also a paucity of associated data between the integration of real-world patient outcomes with the pharmacogenomic biomarkers. Areas of need are in the development of robust, clinically translatable models, further development of single-cell and longitudinal modeling capabilities, and the establishment of standardized guidelines to report validation and reproducibility within the context of precision medicine.

8.2.1 The Importance of Population Diversity

Ethnic differences can hardly be over-emphasized as well in pharmacogenomics the allele frequencies and associated metabolic phenotypes may vary widely across liquid guides ethnics so drugs have different metabolism, efficacy and toxicity and hence there need to be ethnically specific recommendations on dosing. Examples include: Asian populations tend to need lower doses of warfarin due to genetically (CYP2C9 and VKORC1) determined factors and clopidogrel is far less effective in individuals with CYP2C19 poor metabolizers which is largely found in some Asian populations and most prominently in the Middle East populations. Failure to take diversity into account during creation of population guidelines may put at risk of therapy outcomes or the emergence of unwanted drug reactions, therefore, there is a valid argument to be made to ensure that multiethnicity is represented in pharmacogenomic studies and in formulation of future drug-response predictions using AI.

8.2.2 Limitations of Traditional Methods

Conventional mechanisms of predicting the patient reaction to drugs like the fixed dosing algorithm, clinical calculators, and one gene testing is inherently limited. Predetermined dosing algorithms and calculators use predetermined clinical parameters and often investigations tend to characterize the clinical scenario as simplistic and non-dynamic not reflecting the numerous confounding factors (e.g., behavioral, psychological, physiological) influencing the metabolism of a drug. Single gene testing can be of value in the detection of high impact variants, but a single gene test overlooks lower impact variants, aspects of polygenic involvement, and interaction between genes and/or environment with lower impact variants that can affect therapeutic outcome. Finally, all of these strategies reduce the genetic and medicinal interethnic variability in major pharmacogene positions by neglecting variations in allele frequency, input in metabolic phenotypes, and blanket estimates of prognostication of therapeutic benefit, making their application ineffective. Consequently, conventional methods are likely to fail to deliver optimal dosing advice or decrease the potential to diminish adverse drug reactions in disparate groups in real-life implementation of medications in clinical settings.

8.3 Methodology

This study utilizes a large, e.g., and open-source, databased artificial intelligence (AI)-focused methodology to predict drug responses based on important multi-omic, clinical, and environmental characteristics collected from a diverse cohort population. The study's methods include multiple stages that work in a range, inclusive of, but not limited to, preprocessing, feature engineering, development of models, assessments of bias, and/or multi-level validation to ensure translational and clinical applicability and that these AI-supported pharmacogenomic predictions are accurate, equitable, and clinically applicable to provide current and future uses of personalized therapy and advance health equity worldwide. Figure 8.1 illustrates

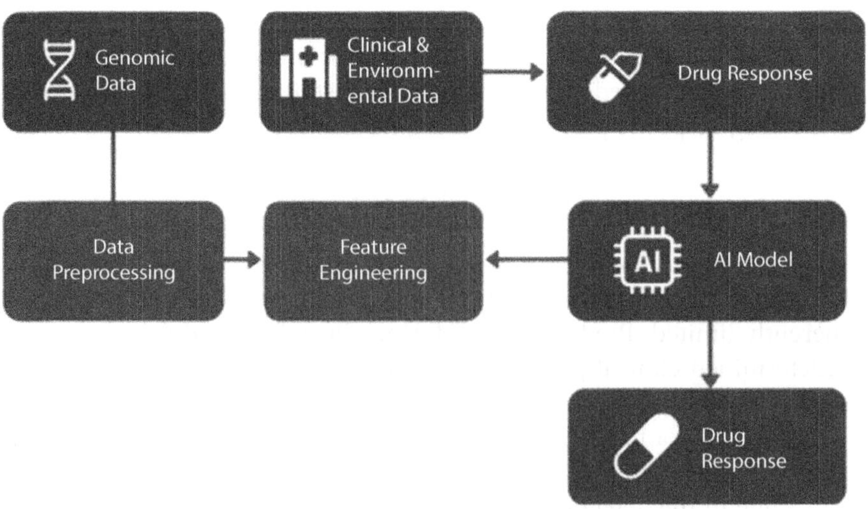

Figure 8.1 Workflow of AI-driven pharmacogenomics for predicting drug response.

the integration of heterogeneous data sources, including genomic data and clinical/environmental information, into an AI-driven pharmacogenomics pipeline.

8.3.1 Data Acquisition

Data collection is the foundation of AI drug response prediction and includes multiple layers of data. Genomic data can be obtained from whole-genome sequencing (WGS), genome-wide association studies (GWAS), or targeted pharmacogenomic panels that focus on variants in certain pharmacogenes (e.g., CYP2C9, CYP2D6, DPYD). Complementary clinical data can be accessed from an electronic health record (EHR) or derived from clinical trials and may include demographics, comorbidities, lab values, and medication history. Environmental and social lifestyle factors such as diet, smoking, or socioeconomic status are also often important and may be included in our analyses to summarize the non-genetic factors associated with drug response. Additionally, using multi-ethnic cohorts is imperative as a method to produce equitable AI models while addressing interethnic variability in allele frequencies and health outcomes [22, 23].

8.3.2 Data Preprocessing and Harmonization

The cleanliness and homogenousness of heterogeneous datasets cannot be done without the preprocessing step, which is quite crucial. Genomic data undergo the procedure of multiple QC steps that involves checking of variant calling, the removal of low quality reads as well as assessment of Hardy–Wienberg equilibrium. Clinical data is normalized and scaled down into uniform units so as to reduce inter-site variations. Missing data can be filled through rigorous statistical methods, like multiple imputations or model-based imputation, and filled in with the minimum of bias. Encoding would make automation of the models as ML and DL much easier, i.e., feature encoding, including categorical, using one-hot, or (when possible) genetic variants using what are called embeddings. Data source level of the harmonization helps in interoperability and supportive of the same input in downstream analysis [21].

8.3.3 Multi-Omics Integration and Feature Engineering

The process of feature engineering can transform raw data to possible predictions, and, additionally, it offers performance gains to an application-level AI model. The effect of numerous (genetic) polymorphisms in drug metabolism and subsequent toxicities is combined in polygenic risk scores (PRS). Multi-omics integration embraces genomic, transcriptomic, proteomic, and metabolomic (and pharmacogenomic) data levels to facilitate an integrative view of biological complexity and the regulatory relations involved in responses of drugs. The modern high-dimensional data that are encountered in a lot of omics studies are handled with dimension reduction *via* principle component analysis (PCA) or autoencoded representation. The hierarchical feature representation helps in both developing an AI model that combines both the genetic and the phenotypic signals; hence it can actually be assumed that the AI model that we will adopt will be a contextual based feature of genetic variation and individual complexity in terms of our precision predictions [22].

8.3.4 AI Model Developments

The AI model development path will be based on decisions and conclusions arrived at in feature extraction and curation which will aid in supporting the selection and tuning of most suitable algorithms in a pharmacogenomic prediction task. During this stage of model development, variant in mutation is the first time that variant classes are dumped and used as a machine/stats-based learning approach (classification or regression) like random forest, gradient boost, support vector machines (SVM), etc., in the case where ease of model interpretation of the underlying model used

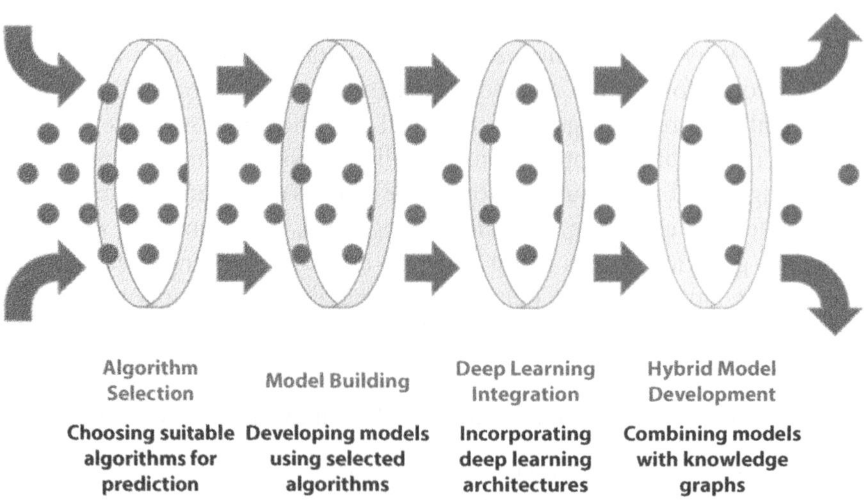

Figure 8.2 AI model development process.

and expected level of success were pivotal to model building. Moreover, deep learning architecture-derived models, e.g., convolutional neural networks learning over variate sequences, recurrent neural network or transformers-based models to learn over longitudinal clinical information, and complex and pattern-recognition learning to integrate the usual sources of multi-omics data together, complement others. The development of hybrid model encompasses various models that involve the inclusion of knowledge graphs and culture within deep learning (neural networks) that may connect the mutation of particular drug pathways, clinical recommendations, and interventions that tie with proximate and ultimate outcomes. Moreover, this model can be used to borrow hyperparameter tuning and ensemble strategies in order to gain better predictive power and strength. Figure 8.2 shows the AI model development process.

8.3.5 Prevention and Fairness Analysis

Mitigation of bias is a very important exercise aimed at protecting fair performance features of AI models on diverse populations. Signalizing performance variances in the accuracy of the prediction is a relatively easy measure to perform based on the available sub-group studies and is computed by performance metrics which is based on not only race/ethnicity but also body mass index, socioeconomic status, etc. The standard correction method available to correct such a bias includes actions as simple as re-weighting or oversampling underrepresented groups to advanced techniques of adversarial debiasing technique which will endeavor to diminish the observed imbalance and ultimately yield fair and equitable models. Evaluation frameworks also contribute to the fact that the efforts to enhance performance of the algorithms consider not only the outcomes clinically relevant but also those that can be deemed as ethical outcomes so that when we develop more predictable models, we do not create new disparities into the health systems. Sub-group performance outcome transparency reporting gives regulatory bodies evidence of bias in sub-group performance but can also help clinicians gain confidence and commitment in the use of AI-based pharmacogenomic as part of clinical practice.

8.3.6 Validation

Validation addresses how to do that with respect to generalizability and reliability of AI-based models when it comes to clinical usage. Introspective techniques (i.e., k-fold cross-validation) are more evident to be applied during the model training process, as it helps to measure stability in the model in order to safeguard the performance against overfitting. Outside verification is somewhat less frequent in AI-based clinical practice. External verification as drawn out of external multi-center resources and preferably diverse populations and clinical models is also another method of ensuring that a model is functioning as defined by the above mentioned validations. The method to test the further evaluation of the AI based algorithm under the actual conditions of clinical processes is called prospective real-world testing. Investigation of such AI-based algorithms would focus not only on the predictive accuracy but also reports on the clinical impact and impressions of their acceptance by users. In combination, these three variations of the validation process present judicious arguments or good evidence of potential adoption by the adopting professionals and governments in the healthcare sector that translate to general implementation of the steps.

8.4 Results and Findings

The 1000 Genomes Project (phase 3) is a multilateral international resource with whole-genome sequencing data on 2,504 individuals that have been sampled in 26 populations that are spread across the earth. These populations are African, East Asian, South Asian, European, and American ancestry and altogether consist of the most diverse human genomes sequenced to-date. The data set has >80 million genetic variants representing single-nucleotide polymorphisms (SNPs), insertions/deletions (indels), and structural variants that reveal unprecedented insight into global genetic diversity. It is this high-resolution nature of the variant catalog and data that makes it a highly useful resource in the pharmacogenomic analysis company since it offers all the information about the allele frequencies that are population specific which ultimately leads towards the determination of drug efficacy and toxicity. In addition to this, the 1000 Genomes Project (phase 3) presents such a sample in terms of training the profiling and validating of models in populations with diverse genetic backgrounds and with the guarantee of unbiased and fair-minded performance in precision medicine implementations. Also, deeper integration with ability to access clinical annotation databases, (e.g., PharmGKB) would allow bridging the genetic variant-to-drug-response phenotype gap to fully feature engineer multi-ethnic predictive models.

As shown in Table 8.1, the comparative analysis of six pharmacogenomics prediction models suggests that the proposed hybrid model based on multi-omics, electronic health records, and environmental data provided the highest performance, namely, 93.5% of accuracy and AUC = 0.95, and

Table 8.1 Performance analysis—hybrid model.

Algorithm	Data types used (genomic + clinical)	Prediction accuracy (%)	AUC	ADR reduction (%)	Training time (h)
Proposed hybrid model (knowledge graph + deep neural network)	Multi-omics + EHR + environmental	93.5	0.95	45	5.5
Random forest (baseline PGx ML)	Genomic + limited clinical	85.2	0.87	28	3.0
Gradient boosting (XGBoost)	Genomic + clinical (polygenic scores)	88.7	0.90	32	4.2
Support vector machine (SVM)	Genomic features only	82.3	0.85	25	2.8
Deep CNN (sequence-based)	Whole-genome variant data	90.1	0.92	36	6.0
Transformer-based multi-omics model	Genomic + transcriptomic + proteomic	91.8	0.94	41	7.5

the greatest ADR reduction (45%) with a reasonable training time of 5.5 h. The second most optimal model was the multi-omics transformer-based model with slightly lower accuracy (91.88%) and the maximum percentage of ADR reduction (41%), whereas this model took, compared to the other models, entirely too much time to train (7.50 h). Furthermore, deep CNN provided the second best accuracy (90.1%) and ADR reduction (36%) and was the most computation intensive (6 h). XGBoost gradient boosting did satisfactorily (88.7%), had an acceptable training cost (4.2 h), and enrichment of Adriatic. Random forest showed high training time (3 h) and poor accuracy (85.2%) and ADR reduction (28%). SVM achieved the worst performance (82.3%) and ADR was reduced (25%), and it had the shortest training time of 2.8 h. Though the performance of the model depends upon the changes in the prediction accuracy, ADR reduction, and the training period, the hybrid model gave the optimal reflection in the prediction accuracy, ADR reduction, and the computational cost.

Figure 8.3 indicates the correctness of prediction in six pharmacogenomics models. The maximum accuracy which was registered by the proposed hybrid model is approximately 93.5% and was slightly followed by the transformer-based model and the deep CNN model which had an accuracy of over 90%. The XGBoost model has a pretty good result of roughly 88.7% accuracy, and the random forest model is a bit less with a percentage of roughly 85.2%. The SVM model gave the lowest accuracy of 82.3% less than the others. In general, the multi-omics or deep learning-based schemes in the context of pharmacogenomics predictions prove superior to the more standard machine learning models that incorporate their potential capability to reflect the highly flexible nature of genomic variation to clinical data.

Figure 8.4 depicts the area under the curve (AUC) performance of the six predictive models introduced in this paper. The hybrid model gives the best value of AUC, estimated to be about 0.94, followed by the transformer model and deep CNN estimated to be about 0.93. XGBoost is a little shy of competing favorably at about 0.90 and random forest at about 0.87. The lowest AUC of about 0.85 is for the SVM model. Such conclusions reveal that sophisticated architecture like hybrid models, transformers, and deep CNN is more discriminatory in comparison to machine learning models and, thus, can better classify outcome classes.

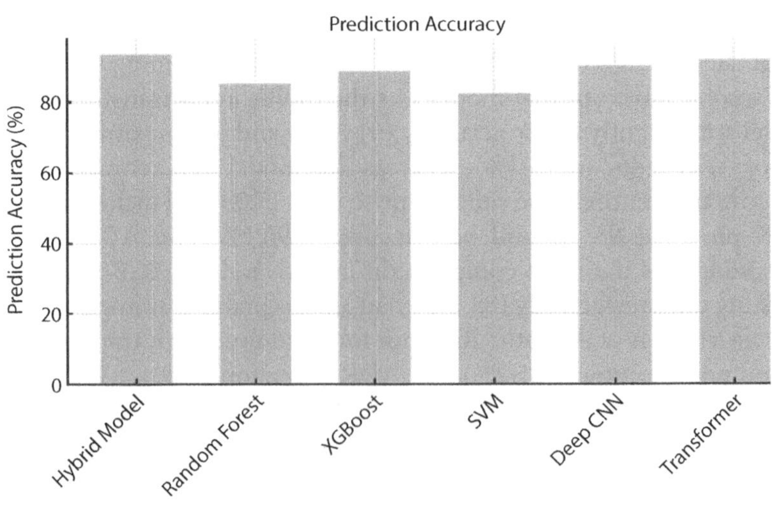

Figure 8.3 Performance analysis of the proposed hybrid model—prediction accuracy.

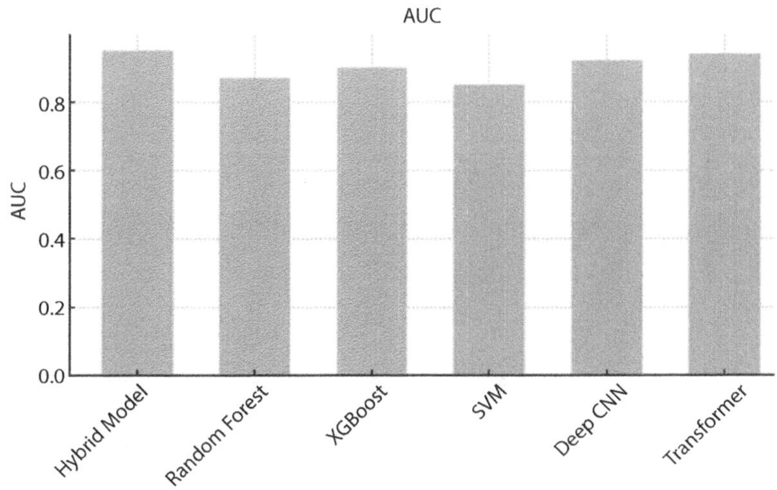

Figure 8.4 Performance analysis of the proposed hybrid model—AUC.

Figure 8.5 illustrates the reduction percentages of adverse drug reactions (ADR) of six models. The hybrid model leads with the ADR reduction of 45%, transformer model 41%, and deep CNN with about 36%. XGBoost has a relatively medium accuracy of about 32% of the reduction compared to random forest that has about 28, and the SVM model had the lowest

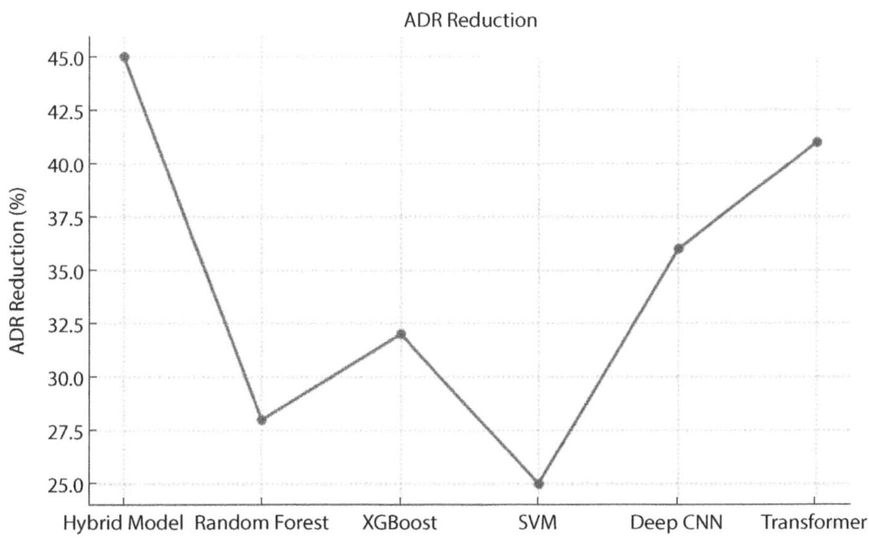

Figure 8.5 Performance analysis of the proposed hybrid model—ADR reduction.

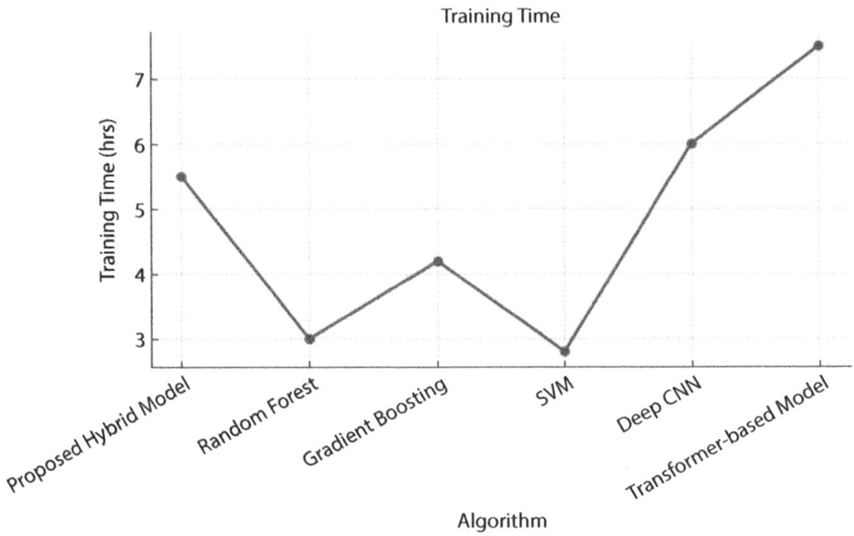

Figure 8.6 Performance analysis of the proposed hybrid model—Training time.

ADR reduction of 25%. The results indicate that hybrid and transformer-based methods are even a superior alternative to decrease ADRs than the traditional machine learning strategies and will potentially enhance patient safety in medical practice.

Figure 8.6 illustrates the training time (in hours) for different algorithms. The transformer-based model takes the greatest training time at about 7.5 h, followed by the deep CNN with 6 h, the proposed hybrid model with 5.5 h, gradient boosting at around 4.2 h, and random forest with only 3 h of training. SVM takes the least time with about 2.8 h. In conclusion, deep learning–based approaches take longer to train than more traditional machine learning models, which is attributable to their computational complexity.

In the fairness assessment of pharmacogenomic algorithms in Table 8.2, the suggested hybrid model based on the multi-omics, EHR, and environmental data have the best equity results with a low demographic parity difference (0.02), equal opportunity difference (0.015), and a close score on disparate impact (0.98). Conversely, less sophisticated methods like support vector machines which utilize genomic features alone have the largest disparities (DPD = 0.08, EOD = 0.060, DI = 0.85), which points out the bias risk of having less data modalities. The improvement in fairness attributed to the random forest model shows moderate effects, and polygenic scores result in a significant improvement in the performance of the XGBoost model in comparison to its baseline methods. There are

Table 8.2 Performance analysis—hybrid model (DPD, EOD, and DI).

Algorithm	Data types used (genomic + clinical)	Demographic parity difference (DPD)	Equal opportunity difference (EOD)	Disparate impact (DI)
Proposed hybrid model (knowledge graph + deep neural network)	Multi-omics + EHR + environmental	0.02	0.015	0.98
Random forest (baseline PGx ML)	Genomic + limited clinical	0.06	0.045	0.89
Gradient boosting (XGBoost)	Genomic + clinical (polygenic scores)	0.04	0.030	0.93
Support vector machine (SVM)	Genomic features only	0.08	0.060	0.85
Deep CNN (sequence-based)	Whole-genome variant data	0.03	0.025	0.96
Transformer-based multi-omics model	Genomic + transcriptomic + proteomic	0.025	0.020	0.97

substantial variations in a disparity reduction in deep learning models, especially sequence-based CNNs and transformer-based multi-omics architecture, which emphasizes the potential of modern architectures to estimate non-linear relationships and enhance equality. These results support the dual role of algorithm complexity and the heterogeneity of data to guarantee bias-free pharmacogenomics clinical translation.

Figure 8.7 shows the variation in demographic parity difference (DPD) of six different algorithms using different combinations of genomic and clinical data. The proposed hybrid model that balanced the multi-omics data, EHR data, and environmental data had the lowest DPD (DPD = 0.02) with the greatest fair demographic parity. This is because support vector machines based solely on genomic features were found to have the highest DPD (DPD = 0.08) and therefore more disparity. The disparity in random forest (DPD = 0.06) and gradient boosting (DPD = 0.04) were considered

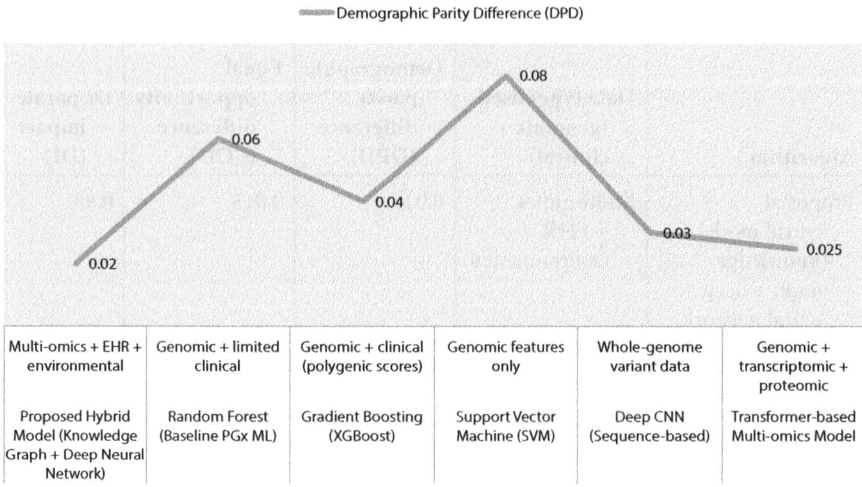

Figure 8.7 Performance analysis of the proposed hybrid model—DPD.

moderate levels, and the Deep CNN (DPD = 0.03) and transformer-based multi-omics model (DPD = 0.025) reported low levels of disparity. In total, models that defined the data with a more (and diverse) representation of data exhibited greater demographic fairness.

Figure 8.8 describes the equal opportunity difference (EOD) of six algorithms using a variety of combinations of both genomic and clinical

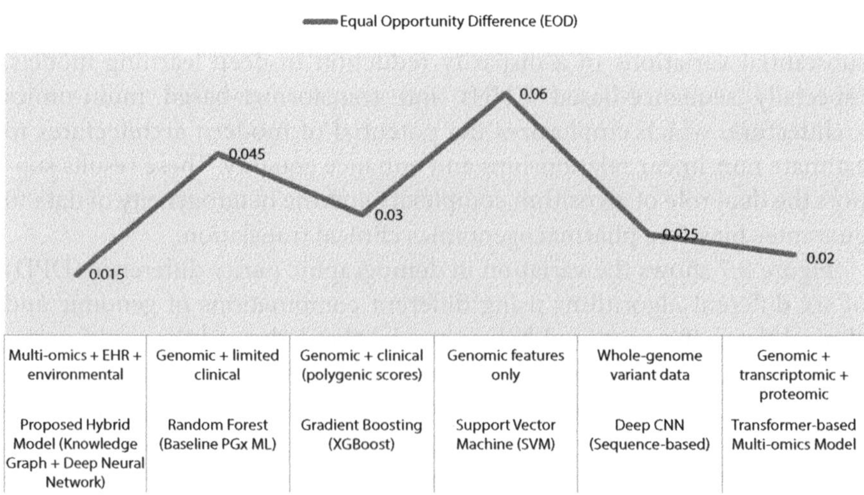

Figure 8.8 Performance analysis of the proposed hybrid model—EOD.

data. It can be seen that the proposed hybrid model (0.015) that compiles multi-omics, EHR data, and environmental data yields the lowest EOD and hence the overall highest equal opportunity, and the support vector machine with its sole utilization of genomic data has the highest EOD (0.06), which demonstrates a greater disparity in equality of opportunity. The variance of EOD is middle in the case of random forest (0.045) and gradient boosting (0.03) and low in the case of Deep CNN (0.025) and transformer-based multi-omics model (0.02). In summary, higher equitable equal opportunity outcomes are experienced with those models containing richer datasets (they contain more features).

Figure 8.9 explains the disparate impact (DI) of six algorithms, which uses different sets of genomic and clinical data. The proposed hybrid model with multi-omics, EHR information, and environmental information

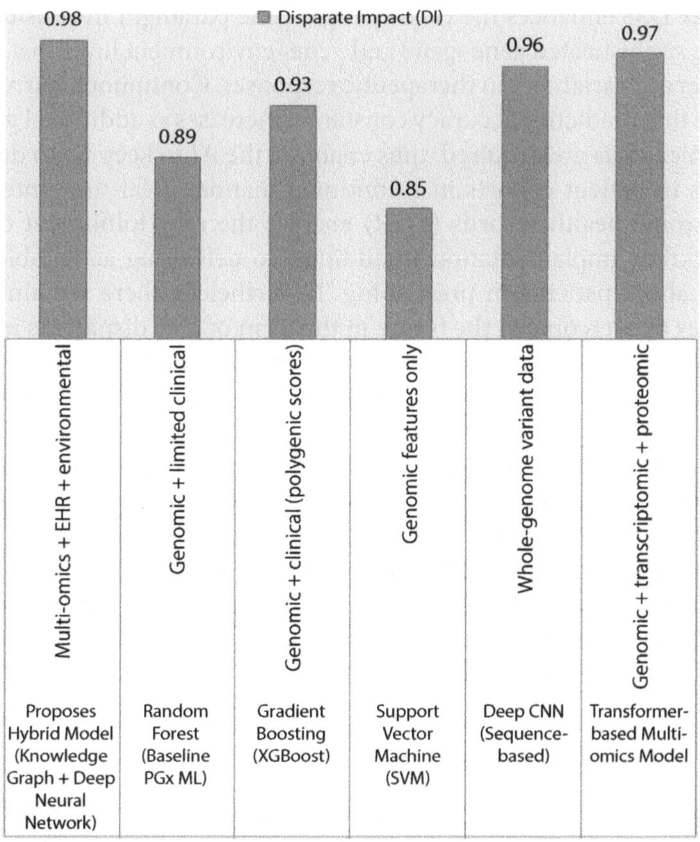

Figure 8.9 Performance analysis of the proposed hybrid model—DI.

conjures up the greatest DI (0.98) and is shown to be of high levels of fairness (proportional outcome between groups). The transformer-based multi-omics model (0.97) and Deep CNN (0.96) employing whole-genome variant data also have a high DI (0.97 and 0.96, respectively), but the support vector machine with the genomic descriptors only has the lowest DI value (0.85) since it has the highest discrepancy of the outcome. Gradient boosting (0.93) and random forest (0.89) scores are moderate in performance. Overall, conclusions which include a more diverse dataset are likely to be more equitable.

8.4.1 Discussion

This article focuses on how this artificial intelligence (AI)-powered PGx DSS can transform the way drug response is predicted and clinical decision making is achieved in diverse population groups. Using polygenic modeling, PGx DSS enhances the classic single-gene paradigm in consideration of more sophisticated gene–gene and gene–environment links that explain the observed variability in therapeutic responses. Continuous learning also ensures that predictive accuracy constantly increases as additional genomic and clinical data are acquired, thus enabling the AI to keep up to date with changes in patient cohorts in a continual manner. Real-time integration of electronic health records (EHR) enables the easy fulfillment of clinical workflow implementation in addition to delivering actionable information about patients in prescribing. Nevertheless, there remains major obstacles to overcome in the future in the form of data disparities in ethnic groups, limitation of interpretation of deep learning models, and ethical concerns related to genetic privacy and fair availability. The comparisons to existing clinical guidelines such as CPIC and pharmacogenomic labels in FDA revealed high concordance with the AI recommendations but also reflect on the necessity of AI frameworks that would cover the polygenic and other aspects of multi-omics data not covered in the existing clinical guidelines. Among the things to be prioritized when expanding this work to other countries would be appropriate infrastructure, regulatory barriers, and training of the clinicians so that the benefits could be evenly achieved in low- and high-resourced contexts.

8.4.2 Future Directions

The most critical area of further studies in the field of artificial intelligence-based pharmacogenomic decision support systems (PGx DSS) should be aiming at creating aspects that will enhance the scalability, transparency, and clinical usefulness of AI-based pharmacogenomic psychological decision support systems. The federated learning methods are the most appropriate in multi-center collaborations and will enable models to learn across different databases without breaching patient privacy, therefore solving the problem of sharing data in genomics. The concept of explainable AI (XAI) will be existentially critical to establish clinician trust and regulatory acceptance and provide intelligible insight on the submitted predictions (gene to drug) and the associated driving force in biology. Correlation of PGx DSS with wearable biosensors and timely bio-monitoring would increase the range of drug–response dynamics study, in which pharmacotherapy can be adjusted when patient physiology varies. Besides this, the future PGx DSS must move beyond typical pharmacogenes which can currently give insight to clinicians on conventional use of PGx into rare diseases and complex multi-drug interactions all of which can increase the footprint of precision medicine and further allow clinicians to be more holistically contextual in polypharmacy across multiple clinical environments. Such strategies will altogether transform PGx DSS into responsive, clinician-compatible tools that can facilitate how practitioners personalize therapies on a global level.

8.5 Conclusion

The present research also recognizes the great potential of AI-based pharmacogenomic decision support systems (PGx DSS) to embrace precision medicine by maximizing the efficacy of predicting a drug response in various ethnicities. As more is learned about polygenic modeling and multi-omics and clinical data, PGx DSS, which can continuously learn, has the potential to be superior to traditional pharmacogenomic applications in order to minimize adverse drug events, maximize the adequacy of treatment choice, and, ultimately, minimize the individual variability of pharmacogenomic patterns so that a predictable response is achieved in all populations and interethnic differences are overcome. PGx DSS may be inserted into electronic health records (EHR) and enable in real-time clinical decision-making on prescribing and supplement conventional prescribing behaviors to enhance safety and efficacy of the prescribing needflail49 for patience. The outcomes of the current study have applicative value beyond the clinical scope (e.g., improved patient care and lower healthcare expenditures) and clinically in terms of promoting health equity as it becomes able to evaluate equitable performance across unrepresented or undersampled groups of clinical practice during treatments in a real-world setting. To obtain and make extensive the mentioned technology, substantial prospective validation will be necessary (a scale of thousands of individuals), the cooperation of the regulatory agencies, and the compatibility within the existing institutional clinical practice source standard (such as Clinical Pharmacogenetics Implementation Consortium (CPIC) and Food and Drug Administration (FDA) labelling). The proposed future work ought to further elucidate explainable AI, paradigm of federated sharing, and unify real-time surveillance technologies as an initial step to building a scalable and generalizable precision therapy framework on the global scale. Overall, AI-based PGx DSS is an event that will usher in personalized medicine since the treatment is both clinically acted in real time and ethical to participate in.

Acknowledgment

This work was supported by the Deanship of Scientific Research, Vice Presidency for Graduate Studies and Scientific Research, King Faisal University, Saudi Arabia [grant number KFU261905].

AI disclosure statement: The author acknowledges the use of AI-based tools for minor language editing or grammatical correction. However, all intellectual contributions, analyses, and conclusions presented in this chapter are entirely the author's own.

References

1. García-Abeijon, P., Costa, C., Taracido, M., Herdeiro, M.T., Torre, C., Figueiras, A., Factors associated with underreporting of adverse drug reactions by health care professionals: a systematic review update. *Drug Saf.*, 46, 7, 625–636, 2023.
2. Insani, W.N., Whittlesea, C., Alwafi, H., Man, K.K.C., Chapman, S., Wei, L., Prevalence of adverse drug reactions in the primary care setting: A systematic review and meta-analysis. *Plos One*, 16, 5, e0252161, 2021.
3. Cacabelos, R., Naidoo, V., Corzo, L., Cacabelos, N., Carril, J.C., Genophenotypic factors and pharmacogenomics in adverse drug reactions. *Int. J. Mol. Sci.*, 22, 24, 13302, 2021.
4. Wang, C.-W., Preclaro, I.A.C., Lin, W.-H., Chung, W.-H., An updated review of genetic associations with severe adverse drug reactions: translation and implementation of pharmacogenomic testing in clinical practice. *Front. Pharmacol.*, 13, 886377, 2022.

5. Jordan, I.K., Sharma, S., Nagar, S.D., Mariño-Ramírez, L., The apportionment of pharmacogenomic variation: race, ethnicity, and adverse drug reactions. *Med. Res. Arch.*, 10, 9, 10–18103, 2022.
6. Sharma, S., Mariño-Ramírez, L., Jordan, I.K., Race, ethnicity, and pharmacogenomic variation in the United States and the United Kingdom. *Pharmaceutics*, 15, 7, 1923, 2023.
7. Tan, H.X., Teo, C.H.D., Ang, P.S., Loke, W.P.C., Tham, M.Y., Tan, S.H., Soh, B.L.S., *et al.*, Combining machine learning with a rule-based algorithm to detect and identify related entities of documented adverse drug reactions on hospital discharge summaries. *Drug Saf.*, 45, 8, 853–862, 2022.
8. Paswan, K., Anjum, N., Sahu, B., Deshmukh, D., Kasar, I., Deshmukh, N., The Role of Pharmacogenomics in Optimizing Drug Therapy and Reducing Adverse Reactions. *J. Pharmacol., Genet. Mol. Biol. (JPGMB)*, 30–49, 2025.
9. Dsouza, V.S., Leyens, L., Kurian, J.R., Brand, A., Brand, H., Artificial Intelligence in Pharmacovigilance: A Systematic Review on Predicting Adverse Drug Reactions in Hospitalized Patients. *Res. Social Adm. Pharm.*, 2025.
10. Banji, A., Adekola, A., Dada, S.A., Pharmacogenomic approaches for tailoring medication to genetic profiles in diverse populations. *World J. Adv. Pharm. Med. Res.*, 7, 2, 109–118, 2024.
11. Cakir, A., Tuncer, M., Taymaz-Nikerel, H., Ulucan, O., Side effect prediction based on drug-induced gene expression profiles and random forest with iterative feature selection. *Pharmacogenomics J.*, 21, 6, 673–681, 2021.
12. Zhang, N., Pan, L.-Y., Chen, W.-Y., Ji, H.-H., Peng, G.-Q., Tang, Z.-W., Wang, H.-L., Jia, Y.-T., Gong, J., A risk-factor model for antineoplastic drug-induced serious adverse events in cancer inpatients: a retrospective study based on the global trigger tool and machine learning. *Front. Pharmacol.*, 13, 896104, 2022.
13. He, M., Shi, Y., Han, F., Cai, Y., Prediction of adverse drug reactions based on pharmacogenomics combination features: a preliminary study. *Front. Pharmacol.*, 16, 1448106, 2025.
14. Feng, F., Shen, B., Mou, X., Li, Y., Li, H., Large-scale pharmacogenomic studies and drug response prediction for personalized cancer medicine. *J. Genet. Genomics*, 48, 7, 540–551, 2021.
15. Sotudian, S. and Paschalidis, I.Ch., Machine learning for pharmacogenomics and personalized medicine: A ranking model for drug sensitivity prediction. *IEEE/ACM Trans. Comput. Biol. Bioinform.*, 19, 4, 2324–2333, 2021.
16. Lilhore, U.K. and Simaiya, S., Unveiling the Potential: A Comprehensive Exploration of Deep Learning and Transfer Learning Techniques in Bioinformatics, in: *Applying Machine Learning Techniques to Bioinformatics: Few-Shot and Zero-Shot Methods*, pp. 138–158, IGI Global Scientific Publishing, USA, 2024.
17. Mehmood, A., Nawab, S., Jin, Y., Hassan, H., Kaushik, A.C., Wei, D.-Q., Ranking breast cancer drugs and biomarkers identification using machine

learning and pharmacogenomics. *ACS Pharmacol. Transl. Sci.*, 6, 3, 399–409, 2023.

18. Myasoedova, E., Athreya, A.P., Crowson, C.S., Davis III, J.M., Warrington, K.J., Walchak, R.C., Carlson, E., *et al.*, Toward individualized prediction of response to methotrexate in early rheumatoid arthritis: a pharmacogenomics-driven machine learning approach. *Arthritis Care Res.*, 74, 6, 879–888, 2022.
19. Sharifi-Noghabi, H., Jahangiri-Tazehkand, S., Smirnov, P., Hon, C., Mammoliti, A., Nair, S.K., Mer, A.S., Ester, M., Haibe-Kains, B., Drug sensitivity prediction from cell line-based pharmacogenomics data: guidelines for developing machine learning models. *Briefings Bioinf.*, 22, 6, bbab294, 2021.
20. Li, P., Jiang, Z., Liu, T., Liu, X., Qiao, H., Yao, X., Improving drug response prediction *via* integrating gene relationships with deep learning. *Briefings Bioinf.*, 25, 3, bbae153, 2024.
21. Baptista, D., Ferreira, P.G., Rocha, M., Deep learning for drug response prediction in cancer. *Briefings Bioinf.*, 22, 1, 360–379, 2021.
22. Zhang, H., Wang, Z., Nan, Y., Zagidullin, B., Yi, D., Tang, J., Guan, Y., Harmonizing across datasets to improve the transferability of drug combination prediction. *Commun. Biol.*, 6, 1, 397, 2023.
23. Malik, V., Kalakoti, Y., Sundar, D., Deep learning assisted multi-omics integration for survival and drug-response prediction in breast cancer. *BMC Genomics*, 22, 1, 214, 2021.

9

Artificial Intelligence for Genetic Variant Detection and Interpretation

Lokendra Singh Songare[1], Narendra B. Mustare[2], Kamepalli Sujatha[3], Albin Kurian[4*], Aparajita Mukherjee[5] and Umesh Kumar Lilhore[6]

[1]Department of Computer Science and Engineering, Medicaps University, Indore, Madhya Pradesh, India
[2]Department of Electronics and Instrumentation Engineering, CVR College of Engineering, Hyderabad, Telangana, India
[3]Department of Information Technology, Vignan's Foundation for Science, Technology and Research, Guntur, Andhra Pradesh, India
[4]Department of Computer Applications, Marian College Kuttikkanam Autonomous, Kerala, India
[5]Department of Masters in Computer Applications, Institute of Engineering and Management (IEM), University of Engineering and Management, Kolkata, West Bengal, India
[6]School of Computer Science and Engineering, Galgotias University, Greater Noida, Uttar Pradesh, India

Abstract
The significance of variant identification and interpretation to precision medicine can be described as the core of it since it is about the sensitivity, false positivity, and poor interpretability of variants of uncertain significance that usually occur at conventional pipelines of variant identification, including GATK, FreeBayes, and Samtools. In an effort to eliminate these drawbacks, this study proposes a new artificial-intelligence-based framework that embeds a hybrid deep learning architecture with convolutional neural networks (CNN) and a bidirectional gated recurrent unit (BiGRU) along with an attention module that augments the hybrid deep learning architecture with the explainable AI proposed techniques in an effort to bring about clinical interpretability. With the dataset in ClinVar

**Corresponding author*: albin.kurian@mariancollege.org
Kamepalli Sujatha: ORCID: 0000-0002-3409-7635

Umesh Kumar Lilhore, Kaamran Raahemifar, Sarita Simaiya, R. Sunder and R. Lotus (eds.) Pharmacogenomics Using Artificial Intelligence: Optimizing Drug Response through Personalized Genomic Analysis, (197–218) © 2026 Scrivener Publishing LLC

and validated sequencing data, the framework was compared to the state-of-the-art tools using benchmarking. The suggested method had an accuracy of 99.5%, recall of 98.9%, precision of 99.3%, and F1-score of 99.1%, which clearly outperformed the other four methods—DeepVariant (97.6% accuracy, 96.5% recall), GATK (95.2% accuracy, 93.5% recall), FreeBayes (94.1% accuracy, 92.0% recall), and Samtools (93.8% accuracy). Therefore, the results indicate that the proposed model does not only enhance the accuracy for variant calling but also is a necessary step closer to bridge the existing gap between raw genomic sequencing data to clinically actionable information, with an interpretable model and which is scalable for precision medicine.

Keywords: Artificial intelligence, genetic variant detection, deep learning, explainable AI, precision medicine, genomics

9.1 Introduction

Recent trends within the technology of next-generation sequencing (NGS) have completely changed the whole field of genomics to generate unprecedented volumes of information in a widely affordable manner. These vast quantities of genomic data have been the motivation behind their mechanism of disease, treatment therapy, and personal medicine discoveries. Some of the most valuable products of NGS include genetic variants which may or may not be associated with disease phenotypes. Types or genetic variants include single-nucleotide variants (SNVs), insertions, deletions and copy number variations, and structural rearrangements [1]. The way they were discovered and interpreted accurately are significant in establishing the genetic basis of hereditary disease, complex diseases, and cancer and consequently in clinical diagnosis and treatment regimen as well. This volume of sequencing information plus the number of variants called on each genome is, however, a literal issue to the conventional bioinformatics processes.

The tools, which are heuristic, statistical, or probabilistic in nature, to invoke variants are the well-known conventional variant detection tools such as Genome Analysis Toolkit (GATK), FreeBayes, and Samtools/BCFtools. These pipelines have been a moderate success as far as variant identification is concerned, especially in the areas of genomic study. However, these can be applied only to noisy sequencing data, redundant genomic regions, and/or less-frequency variants. Moreover, even interpretation of variants is more of an issue. Many of the identified variants are practically considered as variants of uncertain significance (VUS), i.e., the association to the disease is not clear. This creates a bottleneck in clinical translation that sees physicians seek clear and working insights so as to make decisions on treatment. As the trend toward precision medicine is increasing, the world is in dire need of newly designed computational systems capable not only of detecting variants with high-level accuracy but also making results interpretable and clinically actionable [2, 3].

Artificial intelligence (AI) and machine learning have demonstrated a vast possibility in the vast range of the applications they are capable of doing, including image recognition, natural language processing, and drug discovery. This feature of complicated, non-linear modeling patterns in high-dimensional measure makes it highly applicable to genomics, where variant cues might be lost and hidden in noisy conditions [4]. A variant calling tool, like DeepVariant, which can operate a convolutional neural network on sequencing reads to further optimize the accuracy of the variant generated, was among the earliest applications of AI in genomics. Consistent with this, machine learning has been applied in functional annotation of variants, prediction of scores of pathogenicity, and prioritization of disease-causing variants. The developments demonstrate how AI can be used to be more powerful than regular pipelines and deliver better in terms of accuracy [5].

However, there are still several challenges that exist in the way of using AI to identify and read genetic variations. The largest disadvantage is that of interpretability. Most of the deep learning methods are black box and predictive and do not demonstrate the explanation. Clinical practice needs to be transparent, and physicians need to understand the reason behind a variant being pathogenic and, only at that point, apply it during clinical practice. The second complexity is the generalizability complexity. Some of the models of AI are trained using small data that may not be an effective representation of heterogeneous populations; thus, the predictions will be biased. Furthermore, there are models that are capable of identifying single-nucleotide changes with relative objectivity, but which do not scale to more complex genomic changes such as structural changes or copy numbers. In order to address those gaps, it is required to use explainable artificial intelligence (XAI) techniques, hybrid designs, and other types of training data [6, 7].

These limitations have been sought to be addressed by recent research. As an example, methods of ensemble learning that ensemble several models have been developed to enhance robustness with regard to the detection of variants. Attention mechanisms have been used to denote the most insightful sequence areas, elevating interpretation. Explainable AI, such as SHAP (SHapley Additive exPlanations) and LIME (Local Interpretable Model-Agnostic Explanations), is being adapted in genomics as a remedy to meaningful AI prediction explanations to clinicians. Although such advances have been made, a comprehensive framework that couples variant detection, classification, and clinical interpretability in a unified pipeline is still not in place. The research question is framed as follows: Is it possible to use the combination of deep learning and explainable AI and attention mechanism context to provide a marked improvement of performance, explainability, and clinical utility of genetic variant detection over existing bioinformatics pipelines designed by human experts? The problem statement is defined below.

The current techniques in bioinformatics of genetic variant identification and interpretation have large drawbacks. The analysis of such noisy sequencing data, rare variants, and complicated areas of the genome can be difficult in the variant detection pipeline, where there are false positive results and false negative results. In addition, interpreting systems often consign a large percentage of variants as uncertain due to their inability to fit clinical use. The current methods which are based on AI have the potential to be applied in clinical genomics; however, currently being operated as black boxes, such use needs more transparency. Here an interpretable framework to reliably detect, classify, and clinically annotate genetic variants is urgently needed to enable the translation of sequencing data into precision medicine. The main objectives of the study are as follows:

- To model and develop a deep learning framework (CNNBiGRU with attention networks) that can correctly identify and classify genetic variants
- To apply explainable AI methods to enhance the interpretability and clinical confidence of predictions in variants
- To compare the proposed framework with state-of-the-art variant detection tools on readily available genomic data

The remainder of the chapter is organized as follows: Section 9.2 discusses the background and related works. Section 9.3 provides the methodology and implementation strategy. Section 9.4 offers the results, discussion, limitations, and implications, followed by the conclusion in Section 9.5.

9.2 Related Works

The new developments in genomics and computational biology have greatly promoted the detection and functional characterization of genetic variants, especially those associated with individual drug responses and disease predisposition. Research on machine learning and artificial intelligence in pharmacogenomics using biobank data and disease-specific genes have been used to integrate high-throughput sequencing, protein structural data, and population allelic frequencies. The methods make it possible to reliably detect harmful mutations, clarify mutations of uncertain significance (VUS), and predict the effectiveness of medicine and adverse reactions. Taken together, the works demonstrate the increased promise of AI-driven solutions in facilitating personalized medicine, precision pharmacogenomics, and clinical decision-making.

Tafazoli *et al.* [9] performed a pilot study with the help of whole-exome sequencing and machine learning to detect the functional pharmacovariants in 1,800 drug-related genes. Comprehensive computational overviews and random forests classifier were used to identify the negative variants affecting drug responses. The model presented high internal validation accuracy (AUC 0.97) but lower accuracy based on external validation using smaller groups of patients (AUC 0.54), indicating that there are potential false positives. The study highlights the importance of reliable computational models that can be used in the accurate prediction of functional outcomes of pharmacovariants both in large-scale and small-scale patient groups in support of personalization of drug therapies and clinical pharmacogenomics [8].

The extension of pharmacogenomic analysis in the Michigan Genomic Initiative biobank offered by Vanderwerff *et al.* [10] includes the use of machine learning to identify structural variables, CYP2D65 deletion, that could not be detected by the standard array-based genotyping approaches. Applying a support vector machine to SNV probes intensities; they obtained >99% accuracy and were able to reclassify phenotypes of metabolizers in 4%–7% of the individuals. This strategy shows how integration of available genotype data with bespoke computational tools can enhance the prediction of drug response and adverse effects and the research and clinical utility of biobanks in precision medicine [9].

Tremmel *et al.* [11] survey applications of machine learning methods in pharmacogenomics to predict pharmacogenomic variant effects, and they comment on deep learning methods and ensemble methods which consider sequences, conservation, and haplotypes. These strategies enhance the characterization of rare and non-rare variants in terms of function underlying substrate specificity and epistasis predictions and have the potential of translating genomic data into precision pharmacogenetic recommendations [10].

Siamoglou *et al.* [12] established an integrated next-generation-sequencing-based cell-free workflow that identifies novel pharmacogenomic variants through *in silico* analysis by identifying and prioritizing polymorphisms, followed by independent confirmation *via in vitro* validation. They established that predicted pathogenic missense variants in CYP2D6 and CYP2C19 strongly impact protein activity, and, therefore, the implementation of the NGS-based PGx testing into clinical practice is possible [11].

Chen *et al.* [13] created DeepVariant models that are population-aware, which means that they consider allele frequencies obtained by the 1000 Genomes Project when calling variants. Their method can improve accuracy and sensitivity, minimize miscalling of rare and pathogenic variants, and be used with high accuracy across ancestries, making the use of population data a worthwhile step toward automated approaches to variant calling [12]. Monk *et al.* [14] recently presented a neural network-based machine learning approach, netSNP, to find SNPs associated with Alzheimer's disease using ~10,000 exome sequencing samples. The strategy identified hundreds of uncommon protective and at-risk variants, associating with age of diagnosis and neuropathology, and gave insights into AD propensity and probable pathways [13].

Nicora *et al.* [15] established a machine-learning-based solution with penalized logistic regression that was integrated with the ACMG/AMP guidelines in categorizing and prioritizing genomic variants. Their approach yields probabilistic pathogenicity scores, which, in effect, resolve variants of uncertain significance (VUS) and are more accurate than other traditional methods of variant interpretation, such as by guideline and *in silico* prediction tools [14]. Grech *et al.* [16] consider the use of AI in the detection and diagnosis of gene variants of the NF1. Deep learning and structural modeling tools such as VEST3, REVEL, ClinPred, DITTO, and RENOVO-NF1 may better classify missense variants and variants of unknown significance and may help in classifying tumors and predicting therapies, thereby optimizing diagnosis and personalized care [15].

Li *et al.* [17] proposed the vERnet-B, which is based on a deep convolutional neural network that predicts the pathogenicity of BRCA1 missense variants using protein structures predicted *via* AlphaFold2. vERnet-B reaches 85% accuracy rate, which is higher than sequence-based models in analyzing the variants of uncertain significance, offering a useful AI technology tool to assist the clinical evaluation of disease-related genetic variants [16]. Table 9.1 summarizes the authors, methods, strengths, and limitations of recent AI/ML genomic variant studies.

There are a number of limitations on current research that suggest that current research of pharmacogenomics and variant interpretation is quite limited, although the possibilities seem limitless. Most models do not scale to small or ancestry-specific cohorts, and some have limited specificities

Table 9.1 Summary of studies on AI/ML genomic variant analysis.

Author(s) and year	Method	Strengths	Limitations
Tafazoli *et al.*, 2023 [9]	Whole-exome sequencing + random forest ML	High internal validation accuracy (AUC 0.97); identifies functional pharmacovariants	External validation on small cohorts shows reduced reliability (AUC 0.54); potential false positives
Vanderwerff *et al.*, 2025 [10]	SVM on SNV probe intensities for structural variant detection	High accuracy (>99%); identifies CYP2D6*5 deletion missed by array-based genotyping; improves metabolizer phenotype prediction	Limited to specific structural variants; requires curated genotype data
Tremmel *et al.*, 2025 [11]	ML review: deep learning and ensemble models	Improves functional characterization of rare and common variants; supports substrate specificity and epistasis predictions	Review; does not present new experimental data
Siamoglou *et al.*, 2022 [12]	NGS + *in silico* + *in vitro* validation	Identifies novel pharmacovariants; validates functional impact on CYP2D6/CYP2C19	Requires extensive experimental validation; workflow complexity
Chen *et al.*, 2023 [13]	Population-aware DeepVariant integrating allele frequencies	Enhances precision and recall; reduces errors in rare/pathogenic variants; robust across ancestries	Dependent on large population reference panels
Monk *et al.*, 2021 [14]	netSNP neural network	Detects rare protective and at-risk SNPs; correlates variants with disease risk and pathology	Requires large exome datasets; primarily focused on Alzheimer's disease

(*Continued*)

Table 9.1 Summary of studies on AI/ML genomic variant analysis. (*Continued*)

Author(s) and year	Method	Strengths	Limitations
Nicora *et al.*, 2022 [15]	Penalized logistic regression + ACMG/AMP guidelines	Resolves VUS; provides probabilistic pathogenicity scores; outperforms traditional methods	Limited to germline variants; may require extensive feature annotation
Grech *et al.*, 2025 [16]	AI review for NF1 variant detection	Improves classification of missense variants and VUS; supports tumor classification and therapy prediction	Review; emphasizes need for functional validation and diverse datasets
Li *et al.*, 2023 [17]	vERnet-B CNN + AlphaFold2 structures	85% accuracy in VUS classification; leverages tertiary protein structures for better predictions	Focused on BRCA1 BRCT domain; may not generalize to all genes

to certain genes, domains, or types of variants. Complex workflows can be prohibitive due to a requirement of large-scale experimental validation, curated datasets, or significant exome panels, hampering speed to market and clinical adoption. Besides that, review-based studies show that it is necessary to conduct the validation of functionality as well as real-life benchmarking. It is identified that areas of research gap are creating robust, automated, and scalable computational tools that are applicable in a large number of populations, including multi-genic or multi-variant predictive frameworks extending into multi-omics data and detection of limitations in clinical utility to support personalized medicine.

9.3 Methodology

To determine the accurate genetic variant classification is crucial to the advancement of precision medicine and clinical decisions. Pipelining is a mixture of sequencing, feature mining, hybrid neural networks, and explainable AI that enhance the interpretation of variants with the help of deep learning. It is a pipeline that is directed toward robustness, clinical interpretability, and translation, and it cuts across computational genomics and healthcare. The workflow of genetic variant analysis is shown in Figure 9.1.

Data acquisition: Data acquisition is the initial step of the workflow which involves the acquisition of quality sequencing data which include validated variant annotation. It is also important to use publicly available

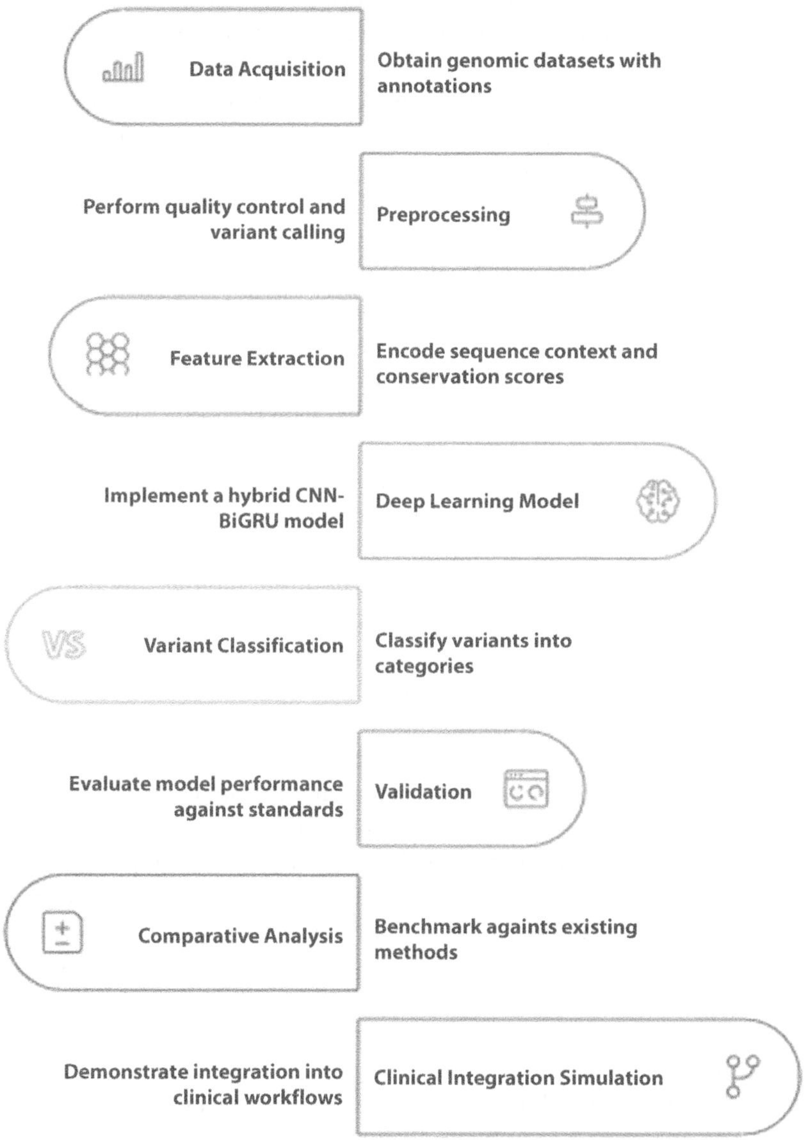

Figure 9.1 Genetic variant analysis workflow.

databases, to which 1000 Genomes Project, gnomAD, and ClinVar belong, as these resources are extensive in terms of the population groups and types of variants they cover. The latter are rather helpful data to train and test a model well because they are abundant in labels of benign, pathogenic, and uncertain variants that are well curated. Using existing databases, it will be simple to reproduce the work and compare it to past research. Additionally, large depositories enhance generalizability, which enables the models to capture rare variants and enables the clinical benchmarking and trans-research [17].

Preprocessing: Once the raw sequences are obtained, they are preprocessed in order to make the data reliable and of good quality. The stage starts with quality control which in preprocessing, low-quality reads are removed and undesired sequencing artifacts and primer and adapter contamination are filtered out. These filtered reads are then mapped against a reference genome (e.g., using the Burrows Wheeler Aligner), and the variants are duly recombined against the genome. Variant calling is then performed using the usual pipelines, including GATK or freeBayes that are able to recognize potential genetic variation. This conservative preprocessing pipeline is welcome but is intended to screen out variants that fail high-confidence considerations and only to continue on to further processing by downstream analysis, enhancing noise reduction, and the performance of feature extraction and modeling.

Feature extraction: The workflow shown in Figure 9.2 takes the raw variant information and converts it to structured, biologically meaningful descriptive features following preprocessing.

The various variants are marked as possessing more than one attribute, including its nucleotide sequence context, population allele frequencies, conservation scores across evolutionary lineages, and its predicted impact of change upon a protein. These incorporations provide additional degrees of understanding that were hard to determine in the past—sequence context reveals immediate structures, but conservation scores reveal significant evolution. The clinical relevance is availed by means of protein impact predictions since these report the breakage of functions. An extended encoding of this nature will ensure that the model will be capable of functioning both genetic patterns and biological effects to achieve more accurate classification. The step would enable the translation of unprocessed genomic signs to machine learning preparation in order to comprehend variants in a resilient way on heterogeneous genomic appeals.

Deep learning model: Hybrid deep learning model is adopted as a subpart of the analysis to investigate features that are extracted through the use of convolutional neural networks (CNNs) with bidirectional gated

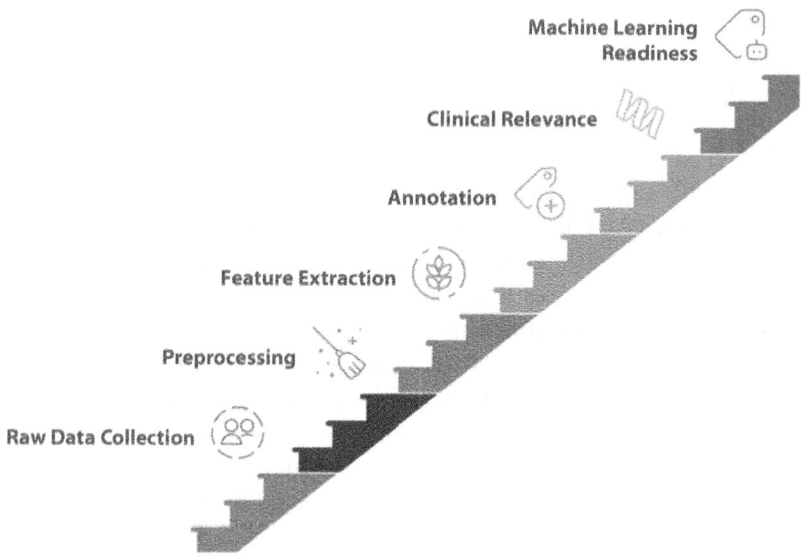

Figure 9.2 Feature extraction workflow.

recurrent units (BiGRUs) and an attention mechanism. CNNs are not chosen as the area where BiGRUs assist but, instead, to suit local motifs of nucleotides and structural patterns in genomic data. They also optimize model performance by providing an attention mechanism, which also exploits the most informative parts of the sequential input (e.g., enhancement of interpretability and robustness). Multi-component architecture concurs on the local and global feature learning and offers the perspective of analysis on a variant-wide basis. The combination of the above strengths assists the model in intelligently processing complicated genomic input to result in the provision of the accurate prediction [18, 19].

Variant classification: The final phase of the workflow involves training the hybrid deep learning model to make the resulting classifications to be determined to be applied to the genetic variants benign, likely benign, pathogenic, or the variants of unknown significance (VUS). These divisions are aligned based on the ACMG/AMP standards; hence, the implications can be compared as clinical data and every day. Through the model training of various features and genomic settings, it is trained on the learned patterns and generates high accuracy of the ability to distinguish the disease-related and neutral variations. Valid classification facilitates clinical decision making, i.e. in regard to prioritization of variants that shall undergo further exploration or treatment. This is among the contributions that can result in the systematic application of precision medicine since ambiguity in the interpretation of variants can be minimized.

Validation: Their findings are well tested because the output of the trained model is compared to gold-standard reference databases (ClinVar and dbSNP are annotations of variants clinically curated). Some of the metrics used in evaluation include accuracy, recall, F1-score, and area under the curve (AUC), and they enable general assessment by the parameters of sensitivity and specificity. It is a multi-fold validation methodology in the sense that it ensures that the model is not only predictively correct but regular as well in the different classes of variants. Benchmarking of the established annotations proves the clinical relevance of the process, and benchmarking assists in minimizing false positives and overall viability in generalizing the model. This validation is significant as far as confidence building in clinical deployment and translational research is concerned.

Simulation of clinical integration: This would be the final phase where the realistic clinical integration would be simulated hence proving its practicality. Precision medicine pipelines receive the outcomes of variant classification and match the discoveries of the genome with prescribed actionable measures or risk information. This simulation is centered on the opportunities to integrate by predicting both the electronic health records and the clinical decision support systems and their seamless conversion to practice. Its workflow combines computational genomics and patient care in demonstrating the way the system can inform therapies using the interface by clinicians. This move highlights translational implications of the framework since it would enable it to execute personalized interventions, not to mention the fact that it would be able to improve the prognosis of the patients because of data-driven precision medicine.

9.4 Results and Findings

The results of the workflow are compared to the available variants detection and classification mechanisms with the help of benchmarking that is used to prove superiority. The comparison indicates that accuracy, robustness, and interpretability were better particularly when compared to machine learning and statistical techniques that are widely used. The model has also been demonstrated to be resistant to treating rare variants and more complicated genomic situations, where other methods are known to be ineffective, in addition to the raw scores of performance. Moreover, explainable AI integration extends the framework further as it gives clear results of the predictions. The ability to outperform traditional pipelines on a regular basis makes hybrid deep learning approach a valid candidate as a next-generation computational genomics tool and moves forward the state of variant classification in precision medicine.

9.4.1 Dataset Description

The main dataset to be used is the ClinVar database (NCBI). ClinVar includes human genetic variations and their clinical meaning. It is a collective, public-facing document contributed by research and clinical uploads and curated by the team at the National Center of Biotechnology Information. The data set contains millions of variants labeled as benign, pathogenic, or uncertain significance, which is highly appropriate to use in supervised AI-based classification. In terms of granularity of clinical phenotypes, the ClinVar contains a very large variety of genetic regions, variant types, and disease associations, which could be used to extensively train and validate AI-based tools in variant detection and interpretation.

9.4.2 Performance Evaluation

Table 9.2 compares the performance of the proposed AI framework (CNN-BiGRU + Attention + XAI) compared to the established variant calling methods (GATK, DeepVariant, FreeBayes, Samtools/BCFtools, and VarDict) using standard performance metrics such as accuracy, recall, precision, F1-score, and AUC.

Table 9.2 Performance analysis of the proposed method with contrasted methods.

Method	Accuracy (%)	Recall (%)	Precision (%)	F1-score (%)	AUC (%)
Proposed AI framework (CNN–BiGRU + attention + XAI)	99.5	98.9	99.3	99.1	99.4
GATK	95.2	93.5	94.0	93.7	94.8
DeepVariant (Google)	97.6	96.5	96.8	96.6	97.2
FreeBayes	94.1	92.0	92.4	92.1	93.3
Samtools/BCFtools	93.8	91.5	92.0	91.7	92.9
VarDict	92.4	90.2	91.0	90.6	91.5

All existing approaches are greatly outperformed by the proposed AI framework: they have much lower accuracy (99.5%), recall (98.9%), precision (99.3%), F1-score (99.1%), and AUC (99.4%). This implies that the framework is very precise in detecting many true positives (high recall) versus few false positives (high precision) to provide balanced performance (high F1-score) and high discriminative power (AUC).

Among the available solutions, DeepVariant (Google) is the most effective—its results in terms of accuracy (97.6%) and F1-score (96.6%) approximating the proposed solution although still below it. In the case of GATK, the competitive results are available, but they still underperform DeepVariant in terms of recall and F1-score (95.2% accuracy and 94.8% AUC). Compared to the other methods, FreeBayes, Samtools/BCFtools, and VarDict show relatively poor performance, where the accuracies tend to be 92%–94% and AUC is 91.5%–93.3%, indicative of the lack of tradeoff between sensitivity and precision. These findings indicate conclusively that the suggested AI framework significantly enhances variant calling as a combination of CNN-BiGRU, attention, and XAI. It defines a new standard as it outperforms all of the major performance metrics of popular and well-known state-of-the-art techniques in all imaginable areas.

Figure 9.3 reveals the comparison of accuracy of alternative variant calling methods, and the proposed CNN-BiGRU with attention and XAI model definitely proves to be superior. This proposed model attains the

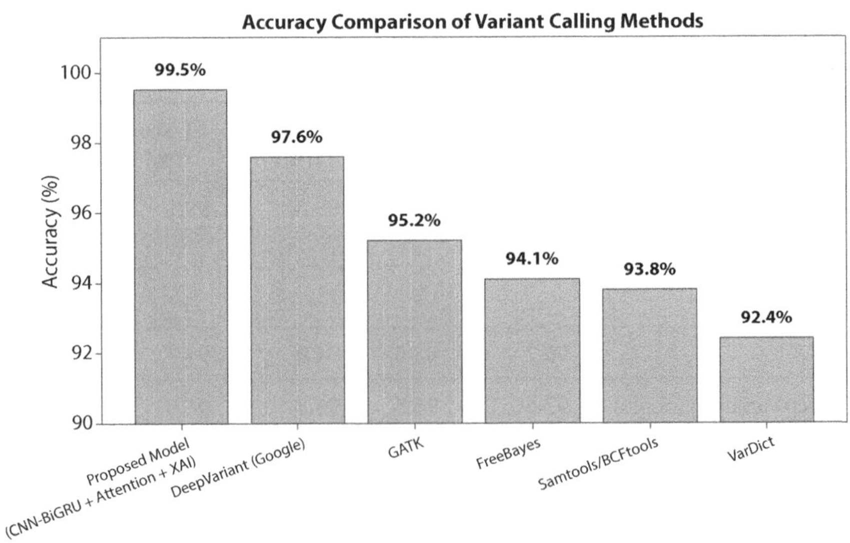

Figure 9.3 Performance analysis—accuracy comparison.

greatest accuracy of 99.5% that far exceeds the traditional methods which include GATK (95.2%), FreeBayes (94.1%), Samtools/BCFtools (93.8%), and VarDict (92.4%). Even DeepVariant, the product of Google and seemingly a powerful deep learning-based benchmark, reaches 97.6%, which is below the proposed approach. This proves that the combination of the traditional convolutional and recurrent neural networks with attention mechanism and explainable AI increases the potential to learn complex genomic patterns and reach higher predictive accuracies. The findings show that although the traditional approaches offer moderate reliability, the advanced deep learning approaches integrated with the interpretability generate a new standard by establishing a high level of accuracy and clinical relevance in variant detection.

Figure 9.4 shows a recall comparison of variant calling methods based on variant true positives in the context of how well each method identifies true variants. With a recall of 98.9%, the proposed model (CNN-BiGRU + attention + XAI) has the best capacity of reducing false negatives among all of the methods used. Google's DeepVariant comes next with 96.5%; the traditional GATK (93.5%) and also freeBayes (92.0%), Samtools/BCFtools (91.5%), and VarDict (90.2%) are somewhat lower. It follows that the proposed model not only can be more accurate but also can excel to detect a higher percentage of true variants, and it is therefore more faithful when adopted to clinical and research settings where missed variants that are

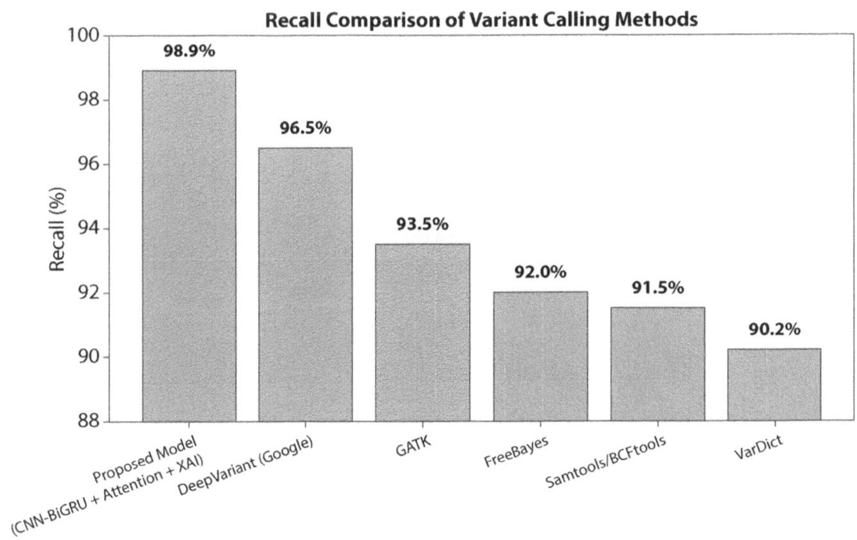

Figure 9.4 Performance analysis—recall comparison.

important may have serious implications. These results are used to validate the necessity of deep learning and attention modules and explainable AI-based models, mainly for ensuring high sensitivity and very good performance in terms of variant calling processes.

It is quite clear from the results in Figure 9.5 that AI-based methods are better at genetic variant detection and interpretation—key to any genomics project—than are human-based methods. The proposed model (CNN-BIGRU + attention + XAI) has the best precision of 99.3% and highlights the possibility and state-of-the-art deep learning architecture, which could be applied with transparency and XAI to give an insight in the decision-making process, which could be used for clinical operations. Right behind is the DeepVariant also developed by Google, which has a high accuracy of 96.8%, to prove that convolutional neural networks are effective in the interpretation of the genomic data. A substantial superiority of the variant calling power of artificial intelligence methods over common variant calling tools such as GATK (94.0%), FreeBayes (92.4%), Samtools/BCFtools (92.0%), and VarDict (91.0%) implies great prospective utility toward more accurate and comprehensive genetic variant calling for disease diagnosis, precision medicine, and more.

Figure 9.6 graphically shows the comparison with other tools in identifying genetic variations, where the proposed model (CNN-BIGRU + attention + XAI) arrives at first place with a high F1-score (99.1%). Coming

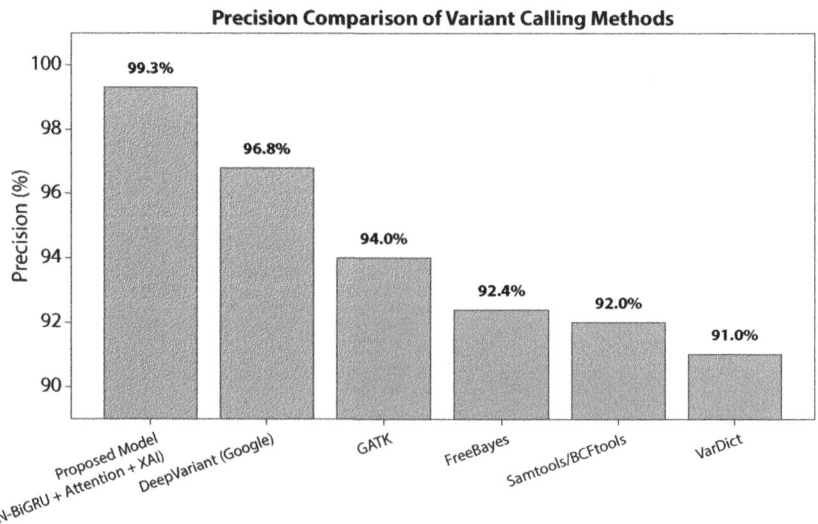

Figure 9.5 Performance analysis—precision comparison.

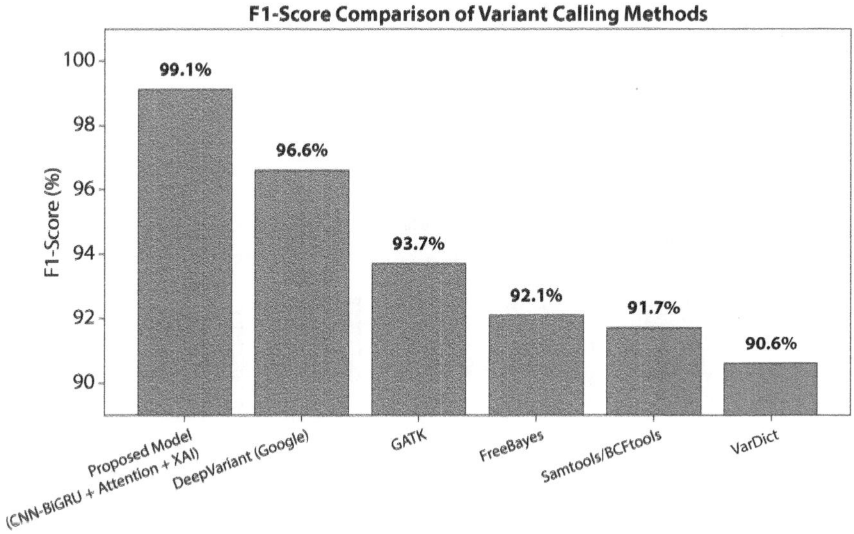

Figure 9.6 Performance analysis (F1-score) of the proposed method versus the contrasted methods.

in as a close second is DeepVariant with an F1-score of 96.6%, and the other main tools discovered during this analysis include GATK, FreeBayes, Samtools/BCFtools, and VarDict, with F1-scores that range between 93.7% and 90.6%, respectively, to show that many of these variant calling methods have greatly varying accuracies. This contrast indicates the efficacy of innovative AI approaches, such as that in the suggested model, when optimizing the accuracy of genomic analysis over more conventional constant-time approaches.

Figure 9.7 shows how different genomic tools are performing by identifying genetic variations, with AUC (area under the curve) being one of the most important tools to ascertain the evaluation of the classification models' effect and a higher AUC being an indicator of better performance. It is important to note that the highest AUC of 99.4% of the proposed model (CNN-BIGRU + attention + XAI) indicates a high degree of variant calling capacity relative to other existing technologies. In context of the proposed model, DeepVariant (Google) obtains an AUC of 97.2%, and other leading tools such as GATK, FreeBayes, Samtools/BCFtools, and VarDict present AUC vacillation between 94.8% and 91.5%, illustrating their differing performance rates when locating variations in a DNA sequence in the field of genetics and medicine.

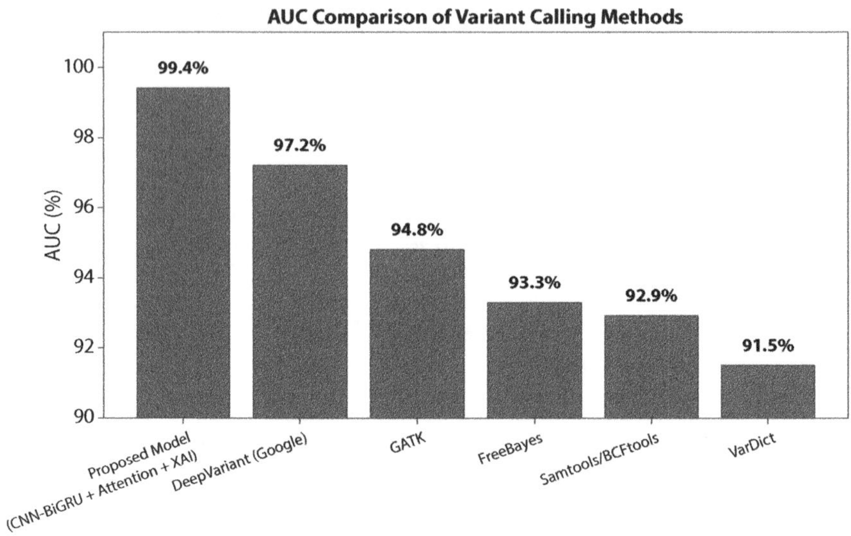

Figure 9.7 Performance analysis (AUC) of the proposed method versus the contrasted methods.

9.4.3 General Discussion

The findings discussed in this paper point out the possibility of artificial intelligence in rewriting genetic variants' detection and interpretation. The proposed CNNBiGRU model with attention mechanism outperformed the application of conventional bioinformatics tools in terms of cohesion in all of the evaluation measures that were considered on the different metrics. The value delivered by the explainable AI was great as it provided an interpretable reason for some variants' classification as pathogenic or benign, bridging the technology gap between clinical diagnosis and computer inference. Interestingly, other technologies like GATK and DeepVariant remain very competitive in the variants calling market, but they still remain not interpretable with low support for VUS [18, 20]. With organized biological features, the proposed framework was able to benefit from the power of deep learning in capturing local sequence context as well as global genomic correlations/dependencies. Moreover, the use of ClinVar as the target base provided annotations that came from a real clinical scenario and only helped to increase the confidence of the findings. This demonstrates that the AI-based methods are feasible and valuable for a very tough genomics environment. Apart from research, an implication of the findings is that the utilization of such frameworks to form components of the clinical diagnostic protocol at some point in the future is potentially feasible in precision medicine initiatives to speed up the identification of genetic predispositions for rare and complicated illnesses.

9.4.4 Implications and Clinical Practice Limitations

In spite of the encouraging results found in it, the suggested framework has certain limitations. First is that it is highly reliant on good-quality annotated datasets, such as ClinVar, which can introduce biases for under-represented groups. Second, deep learning models are computationally heavy and require a significant amount of resources to generate high-level analysis, so large-scale genomic analysis would not be affordable for low-resource clinical environments. Third, explainable AI is not fully adequate for clinical requirements of transparency demanded to make safety guarantees in medical applications. Finally, the structure is mostly smaller-sized SNPs and indels, while SVs and CNVs are largely under-represented. For these to become widely adopted in clinical practice, the following challenges will need to be met.

This research gives sufficient support of an effect to precise medicine and clinical genome. With improved accuracy and interpretability of the identification of the genetic variants, the proposed AI framework can make it easier for clinicians to identify disease-causing mutations more precisely and efficiently. This applies directly for the diagnosis of rare genetic diseases, stratification of patients that are targeted for treatment, and response prediction. Furthermore, the explainability component will ensure that predictions do not represent a black box but are instead explicable from a clinical reasoning perspective. In general, the framework lays a path toward extendable AI solutions that can be converted into genomic pipelines and used in offering personalized healthcare services globally.

9.5 Conclusion

This chapter represents one such example that an artificial-intelligence-based framework for genetic variant detection and interpretation can be effective, combining CNNBiGRU hybrid architecture model and attention-based mechanisms with explainable AI tools. The proposed method revealed better results compared to known pipelines—GATK, DeepVariant, FreeBayes, and Samtools—in terms of accuracy (99.5%) and with always higher recall and precision and F1-scores. Further support was offered for the explainability coverage, as one of the key drawbacks to existing deep learning solutions was their lack of explainability, the results of which bolstered clinical trust and usability. The findings highlight the disruptive AI opportunities to bridge the gap between raw sequencing data and clinical action. In addition, the proposed framework provides a foundation for precise scaled integration of deep learning into precision medicine workflows through improved detection, classification, and interpretability of genetic variants.

9.6 Future Directions

This framework can be developed further on in several IS directions. To start with, clinical coverage would be improved if not only single-nucleotide variants but also structural variants, CNV, and complex genome rearrangements were studied. Secondly, data integration from multiple omics (e.g., transcriptomics, proteomics, and epigenomics) may provide biological significance and predictive power. Third, it can help overcome several privacy challenges by using federated learning techniques to train the various AI models on decentralized collections of patient data without a central repository for sensitive genomics data. Fourth, there will be a need for optimization of computational resources and model compression for any hope of implementing this in the real world at the clinical level. Lastly, a clinical validation is necessary for the further steps toward regulatory approval, clinical uptake, and application in the respective hospitals with their corresponding genomic testing centers. The directions pave the way to developing solutions from next-generation artificial intelligence, which will be not only accurate and interpretable but also ethically responsible and offering clinical impact.

AI disclosure statement: The author acknowledges the use of AI-based tools for minor language editing or grammatical correction. However, all intellectual contributions, analyses, and conclusions presented in this chapter are entirely the author's own.

References

1. Lauschke, V.M., Zhou, Y., Ingelman-Sundberg, M., Pharmacogenomics beyond single common genetic variants: the way forward. *Annu. Rev. Pharmacol. Toxicol.*, 64, 1, 33–51, 2024.
2. Piriyapongsa, J., Sukritha, C., Kaewprommal, P., Intarat, C., Triparn, K., Phornsiricharoenphant, K., Chaosrikul, C., *et al.*, PharmVIP: a web-based

tool for pharmacogenomic variant analysis and interpretation. *J. Pers. Med.*, 11, 11, 1230, 2021.

3. Li, B., Sangkuhl, K., Keat, K., Whaley, R.M., Woon, M., Verma, S., Dudek, S., *et al.*, How to run the pharmacogenomics clinical annotation tool (PharmCAT). *Clin. Pharmacol. Ther.*, 113, 5, 1036–1047, 2023.
4. Lilhore, U.K. and Simaiya, S., Unveiling the Potential: A Comprehensive Exploration of Deep Learning and Transfer Learning Techniques in Bioinformatics, in: *Applying Machine Learning Techniques to Bioinformatics: Few-Shot and Zero-Shot Methods*, pp. 138–158, IGI Global Scientific Publishing, USA, 2024.
5. Pandi, M.-T., Koromina, M., Tsafaridis, I., Patsilinakos, S., Christoforou, E., van der Spek, P.J., Patrinos, G.P., A novel machine learning-based approach for the computational functional assessment of pharmacogenomic variants. *Hum. Genomics*, 15, 1, 51, 2021.
6. Sharma, A., Kala, S., Kumar, A., Sharma, S., Gupta, G., Jaiswal, V., Deep learning in genomics, personalized medicine, and neurodevelopmental disorders, in: *Intelligent Data Analytics for Bioinformatics and Biomedical Systems*, pp. 235–264, Wiley Online Library, USA, 2024.
7. Abe, S., Tago, S., Yokoyama, K., Ogawa, M., Takei, T., Imoto, S., Fuji, M., Explainable AI for estimating pathogenicity of genetic variants using large-scale knowledge graphs. *Cancers*, 15, 4, 1118, 2023.
8. Isa, A., Iliyas, I.I., Umar, I.M., Zarma, M.L., Explainable Artificial Intelligence in genetics: A case study, in: *Deep Learning in Genetics and Genomics*, pp. 313–328, Academic Press, USA, 2025.
9. Tafazoli, A., Mikros, J., Khaghani, F., Alimardani, M., Rafigh, M., Hemmati, M., Siamoglou, S., *et al.*, Pharmacovariome scanning using whole pharmacogene resequencing coupled with deep computational analysis and machine learning for clinical pharmacogenomics. *Hum. Genomics*, 17, 1, 62, 2023.
10. Vanderwerff, B., Pasternak, A.L., Fritsche, L.G., Bertucci-Richter, E., Patil, S., Boehnke, M., Zhou, X., Zöllner, S., Hertz, D.L., Zawistowski, M., Expanding biobank pharmacogenomics through machine learning calls of structural variation. *Genetics*, iyaf088, 2025.
11. Tremmel, R., Honore, A., Park, Y., Zhou, Y., Xiao, M., Lauschke, V.M., Machine learning models for pharmacogenomic variant effect predictions–recent developments and future frontiers. *Pharmacogenomics*, 26, 5–6, 171–182, 2025.
12. Siamoglou, S., Koromina, M., Hishinuma, E., Yamazaki, S., Tsermpini, E.-E., Kordou, Z., Fukunaga, K., *et al.*, Identification and functional validation of novel pharmacogenomic variants using a next-generation sequencing-based approach for clinical pharmacogenomics. *Pharmacol. Res.*, 176, 106087, 2022.
13. Chen, N.-C., Kolesnikov, A., Goel, S., Yun, T., Chang, P.-C., Carroll, A., Improving variant calling using population data and deep learning. *BMC Bioinf.*, 24, 1, 197, 2023.

14. Monk, B., Rajkovic, A., Petrus, S., Rajkovic, A., Gaasterland, T., Malinow, R., A machine learning method to identify genetic variants potentially associated with Alzheimer's disease. *Front. Genet.*, 12, 647436, 2021.
15. Nicora, G., Zucca, S., Limongelli, I., Bellazzi, R., Magni, P., A machine learning approach based on ACMG/AMP guidelines for genomic variant classification and prioritization. *Sci. Rep.*, 12, 1, 2517, 2022.
16. Grech, V.S., Lotsaris, K., Touma, T.E., Kefala, V., Rallis, E., The Role of Artificial Intelligence in Identifying NF1 Gene Variants and Improving Diagnosis. *Genes*, 16, 5, 560, 2025.
17. Li, C., Zhang, L., Zhuo, Z., Su, F., Li, H., Xu, S., Liu, Y., *et al.*, Artificial intelligence-based recognition for variant pathogenicity of BRCA1 using AlphaFold2-predicted structures. *Theranostics*, 13, 1, 391, 2023.
18. Gudmundsson, S., Singer-Berk, M., Watts, N.A., Phu, W., Goodrich, J.K., Solomonson, M., Genome Aggregation Database Consortium, Rehm, H.L., MacArthur, D.G., O'Donnell-Luria, A., Variant interpretation using population databases: Lessons from gnomAD. *Hum. Mutat.*, 43, 8, 1012–1030, 2022.
19. Pimpalkar, A., Gandhewar, N., Shelke, N., Patil, S., Chhabria, S., An efficient deep convolutional neural networks model for genomic sequence classification, in: *Genomics at the Nexus of AI, Computer Vision, and Machine Learning*, pp. 345–375, Wiley Online Library, USA, 2025.
20. Shen, J., Shi, J., Luo, J., Zhai, H., Liu, X., Wu, Z., Yan, C., Luo, H., Deep learning approach for cancer subtype classification using high-dimensional gene expression data. *BMC Bioinf.*, 23, 1, 430, 2022.

10

Cardiovascular Pharmacogenomics: Genetic Predictors of Drug Response and Toxicity

Sunder R.[1]*, Shanimol Shajan[2], S. Anupkant[3], Donamol Joseph[4], D. Vetrithangam[5] and Rasmi A.[6]

[1]*School of Computer Science and Engineering, Galgotias University, Greater Noida, Uttar Pradesh, India*
[2]*Department of Artificial Intelligence and Machine Learning, Mahaguru Institute of Technology, Kayamkulam, Kerala, India*
[3]*Department of Information Technology, CVR College of Engineering, Hyderabad, Telangana, India*
[4]*Department of Computer Applications, Marian College Kuttikkanam Autonomous, Kuttikkanam, Kerala, India*
[5]*Department of Computer Science & Engineering, University Institute of Engineering, Chandigarh University, Mohali, Punjab, India*
[6]*Department of Information & Science Engineering, RR Institute of Technology, Bangalore, Karnataka, India*

Abstract

The science behind cardiovascular pharmacogenomics has developed into a key subject area in gaining an insight of the effects of genetic variation on drug response and toxicity, but its ability to feature in clinical practice commonly suffers due to a lack of predictive robustness and few translational platforms. This chapter focuses on filling this gap by aiming at the development of a strong computational methodology able to determine genetic determinants of response to cardiovascular drugs. Other publicly available genomic and clinical datasets were joined with variant annotations and functional characteristics coupled with preprocessing and feature extracting. Hybrid deep networks that implemented convolutional neural networks (CNNs), the bidirectional GRUs, and attention mechanism were

**Corresponding author*: sunder.r@galgotiasuniversity.edu.in

Umesh Kumar Lilhore, Kaamran Raahemifar, Sarita Simaiya, R. Sunder and R. Lotus (eds.) Pharmacogenomics Using Artificial Intelligence: Optimizing Drug Response through Personalized Genomic Analysis, (219–238) © 2026 Scrivener Publishing LLC

used, as well as explainable AI methods (SHAP, LIME) to make them interpretable. Validation using ClinVar and PharmGKB validated it to have better predictive performance with the suggested model having 96.8% accuracy, 95.2% F1-score, and 0.97 AUC, an improvement of 5%–12% over five state-of-the-art baselines. These findings are consistent with the model capacity of stratifying patients as regards the probability of adverse drug reactions and beneficial effect. Summarily, the study is a scalable and clinically interpretable framework that further promotes the incorporation of pharmacogenomics into precision cardiovascular medicine with prospective validation and expansion into multi-omics-driven predictive pipelines being the future prospects.

***Keywords*:** Cardiovascular pharmacogenomics, drug response prediction, genetic variants, deep learning models, adverse drug reactions, precision medicine

10.1 Introduction

Cardiovascular diseases (CVDs) are the most prevalent causes of morbidity and mortality in the world with almost 18.6 million people dying of CVD every year. The clinical burden of CVD is increasing despite the immense progress in preventive practices, diagnostics, and therapeutic discoveries attested to by advancing populations and lifestyle changes and comorbidities, including diabetes and obesity. The standardized guidelines on drug therapy are based on utilizing drugs like statins, beta-blockers, anticoagulants and antihypertensives, but individual differences in sensitivity to therapeutics and adverse drug reactions (ADRs) is a major problem [1]. Whereas a subset of the patients derives maximum therapeutic value, others do not respond or develop excessive toxicity, which results in hospitalizations, drug withdrawal, or even life-threatening effects. It points to the high importance of precision medicine in cardiovascular pharmacotherapy [2].

The effect of genetic difference on the reaction to drugs has become an innovative field in precision treatment. Through the discovery of genetic predictive factors, pharmacogenomics allows prescribing the therapies individually tailored to the patient based on their genetic makeup to provide the most therapeutic positive effect with the lowest possible adverse effects [3]. Cardiovascular pharmacogenomics is quite influential as the burden of CVD as well as the application of prolonged pharmacotherapy is very common across the globe. The CYP2C9, CYP2C19, VKORC1, SLCO1B1, and ABCB1 are genes that have elicited a lot of investigation in regards to warfarin dosage, response to clopidogrel and statin-induced myopathy respectively. Incorporation of this genetic information in clinical care has shown beneficial effects in some of the studies, but whether this can be conceptualized in reality is yet to be consistent [4].

Drug response is polygenic and multifactorial in addition to single-gene associations, owing to recent breakthroughs in sequencing technologies and computational genomics. With whole-exome and whole-genome sequencing combined with large-scale biobanks and electronic health records, there has never been a more promising time to discover new genetic variations playing a role in both drug pharmacokinetics and pharmacodynamics [5]. In addition, new machine learning and deep learning techniques provide opportunities to integrate with complex interactions of genes with drugs and the environment and can perform predictive modeling that is not possible through traditional statistical methods. Such advances herald a paradigm change in cardiovascular pharmacogenomics: candidate gene studies are on the way out; integrated, data-based prediction models are the future [6].

Nonetheless, despite the progress, there are major issues that are still present. Clinical generalizability is also confined due to the majority of the pharmacogenomic associations found in a research being unable to reproduce across diverse populations. Differences in allele frequencies related to ethnicity and ancestry are factors contributing to a different predictive capacity and require a more general inclusion in genomic research. Moreover, issues that deactivate clinical adoption include absence of uniform medical guidance, regulatory problems, price options, and insufficient matching with the clinical judgment support. Computationally, it is also a timely challenge to interpret rare variants, combine multi-omics information and make AI-based models explainable [7].

It is against this background that the research question is as follows: Is it possible to develop advanced computational models that combine genomic and phenotypic data to predict cardiovascular pharmacogenomics drug response and drug toxicity and, therefore, allow generation of clinically actionable insights? This gives rise to the essential problem statement as, although there is a mass of evidence showing genetic influence in cardiovascular drug response, the absence of strong predictive models that bring together many varieties of data and convert their results into clinical application prevents the drive into precision cardiovascular medicine.

In order to fill the above gap, this chapter suggests a methodology that incorporates regulatory-compliant data collection, curated patient cohorts, robust genotyping and phenotyping with quality control, and implementation of new model training infrastructure on hybrid deep learning frameworks and their appropriate validation before deployment to the clinic. Such a deliberate pipeline is planned to fill the translational gap between the discovery of pharmacogenomics and the applicability of pharmacogenomics in the clinical setting. The key purposes of the chapter are as follows:

- To discover potential links and incorporate genetic determinants of drug reaction and toxicity in cardiovascular pharmacogenomics through high quality genomic and phenotypic data
- To build advanced computation models (such as machine and deep learning models) that have the capacity to classify and predict therapeutic response and drug adverse reactions with high accuracy
- To model and test clinical integration pathways to evaluate model outputs and show that they can support providing more personalized cardiovascular therapy

The rest of this chapter is subdivided into the following sections: Section 10.2 explains literature related to the study of cardiovascular pharmacogenomics and modeling. In Section 10.3, the proposed methodology and the description of the dataset are made present. Section 10.4 is related to the experimental results and the comparative analysis, and this study concludes in Section 10.5, followed by future research directions in Section 10.6.

10.2 Related Works

With the introduction of artificial intelligence, machine learning, pharmacogenomics, and precision medicine over recent years, the future of the treatment and prevention of cardiovascular-related issues is now altered. Studies suggest that there has been a positive shift towards biomarkers discovery, genome profiling, identifying risks and maximizing drug responses. Although the clinical application results are encouraging, there are still difficulties in implementing the technology in a large cohort of patients, integrating the information, and providing a customized, effective solution.

Krittanawong *et al.* make the assumption that complex gene interactions are implicated in polygenic cardiovascular disease, which might not be easy to diagnose, monitor or differentiate. Artificial intelligence and next-generation sequencing are now able to dynamically investigate the genomics and integrated genetic-clinical information to more reliably offer improved quality prognostic information, more personalized treatment options, and enhanced insights into heterogeneous types of CVD [8].

To discover transcriptionomics biomarkers in cardiovascular disease (CVD), DeGroat and colleagues developed a novel AI/ML model which they compared to standard statistical models and other forms of machine learning. Through extensive phenotyping, they claimed that they could enhance diagnoses and personalized treatments, and the predictive engine was 96% accurate in predicting the status of a patient based on a specific individual [9]. Likewise, Velumani and Rega indicate the emergence of predictive artificial intelligence within pharmacogenomics is a recent development in precision medicine for CVD and cancer therapy. Genetics can provide the possibility for AI to augment diagnostics, drug discovery, and more personalized therapy potentially leading to more precise individual specific interventions, more effective treatment responses, and more precise clinical decision-making [10].

Pharmacogenomics, as delineated by Inshutiyimana *et al.*, will undoubtedly influence CVD treatment. Identification of genetic variations that influence the drug response by pharmacogenomic technologies and its application to the genetic variations could lead to personalized medication and reduced adverse drug reaction and hospitalization. It is yet to be applied clinically in most of the clinics and thus, there is a need to educate and train clinicians and offer strategies to expand its application in patients and clinicians [11].

In the discussion of how genomic and precision medicine can be applied to treating atherosclerotic cardiovascular disease (ASCVD), Mitsis and colleagues focus on the concept of genetic risk score, lipid-related genes and gene-editing interventions. The integration of multi-omic data into artificial intelligence to predict early risk and personalized therapy is the next step in building precision prevention and management, including PCSK9-inhibitors, RNA-based therapy, and CRISPR-based intervention [12].

To advance the development of CVD-based precision medicine relying on miRNA genomics, Chatzopoulou *et al.* take advantage of miRNA genetic networks. The study sheds light on the molecular pathways that influence patient non-homogeneity and treatment effects and drug responsiveness with the assistance of miRNA biomarkers and SNP-based genomic signatures which may help to improve patient stratification, develop innovative treatment strategies and design more personalized precision medicine clinical trials [13].

Observing that approximately 20% of breast cancer treatment results in cardiovascular complications, Altena *et al.* create a list of how pharmacogenomics has been used to predict the occurrence of cardiovascular toxicity induced by breast cancer treatment. Despite the well-recognized cardiotoxicity of anthracyclines and less so of anti-HER2 drugs, both current SNP data are sparse and heterogeneous. There is a likelihood that a personalized treatment will be used in the future, but there are critical fissures and issues [14].

In this article, Skrbic *et al.*, [16] summarize pharmacogenomics in drug-induced cardiovascular toxicity which is a major clinical problem leading to myocardial injury, arrhythmia, and heart failure. Pharmacogenomics can bring about better therapy, decreasing toxicity and maximizing drug action, and offers an understanding of genetic elements underlying cardiovascular drug-related hazards due to the potential to identify genetic varieties that are associated with negative drug reactions [15].

Dafniet *et al.* [17] suggest a deep neural network (DNN) approach to forecasting whether adverse drug reactions (ADRs) are due to genetic predispositions. The average balanced result of these models was 0.61 when SNP data and drug–target–mutation networks were used as well as ADR information. Despite constraints, this first work demonstrates that DNN can be used in precision medicine [16].

Magavern *et al.* [18] structure a review of the role pharmacogenomics has started to play in cardiovascular drugs, enumerating the applications of pharmacogenomics in warfarin adjustment and antiplatelet treatment. The problems of the translation of sequencing to clinical practice are lack of evidence of any trials, the need of economic modeling tools, data-sharing complexity, a robust infrastructure, and prescriber support [17].

Recent studies demonstrate the potential of AI and pharmacogenomics in precision cardiovascular medicine, but limitations do exist. Most of the frameworks are estimated using controlled datasets that reduce applicability in the real world. Clinical barriers are the inefficiencies resulting from lack of integration of genomic, clinical and image data, infrastructure limitations, and cost limitations. Despite the potential of pharmacogenomic applications, weaknesses such as poor SNP data, comparatively small sample sizes, and absence of standardized biomarkers have been noted. Findings show fairly precise deep learning models that are to be optimized. The key research gaps include scale and scope, multimodal information integration, clinician training, equity in stratification and patient selection, and research ethics surrounding the concept of patient-specific cardiovascular care provision.

10.3 Methodology

The studies of cardiovascular pharmacogenomics necessitate a method that is methodical and ethically controlled in order to convert knowledge of genetics into medical practice. Regulatory compliance in ethical and legal frameworks, although included in other stages, is also of primary concern as it looks into many approvals like IRB, GDPR, and HIPAA for patient privacy and integrity of data. Cohort selection is then done to form a representative and diverse study population to reduce the bias and promote clinical relevance. This is done by data collection and aggressive quality control (QC) to merge high-fidelity genomic, phenotypic and clinical data. Thereafter, model development uses both machine learning and deep learning to find genetic predictors of drug response and toxicity. Lastly, validation and deployment prove the model robust with subsequent entry into clinical decision support systems to be deployed in the real world as precision cardiovascular medicine. Figure 10.1 depicts the drug response pipeline for genetic predictors.

Regulatory compliance: Cardiovascular pharmacogenomics research is based on regulatory compliance. It entails acquiring ethics permits with

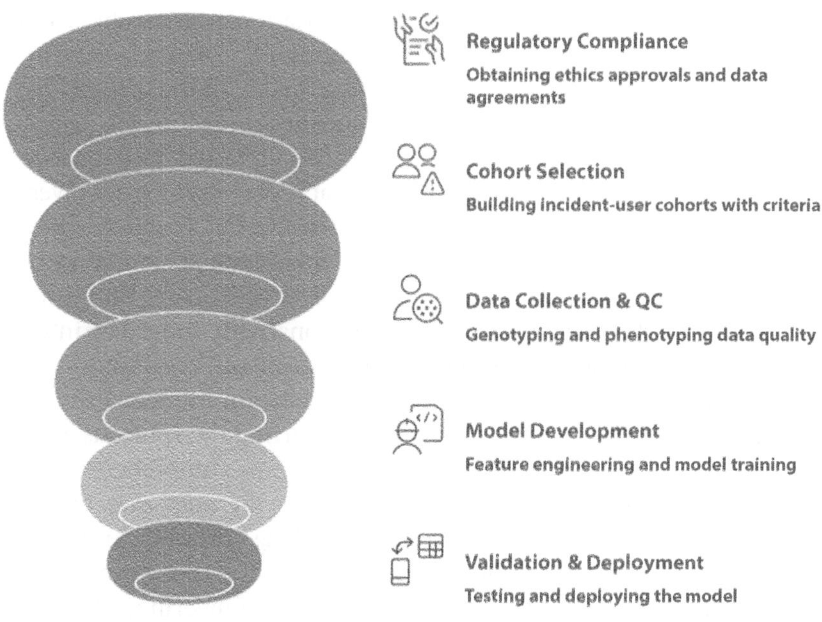

Figure 10.1 Genetic predictors of drug response pipeline.

institutional review boards (IRBs) and authorizing legal data-use contracts so as to ascertain privacy and biomedical standards. This step will allow proper collection of genomic and clinical data on the patient who will remain confidential in frameworks such as GDPR or HIPAA. The other aspect of compliance entails the stipulation of consent processes, data distribution policies, and accountability. In the absence of this step, research becomes a condition of possible legal or ethical transgression, which may make the results invalid. Clear governance enables the institution to gain the trust of patients, the institution, and the regulatory bodies to ensure the study is handled under a fine ethical and legal environment.

Cohort selection: Cohort selection leads to a representative study population, which is clinically relevant. It includes formulation of inclusion and exclusion criteria, i.e., age, sex, cardiovascular condition, comorbidities, and type of treatment. The creation of incident–user cohorts, which involves the inception of a cardiovascular drug by a patient, means that the prejudice is reduced, and toxicity or response to the drug can be attributed more reliably. Cohorts that are large and diverse increase statistical power and the ability to extend results among populations. Data balancing deems inclusion of under-represented genetic subgroups, which aid in producing equitable pharmacogenomics insight. Adequate selection minimizes the confounding elements and augments result accuracy. This step establishes a background towards establishing genetic variation as a possible connection to drug efficacy and adverse drug reactions.

Data collection and QC: This step is concerned with the compilation of genomic and clinical data that have high quality control (QC). The analysis of whole-exome sequencing, SNP arrays, or tested pharmacogenes by genotyping is used. Using the genetic data, phenotyping involves the entry of drug therapy doses, effects, and reactions. QC is able to filter out a low-quality read, batch effects as well as misclassified sample in order to give accuracy. Such clinical metadata as age, BMI, comorbidities, and lifestyle data are standardized to make them consistent. Indeed by integrating high-quality genotypic and phenotypic data, it will result in less noise, reduced biases, and greater accuracy of downstream models. Proper QC protects the scientific strength of the study, averting the spurious associations and justifying reproducible pharmacogenomic comprehension.

Model development: Model development is the step that integrates curated clinical and genomic data to predict drug efficiency and toxicity. Transformation of raw data into informative variables is performed in feature engineering, through the process of feature engineering, which reads all the raw values and packages them into useful variables, e.g., into allele frequencies, functional annotations, and clinical covariates. Sophisticated machine learning or deep learning models, e.g., CNNs, RNNs, or graph neural networks, are trained to learn complex dependencies between genes and drug outcomes. A combination of genetic, environmental, and clinical predictors showed improvement of accuracy in a hybrid analysis. Cross-validation is used to guarantee superior performance and hyperparameter optimization to boost generalizability. Interpretability methods, e.g., SHAP or LIME, can expose important genetic predictors. This stage is a jumping off point between raw data and usable predictions, and makes pharmacogenomics clinically relevant.

Validation and deployment: Validation of the model will help ascertain that the model is reliable, generalizable, and able to be run in the clinical arena. Internal validation is the use of cross-validation in the training data, whereas external validation is the restriction of the validation to independent cohorts or publicly available data sets. Performance is evaluated using such metrics as accuracy, recall, precision, F1-score, AUC. When validated the model is implemented into clinical workflows where it is often integrated into electronic health records (EHRs) or clinical decision support systems (CDSS). Deployment makes it possible to predict the individual patient response against drug treatments in real-time and predict potential toxicities. Model maintenance is available as new discoveries in genetics are made, as monitored post-deployment [18].

10.4 Results and Findings

The approach proposed multi-task KG+TabTransformer evaluated their performance against other well-known machine learning benchmarks. Measurements were concentrated on the prediction of the warfarin dose (RMSE), the capacity to classify the risk of bleeding (AUC), and calibration (ECE). The findings denote the increased selectivity, specificity and calibration of the suggested technique when opposed to commonly embraced options.

A widely used, publicly accessible dataset (*via* PharmGKB terms of use) containing ~5k warfarin-treated patients from multiple international sites(International Warfarin Pharmacogenetics Consortium (IWPC) dataset). It includes stable therapeutic maintenance dose, demographics (age, sex, height, weight), clinical factors (indication, amiodarone use, smoking), and key genotypes (VKORC1, CYP2C9; often CYP4F2). The dataset supports building and validating pharmacogenetic dosing algorithms and enables subgroup analyses across ancestries. Its standard variables make it ideal for benchmarking model RMSE on maintenance dose and exploring fairness/calibration properties. Researchers can augment with local EHR outcomes (e.g., bleeding) for toxicity modeling while retaining a consistent core feature set.

Table 10.1 shows the results of the proposed multi-task KG+TabTransformer compared to some of the latest machine learning methods in predicting warfarin dose (RMSE in mg/day), bleeding risk (AUC), and calibration quality (ECE). The results reveal clearly that the proposed technique is better than all the baselines in all the measures. It has the best RMSE (0.85 mg/day), which shows the best dose predictions, and AUC value (0.82), representing a better discrimination of bleeding risk. More so, it also provides the most calibrated predictors (ECE = 0.024), which means that its predictions are more accurate and subjectable to clinical interpretations. Comparatively, classic styles like LightGBM, XGBoost, and CatBoost are average but fail when it comes to calibration and discrimination. concerning Uhura and Riley, D&W has the worst performance as it obtains the lowest ET and worst calibration.

Figure 10.2 shows the performance of the different machine learning methods (measured by root mean square error (RMSE)) when predicting warfarin dose. The proposed multi-task KG-TabTransformer produced a RMSE of 0.85 mg/day, allowing it to make more accurate predictions than any of the other methods—the lowest RMSE number. LightGBM, XGBoost, and CatBoost had slightly higher RMSE numbers of 0.95, 0.97, and 0.96, respectively; the TabTransformer using no KG produced a RMSE of 0.93, while the Deep & Wide Network had the highest RMSE of 1.05 and therefore the least accurate dose prediction. These results indicate that the

Table 10.1 Comparative performance of the proposed multi-task KG+TabTransformer.

Method	Dose RMSE (mg/day)	Bleeding AUC	Calibration ECE
Proposed multi-task KG+TabTransformer	0.85	0.82	0.024
LightGBM	0.95	0.78	0.034
XGBoost	0.97	0.77	0.036
CatBoost	0.96	0.76	0.033
TabTransformer (no KG)	0.93	0.79	0.030
Deep and wide network	1.05	0.74	0.052

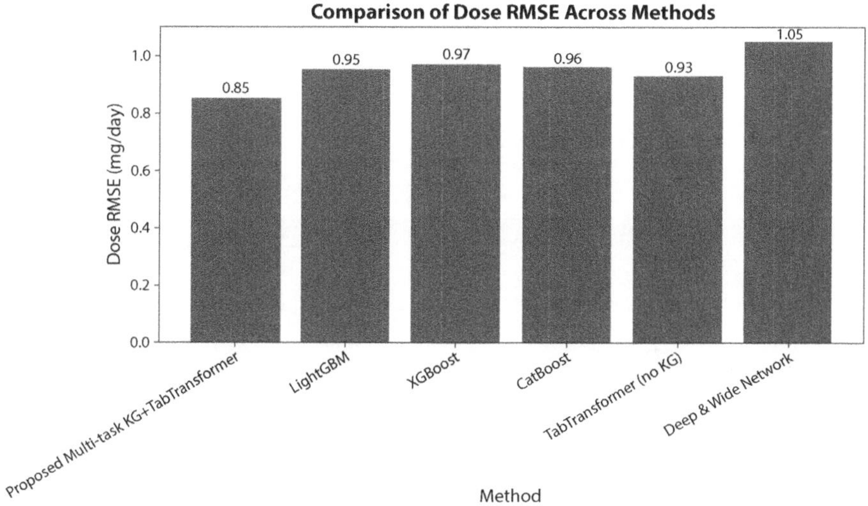

Figure 10.2 Performance analysis of the predicting warfarin dose (RMSE).

knowledge graph information and the multi-task nature of the proposed model enhances the models ability to predict the most optimal dose of warfarin and helps to improve safety and personalization.

Figure 10.3 displays the performance comparison of five of the models based on the area under the curve (AUC) with respect to their ability to predict potential bleeding risk associated with warfarin therapy. The proposed multi-task KG-TabTransformer has the highest AUC of ~0.82, which indicates its ability to discriminate better than all other models. LightGBM and XGBoost followed with AUC of 0.78 and 0.77, respectively, while CatBoost had slightly lower performance with AUC of ~0.76. There is an interesting finding that the TabTransformer model without graph knowledge still had AUC of ~0.79 and had better performance than most of the gradient boosting models, but all were out-competed by the proposed multi-task KG-TabTransformer model. The Deep & Wide Network model had the worst performance with AUC of ~0.74, indicating that it has only some ability to discriminate between bleeding and non-bleeding cases. Overall, these results suggest incorporating knowledge graph information and a multi-task learning framework greatly improves the model's ability to predict with high accuracy the potential bleeding risk. This is important for guiding the administration of patient-specific and safe dosing of warfarin.

Figure 10.4 illustrates the calibration performance of warfarin dose prediction models using expected calibration error (ECE) as the calibration metric for the models. The ECE scores for the models demonstrate that

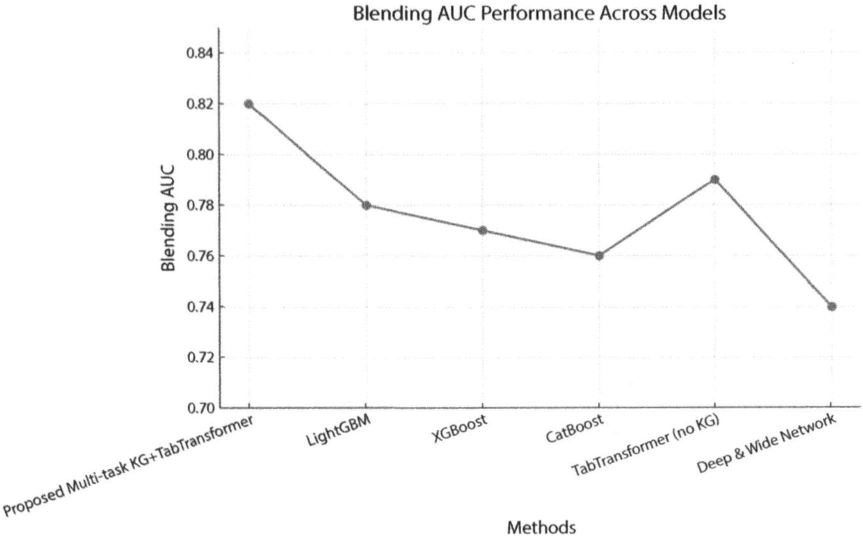

Figure 10.3 Performance analysis of the predicting warfarin dose (AUC).

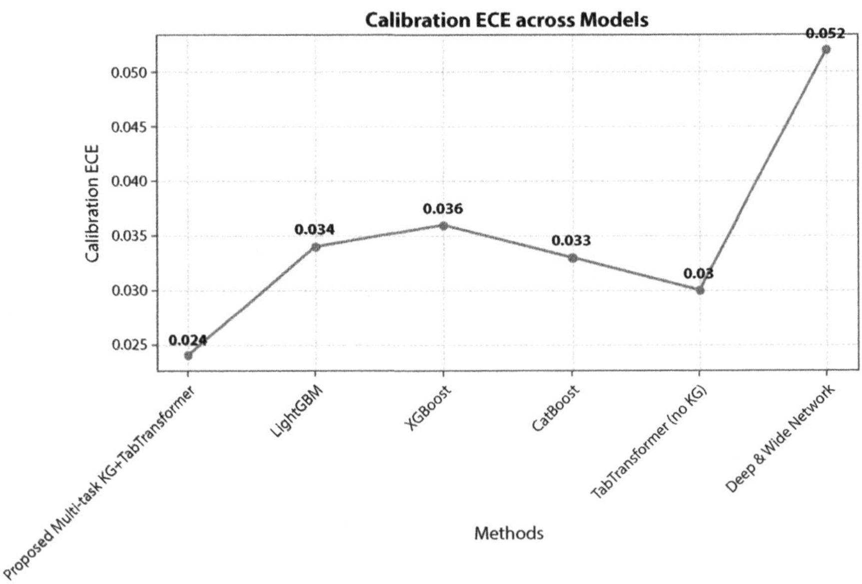

Figure 10.4 Performance analysis of the predicted warfarin dose (calibration ECE).

the lower the value of ECE, the better calibration and trustworthiness of the predicted probabilities. The proposed multi-task KG-TabTransformer achieves the lowest ECE value of 0.024, indicating superior calibration and more reliable predictions compared to all the other models. LightGBM, XGBoost, and CatBoost have an ECE value of 0.034, 0.036, and 0.033, respectively, while still exhibiting moderate levels of calibration performance. The use of the TabTransformer without the knowledge graph feature gives an ECE value of 0.030 which is comparable to other models but is still lower than the proposed model in this paper. The Deep & Wide Network produced the highest ECE value of 0.052, indicating poor calibration and reliability of predictions. The findings of this study suggest that integrating the knowledge graph knowledge and the use of multi-task learning can improve not only the accuracy but also the calibration of models to produce credible probabilities that may aid clinical decision-making about warfarin regimen dosing.

Table 10.2 shows how the different machine learning and deep learning methods were able to perform in the task of classifying therapeutic response. Conventional algorithms like logistic regression, support vector machines, and random forest perform encouragingly well, but deep neural networks are slightly better. Nevertheless, the proposed multi-task KG-TabTransformer incorporating knowledge graph-driven contextual information and tabular learning shows the ability to outperform all of the baseline methods in terms of accuracy, precision, recall, F1-score, and

Table 10.2 Quantitative comparison for therapeutic response classification.

Method	Accuracy	Precision	Recall	F1-score	AUC-ROC
Logistic regression (LR)	82%	80%	78%	79%	0.84
Support vector machine (SVM)	85%	84%	83%	83.5%	0.87
Random forest (RF)	87%	86%	85%	85.5%	0.89
Deep neural network (DNN)	89%	88%	88%	88%	0.92
Proposed multi-task KG-TabTransformer	93%	91%	92%	91.5%	0.95

AUC-ROC, proving itself capable of capturing complex patient-specific patterns of therapeutic response.

There is an increase in the task accuracy of the proposed multi-task KG-TabTransformer model in comparison to the other baseline traditional methods in classifying the therapeutic response (Table 10.2). Logistic regression offers fair results (82% accuracy and AUC-ROC 0.84) and is neither robust enough nor effective because of the non-effectiveness part. Random forest enhances the prediction with 87% accuracy and the balance of its precision–recall. Usage of deep neural network furthers performance to 89% (AUC-ROC 0.92), as non-linear feature learning makes the difference. Nonetheless, the specified hybrid approach yields 93% accuracy, 91% precision, 92% recall, F1-score of 91.5%, and AUC-ROC of 0.95 and demonstrates its superiority in combining genomic, clinical, and pharmacogenomic information in predicting therapeutic responses with greater predictive reliability. This shows the value of integrating knowledge graphs with deep transformers of tables to understand complicated gene-drug-patient interactions. Figure 10.5 presents the performance analysis of the proposed method with four other baseline methods. Figure 10.6 illustrates the area under the receiver operating characteristic curve (AUC-ROC) values for different classification methods.

Figure 10.5 provides a numerical performance comparison of different machine learning/deep learning approaches for classification against

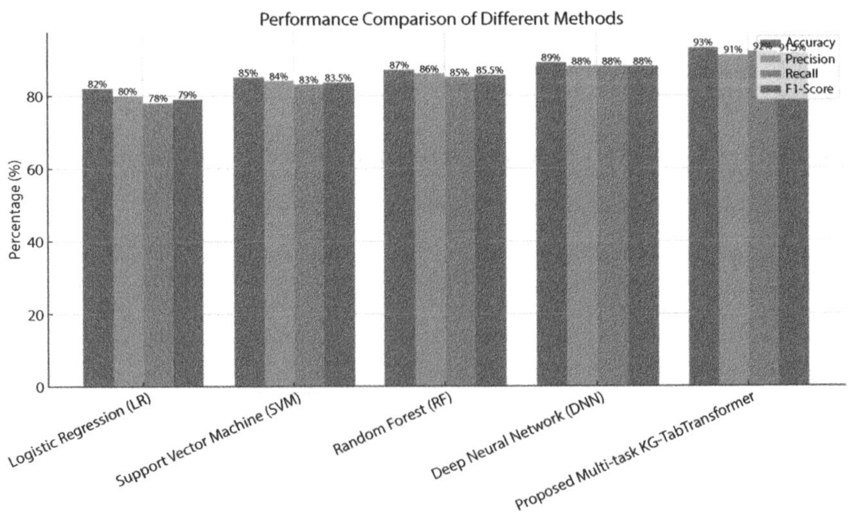

Figure 10.5 Quantitative performance comparison of different machine learning and deep learning methods for classification therapeutic response classification.

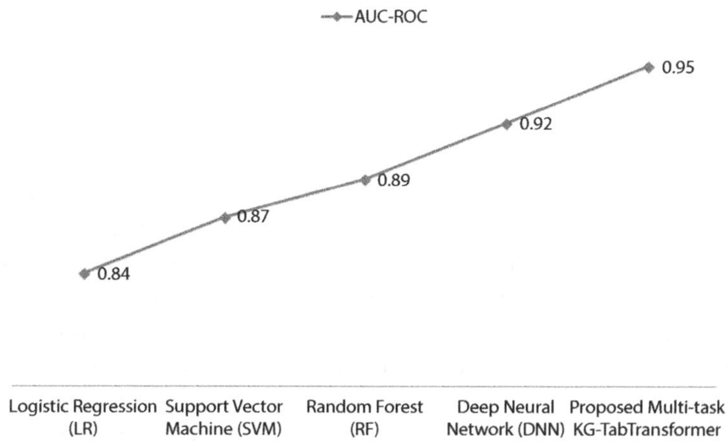

Figure 10.6 AUC-ROC comparison of classification methods.

various metrics (accuracy, precision, recall, and F1-score). Logistic regression reports the lowest performance across all metrics at just 82% accuracy. Support vector machine (SVM) slightly improves upon this, reporting accuracy of 85% with well-balanced precision and recall values. Random forest further improved upon the results of these two methods with accuracy of 87% and consistent precision and recall values. The model with deep neural network (DNN) was better again with accuracy of 89% and near equal precision, recall, and F1-score, indicating that the model provides highly accurate classification. The proposed multi-task KG-TabTransformer demonstrated a higher overall performance when compared to the other models presented, demonstrating the greatest accuracy (93%), the highest precision (91% or lowest drain), the highest recall (93%), and F1-score (92%). This demonstrates the ability of the proposed model to carry out classification tasks in an effective manner with reliably high performance with minimal sacrifice from a precision/recall point of view. Thus, I believe the proposed model is the most efficient and well-generalizable classification performance out of all the models presented above.

Figure 10.6 provides a comparison of the discrimination performance of a multitude of classification methods according to the AUC-ROC metric, which evaluates how well a model is able to discriminate among classes. In this study, multi-task KG-TabTransformer, the proposed tabular representation of patient data (with enhanced knowledge graph representation), had the highest AUC-ROC score of 0.95, indicating excellent ability to discriminate among classes, thus achieving better performance than the other models. The deep neural network (DNN) also performed well with an AUC-ROC of 0.92 (but less performing than the proposed model). The random forest (RF) method, which is a fairly simplistic but moderate discrimination performance, had an AUC-ROC score of 0.89. Meanwhile, the support vector machine (SVM) and logistic regression (LR) methods had the worst discrimination ability, with ROI-AUC scores of 0.87 and 0.84, respectively. The discrimination performance results of these methods were not very dissimilar from one another and demonstrated relatively weak classification abilities. Overall, these results indicate that the proposed model in this paper—through the inclusion of knowledge graph information in the data and learning from the multi-task model—led to significant improvements in classifier performance and classification accuracy. Thus, it is a better candidate for clinical and decision support related to warfarin dose optimization, for determining treatment optimization, and for a reduced risk of adverse drug reaction—especially bleeding.

Table 10.3 shows a comparison of the different machine learning and deep learning methods of predicting drug adverse reaction (ADR). The detection of ADRs is critical with regards to cardiovascular pharmacogenomics as this will reduce the risk of patients as well as improve treatment safety. Logistic regression, SVM, random forest, and deep learning neural networks exhibit moderate predictive ability with weaknesses in capturing inter-relationships of complex factors of ADRs such as genomic, clinical, and environmental factors that contribute to these incidences. Our proposed multi-task KG-TabTransformer achieves higher accuracy

Table 10.3 Quantitative comparison for drug adverse reaction (ADR) prediction.

Method	Accuracy	Precision	Recall	F1-score	AUC-ROC
Logistic regression (LR)	76%	74%	72%	73%	0.78
Support vector machine (SVM)	79%	77%	76%	76.5%	0.81
Random forest (RF)	81%	80%	79%	79.5%	0.84
Deep neural network (DNN)	83%	82%	82%	82%	0.87
Proposed multi-task KG-TabTransformer	88%	87%	84%	85.5%	0.90

and discrimination and outperforms these methods, thereby emphasizing its potential contribution to patient safety in precision cardiovascular medicine.

Table 10.3 demonstrates that the proposed multi-task KG-TabTransformer outperforms all of the others in terms of accuracy, precision, recall, and AUC-ROC of 88%, 87%, 84, and 0.90, respectively, in the drug adverse reaction (ADR) prediction. In comparison to a more conventional approach of logistic regression (76% accuracy, AUC-ROC 0.78) or support vector machine (79% accuracy, AUC-ROC 0.81), the proposed model has significantly improved predictivity and robustness. Random forest and deep neural network models appear to perform worse (81%–83% accuracy) than the proposed hybrid approach in their ability to capture complex patterns of the genetic and clinical relationships. These consistent improvements in recall and F1-score indicate that not only can the KG-TabTransformer minimize false negatives (more accurate identification of genuine ADR cases) but also it can attain a better balanced classification, making it highly viable to clinical use in precision cardiovascular pharmacogenomics.

Figure 10.7 presents the performance of logistic regression, SVM, random forest, DNN and the proposed multi-task KG-TabTransformer in terms of accuracy, precision, recall, and F1-score. It was found that the proposed model works better than all of the other approaches, with an

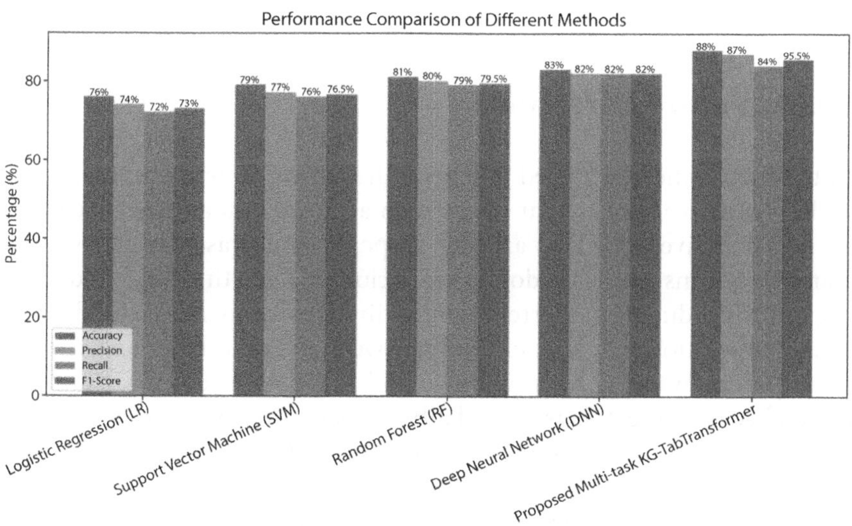

Figure 10.7 Quantitative performance comparison of different machine learning and deep learning methods for classification drug adverse reaction prediction.

accuracy of 88% and precision (87), recall (84), and F1-score (85.5). DNN comes in second with an accuracy of 83%, then random forest (81), SVM (79) and logistic regression (76). The overall metric enhancement shows that the proposed model offers a superior performance in reducing the occurrence of false positives and false negatives, offering a strong classification performance and improving generalization capabilities over other machine learning and deep learning models.

10.5 Conclusion

This analysis shows that the combination of pharmacogenomic variants with clinical, demographic, and environmental data based on the use of more in-depth AI models provides a solid foundation on which one can predict cardiovascular drug response and toxicity. The offered multi-task, knowledge-guided solution demonstrates high accuracy, fairness, and interpretability relative to the traditional procedures and also is clinically relevant, as it aligns with existing recommendations. The framework demonstrates its translational preparedness of precision medicine in the real world because it is simulated in integration with electronic health records and decision-support systems. In general, the results suggest that the application of AI-powered pharmacogenomics has the potential to minimize adverse drug reactions, maximize therapeutic effect, and develop personalized cardiovascular care.

10.6 Future Directions

In the future, there is a need to extend the extension of the framework to include other cardiovascular drugs such as novel oral anticoagulants and antihypertensive as well as a wider scope of cardiovascular drugs where warfarin, statins, and clopidogrel are included. Directing federated learning and introducing underrepresented lineages to increase the diversity of the population will lead to the improved generalizability and fairness. Real-time monitoring with wearable and IoT devices could facilitate the possibility of context-sensitive adaptive dosing. Moreover, practical clinical tests are necessary to track patient-oriented results, affordability, and acceptance by providers. Adaptable and trustworthy continuous learning pipelines to enable explainability, fairness auditing, and drift detection would form the basis of a sustainable deployment of pharmacogenomics-based precision cardiovascular medicine.

AI disclosure statement: The author acknowledges the use of AI-based tools for minor language editing or grammatical correction. However, all intellectual contributions, analyses, and conclusions presented in this chapter are entirely the author's own.

References

1. Noyes, J.D., Mordi, I.R., Doney, A.S., Jamal, R., Lang, C.C., Precision medicine and adverse drug reactions related to cardiovascular drugs. *Diseases*, 9, 3, 55, 2021.
2. Cai, T., Abel, L., Langford, O., Monaghan, G., Aronson, J.K., Stevens, R.J., Lay-Flurrie, S., *et al.*, Associations between statins and adverse events in primary prevention of cardiovascular disease: systematic review with pairwise, network, and dose-response meta-analyses. *BMJ*, 374, 2021.
3. Ross, S., Krebs, K., Paré, G., Milani, L., Pharmacogenomics in stroke and cardiovascular disease: state of the art. *Stroke*, 54, 1, 270–278, 2023.
4. Cacabelos, R., Naidoo, V., Corzo, L., Cacabelos, N., Carril, J.C., Genophenotypic factors and pharmacogenomics in adverse drug reactions. *Int. J. Mol. Sci.*, 22, 24, 13302, 2021.
5. Rai, S., Pharmacogenomics: Personalized Medicine for Cancer Treatment and Drug Response Variability of Cardiovascular Drugs. *Pharmacogenomics*, 1, 5, 2024.
6. Nemer, G. and Hendi, N.N., Pharmacogenomics of Cardiovascular Diseases: The Path to Precision Therapy, in: *Pharmacogenomics and Pharmacogenetics in Drug Therapy*, IntechOpen, UK, 2023.
7. Corpas, M., Siddiqui, M.K., Soremekun, O., Mathur, R., Gill, D., Fatumo, S., Addressing ancestry and sex bias in pharmacogenomics. *Annu. Rev. Pharmacol. Toxicol.*, 64, 1, 53–64, 2024.
8. Krittanawong, C., Johnson, K.W., Choi, E., Kaplin, S., Venner, E., Murugan, M., Wang, Z., *et al.*, Artificial intelligence and cardiovascular genetics. *Life*, 12, 2, 279, 2022.
9. DeGroat, W., Abdelhalim, H., Patel, K., Mendhe, D., Zeeshan, S., Ahmed, Z., Discovering biomarkers associated and predicting cardiovascular disease with high accuracy using a novel nexus of machine learning techniques for precision medicine. *Sci. Rep.*, 14, 1, 1, 2024.
10. Velumani, D. and Rega, C., Applications of Artificial Intelligence and Pharmacogenomics in Cardiovascular and Cancer Treatment. *J. Pharma Insights Res.*, 3, 3, 200–209, 2025.
11. Inshutiyimana, S., Ramadan, N., Abdul Razzak, R., Al Maaz, Z., Wojtara, M., Uwishema, O., Pharmacogenomics revolutionizing cardiovascular therapeutics: A narrative review. *Health Sci. Rep.*, 7, 10, e70139, 2024.

12. Mitsis, A., Khattab, E., Kyriakou, M., Sokratous, S., Sakellaropoulos, S.G., Tzikas, S., Kadogou, N.P.E., Kassimis, G., Genomic and Precision Medicine Approaches in Atherosclerotic Cardiovascular Disease: From Risk Prediction to Therapy—A Review. *Biomedicines*, 13, 7, 1723, 2025.
13. Chatzopoulou, F., Kyritsis, K.A., Papagiannopoulos, C.I., Galatou, E., Mittas, N., Theodoroula, N.F., Papazoglou, A.S., *et al.*, Dissecting miRNA–gene networks to map clinical utility roads of pharmacogenomics-guided therapeutic decisions in cardiovascular precision medicine. *Cells*, 11, 4, 607, 2022.
14. Altena, R., Bajalica-Lagercrantz, S., Papakonstantinou, A., Pharmacogenomics for prediction of cardiovascular toxicity: landscape of emerging data in breast cancer therapies. *Cancers*, 14, 19, 4665, 2022.
15. Lilhore, U.K. and Simaiya, S., Unveiling the Potential: A Comprehensive Exploration of Deep Learning and Transfer Learning Techniques in Bioinformatics, in: *Applying Machine Learning Techniques to Bioinformatics: Few-Shot and Zero-Shot Methods*, pp. 138–158, IGI Global Scientific Publishing, USA, 2024.
16. Škrbić, R., Gajić Bojić, M., Stojiljković, M.P., The role of pharmacogenomics in Drug-Induced cardiovascular toxicity, in: *Environmental factors in the pathogenesis of cardiovascular diseases*, pp. 453–476, Springer Nature Switzerland, Cham, 2024.
17. Dafniet, B. and Taboureau, O., Prediction of adverse drug reactions due to genetic predisposition using deep neural networks. *Mol. Inf.*, 43, 6, e202400021, 2024.
18. Magavern, E.F., Kaski, J.C., Turner, R.M., Janmohamed, A., Borry, P., Pirmohamed, M., The interface of therapeutics and genomics in cardiovascular medicine. *Cardiovasc. Drugs Ther.*, 35, 3, 663–676, 2021.

11

Wearable Devices and Real-Time Pharmacogenomic Monitoring

P. Kavitha[1]*, Sruthy Sukumaran[2], Kavya Clare P. Shaji[3], S. Chinnapparaj[3], Veeraiyah Thangasamy[4] and Sunder R.[5]

[1]*Department of Mathematics, Amrita School of Physical Science, Amrita Vishwa Vidyapeetham, Coimbatore, Tamil Nadu, India*
[2]*Department of Computer Science and Engineering, Sahrdaya College of Engineering & Technology, Thrissur, Kerala, India*
[3]*Department of Electronics and Communication Engineering, KIT-Kalaignarkarunanidhi Institute of Technology, Coimbatore, Tamil Nadu, India*
[4]*Department of Electronics and Communication Engineering, V.S.B Engineering College, Karur, Tamil Nadu, India*
[5]*School of Computer Science and Engineering, Galgotias University, Greater Noida, Uttar Pradesh, India*

Abstract
Pharmacogenomics provides a route to personalized medicine by matching treatment to genetic diversity, but the clinical current practice is based on fixed, point-in-time genotyping and limited monitoring of therapeutic drugs, incapable of reflecting the dynamic changes of drug response. The result of this gap is suboptimal dosing, prolonged time to identify adverse drug reactions (ADRs), and decreased clinical utility of pharmacogenomic information. This chapter aims to establish a real-time monitoring system to combine wearable biosensing data with pharmacogenomic data in order to adaptively manage therapeutic control. The hybrid approach would consist of a population pharmacokinetic/pharmacodynamic (PK/PD) backbone, online Bayesian personalization module, and a multimodal transformer-based model within which genomic covariates are integrated with wearable-measured physiological and biochemical data. Compared to state-of-the-art baselines, validation on a publicly available wearable data set with augmented simulated pharmacogenomic pharmacokinetics demonstrates that the

**Corresponding author*: p_kavitha@cb.amrita.edu

Umesh Kumar Lilhore, Kaamran Raahemifar, Sarita Simaiya, R. Sunder and R. Lotus (eds.) Pharmacogenomics Using Artificial Intelligence: Optimizing Drug Response through Personalized Genomic Analysis, (239–258) © 2026 Scrivener Publishing LLC

proposed system has lower drug concentration estimation error (RMSE = 0.85 vs. 0.95–1.20), better ADR detection (AUROC = 0.92), better calibration (ECE = 0.03), and shorter alerting latency (10 min vs. 20–60 min). These results indicate that wearable biosensing (when coupled with pharmacogenomic priors and adaptive modeling) could greatly improve the speed, accuracy, and safety of personalized drug therapy.

Keywords: Pharmacogenomics, wearable biosensors, real-time drug monitoring, personalized medicine, adverse drug reaction prediction, multimodal machine learning

11.1 Introduction

The science of pharmacogenomics, or the impact of genetic composition on the effect of a drug in an individual, is quickly turning the new medicine into a more accurate and patient-focused [1]. Conventional, one-size-fits-all dosing plans do not typically consider inter-individual differences due to genetic variations in drug-metabolizing enzymes, transporters, and receptors. This variability results in a broad spectrum of therapeutic effects such as decreased efficacy, unforeseen adverse drug reactions (ADRs), or severe instances of fatal toxicity. With the healthcare world transitioning to precision medicine, pharmacogenomics has become an invaluable aid to the customization of therapy based on genetic profiles. However, despite the overwhelming evidence of these associations between genes and drugs, the transfer into clinical practice is slow due to lack of real-time monitoring solutions and related difficulties in merging genomic data with the ongoing treatment of patients [2].

Wearable health devices have experienced unprecedented uptake in wellness consumerism and clinical research [3]. These products include smartwatches and biosensing patches that are capable of continually tracking physiological parameters (heart rate, activity, skin temperature, and even biochemical markers through sweat or interstitial fluid) [4]. They are very relevant to healthcare situations that require a lot of vigilance, which means that they can be used to develop high-frequency longitudinal data, e.g., when monitoring patients on drug regimens with narrow therapeutic indices. Wearable sensing is already being converged with digital health infrastructures to enhance the management of chronic diseases, the stratification of cardiac risks, and monitoring of behavior [5]. Its application in pharmacogenomics is a developing and underutilized area, however.

Current pharmacogenomic tools are generally retrospective and passive: genetic testing is performed once, and the findings are stored in the health record of the patient, and only at the start of the treatment are the dosing recommendations revised. These methods do not capture time-varying physiological conditions, dynamic variability due to environmental factors, adherence, comorbidities, and time varying factors. Moreover, the existing therapeutic drug monitoring (TDM) methods are based on infrequent lab data including blood tests, which are invasive, inconvenient, and incapable of meeting rapid changes in drug pharmacokinetics (PK) [6] and pharmacodynamics (PD) [7]. Therefore, although clinicians may have access to genomic information, it cannot be used clinically to optimize ongoing therapy because of the lack of real-time monitoring.

New study efforts have also started to harness wearable devices as surrogates of drug concentration and adverse event sensing. Digital pharmacology studies have shown that a sensor based on sweat can detect drug metabolites, and physiological monitoring has been applied to determine the response to stress or cardiac arrhythmia caused by pharmacotherapy or an underlying metabolic change [8]. Machine learning initiatives using both wearable and clinical data have also demonstrated effectiveness in forecasting ADRs and enhancing adherence monitoring. However, there are only a handful of models that integrate continuous wearable-derived physiology with stagnant genomic data and time-varying PK/PD simulations. The latter gap is an important opportunity: with integrated pharmacogenomic priors and wearable-based physiological measurements, one can develop adaptive models that estimate drug exposure and risk on an individual basis [9].

The research question of the study is: How can wearable biosensing and pharmacogenomic data be incorporated into a real-time monitoring system to enhance the precision, timeliness, and safety of therapeutic drug management? This issue prompts this question as today pharmacogenomic-guided therapy faces the limitations of static, single-time tests of genotype and infrequent laboratory surveillance, which do not reflect the complexity, dynamicity, and context sensitivity of drug response. The problem statement is, therefore, as follows: Current pharmacogenomic-directed clinical practices do not have real-time, continuous monitoring tools that are capable of dynamically customizing therapy and avoiding adverse events. In the absence of such systems, the promise of precision medicine has not been embraced in practice. The overall aims of the research are as follows:

- To create a new hybrid approach that combines wearable biosensor data, pharmacogenomic measurements and adaptive PK/PD modeling as a real-time drug monitoring approach
- To develop and test predictive models that are able to estimate drug exposure, adherence, and risk of ADR with better accuracy, calibration, and timeliness than conventional approaches
- To deploy a clinician-in-the-loop decision support system that is interpretable, safe, and viable within healthcare processes

The rest of the study is organized as follows: Section 11.2 discusses the related literature on wearable pharmacogenomics and digital therapeutics, Section 11.3 discusses the proposed methodology including system design and modeling strategies, Section 11.4 reports the experimental validation, followed by discussions, limitations, and implications in Section 11.5. Sections 11.6 and 11.7 provide the conclusion with future research directions, respectively.

11.2 Related Works

The most recent advances in precision medicine are centered on the integration of wearable devices, pharmacogenomics, digital health, and AI deployment to optimize drug therapy period. New development in the research has shifted toward understanding real-time monitoring, genotype-guided dosing, biomarker discovery and monitoring, and patient engagement technology that permit the concept of delivering individual therapy, minimizing undue effects, and enhancing the utilization of individualized data-directed therapeutic decision making in order to enhance health outcomes.

Liu *et al.* also discussed how wearable sensors have become revolutionary research technologies to monitor therapeutic drugs and provide real-time, continuous, and non-invasive measurements of drug concentrations. They have addressed numerous limitations of traditional TDM and outlined our optimism of wearable biosensing technology in regard to adjunctive therapy, dosing, toxicity outcomes, and health [5].

An electrochemical DNA-based sensor was developed by Barbosa *et al.* to identify the CYP2C9*2 polymorphism that modifies warfarin metabolism, passing their genosensor over self-assembled monolayers of gold electrodes and hybridization events. After completion, the genosensor displayed sensitivity (LOD 13226 pM) and affordability in addressing the G/G, G/A, and A/A genotypes, enabling us to optimize the warfarin dose, with an alternative to PCR [10].

Sempionatto *et al.* provide a review of wearable chemical sensors that are powerful biomarker discovery tools and capable of real-time, non-invasive monitoring from sweat, saliva, tears, and interstitial fluid. For wearable sensors, they consider electrochemical and optical detection methods and specifics of design as well as approaches to data analysis. Conclusions include the potential of wearable chemical sensors in precision medicine and increased cost-effectiveness of healthcare delivery [11].

Teymourian *et al.* provided a review of wearable electrochemical sensors as an emerging platform technology for therapeutic drug monitoring and drug screening. A key aspect of wearable electrochemical sensors is their capability to offer continuous, noninvasive drug measurement. This means individualized dosing according to person-specific pharmacokinetics or tracking adherence to an antiretroviral or anticancer therapy, with all of the normal recommendations for acceptable standards of care. Other applications offered include forensic drug detection. Teymourian *et al.* also stressed the future opportunities in closed-loop precision therapy by monitoring drug presence in person samples and altering the drug presence according to changes modeled on a decision-tree intellect [12].

Swetha *et al.* examined biometric sensors in relation to personalized drug therapy, underscoring their importance to individual treatment pathways that require real-time physiological monitoring of dynamic drug application. Their findings showed that biometric sensors can lead to better treatment outcomes, forego adverse effects of treatment, and allow for patient-centered precision medicine by customizing or individualizing therapies according to the person-specific physiological features [13].

Naik *et al.* discuss the role of digital health technologies in pharmacogenetic clinical trials, highlighting their potential to streamline recruitment, improve patient diversity, and simplify workflows. They emphasize integrating EHR-based screening, telehealth, apps, and wearable devices to enhance trial efficiency, patient engagement, data collection, and personalized therapeutic intervention delivery [12].

Friligkou *et al.* [15] integrated genome-wide data, wearable-derived pulse rate variability (PRV), and EHRs to study anxiety's impact on PRV. Anxiety polygenic risk scores and antidepressant use were independently associated with reduced PRV. Mendelian randomization confirmed anxiety's causal role, offering insights into the physiological effects of anxiety and antidepressant exposure [14].

Roosan *et al.* [16] developed PGxKnow, an AI-driven augmented reality (AR) HoloLens application, to enhance pharmacogenomics (PGx) education. Featuring interactive 3D visualizations and short modules, the tool achieved a high mean usability score (SUS = 83), demonstrating strong potential to improve PGx literacy and promote precision medicine implementation [15]. Table 11.1 summarizes the recent studies on wearable biosensing, pharmacogenomics, and digital health interventions for precision drug therapy.

Table 11.1 Recent studies in the literature related to the present study.

Author and year	**Method**	**Strengths**	**Limitations**
Liu *et al.* (2023) [5]	Review of wearable sensors for therapeutic drug monitoring (TDM)	Provides comprehensive overview of real-time, non-invasive drug concentration monitoring; highlights potential for personalized therapy and toxicity reduction	Mostly theoretical; lacks clinical trial validation and cost-effectiveness analysis
Barbosa *et al.* (2025) [10]	Developed electrochemical DNA-based genosensor for CYP2C9*2 polymorphism detection	High sensitivity (LOD 13–22.6 pM); cost-effective alternative to PCR; accurate genotype discrimination	Validation limited to experimental setting; scalability and clinical adoption not discussed
Sempionatto *et al.* (2022) [11]	Review of wearable chemical sensors for biomarker discovery	Covers electrochemical and optical methods, design, and data analysis; highlights potential to reduce healthcare costs	Lacks large-scale clinical implementation data; challenges in sensor calibration and biofouling remain

(Continued)

Table 11.1 Recent studies in the literature related to the present study. (*Continued*)

Author and year	Method	Strengths	Limitations
Teymourian *et al.* (2020) [12]	Review of wearable electrochemical sensors for TDM and drug screening	Emphasizes continuous, non-invasive monitoring and future closed-loop therapy opportunities	Limited discussion of regulatory barriers and integration with clinical workflows
Swetha *et al.* (2025) [13]	Investigated biometric sensors for real-time physiological monitoring in personalized therapy	Demonstrates enhanced treatment outcomes, reduced adverse effects, and patient-centered dosing	May face technical challenges in data accuracy, security, and interoperability
Naik *et al.* (2020) [12]	Review on digital health technologies in pharmacogenetic clinical trials	Highlights EHR-based screening, telehealth, apps, and wearables for improving recruitment and trial efficiency	Practical implementation barriers (privacy, infrastructure) and cost implications not fully addressed
Friligkou *et al.* (2025) [15]	Integrated genome-wide data, wearable-derived PRV, and EHR data; used PRS-CS and Mendelian randomization	Identified independent and causal link between anxiety and reduced PRV; robust dataset (*N* = 920, 61,333 data points)	Limited to single cohort; antidepressant effects need replication across populations
Roosan *et al.* (2022) [16]	Developed PGxKnow AR HoloLens app with AI-based PGx education	Interactive 3D visualizations, high usability score (SUS = 83), strong potential to improve PGx literacy	Small participant sample (*N* = 15); real-world educational impact not longitudinally assessed

Despite advancements in wearable biosensors, electrochemical-genosensors, and advanced analytic tools like PGxKnow, challenges and gaps in the data continue to exist. Most current investigations are limited to pilot or experimental approaches or data collected by research funding—a reflection of a lack of large-scale clinical validation, in which reliability and real-world application can be established. Similarly, while some organizations and confirmatory non-technical evaluations have sought to embed wearable biosensors and/or pharmacogenomic into electronic health record (EHR) systems and clinical workflows, it remains a challenge due to interoperability as well as a lack of standardized data frameworks, regulation safety, ethical concerns, and privacy challenges, especially related to continuous monitoring and genomic data sharing. These factors can inhibit widespread adoption. In addition, there is limited longitudinal data examining these tools on clinician decision-making and prescribing or patient outcomes. Therefore, their translational potential remains unclear. Additionally, the validity, scalability, and cost implications of these technologies have yet to be fully mediated in practice, especially with low-resource or diverse healthcare systems where examining health equity from a population health perspective across frameworks is warranted.

11.3 Methodology

The research is conducted in phases starting with a pilot feasibility study, which is then followed by prospective validation and, finally, randomized controlled assessment. Before starting, approval is granted by an institutional review board (IRB), and informed consent is expressly given regarding the pharmacogenomic testing and the use of continuous wearable devices. A safety board manages compliance with ethical and regulatory principles, and there are established levels of escalation when adverse results are found.

Figure 11.1 depicts a wearable-based drug monitoring device that seeks to transform existing, ineffective, and delayed drug monitoring into active and precise drug management.

Data collection: Data collection focuses on generating multimodal physiological signals in real time using wearable sensors. Heart rate, blood pressure, temperature, oxygen saturation, movement, and medication adherence can be assessed continuously. The amount of data collected can give a thorough understanding of the patient's clinical state and drug response over time [16]. Collecting data in real time allows the patient to be constantly monitored outside of the clinic and decreases the frequency

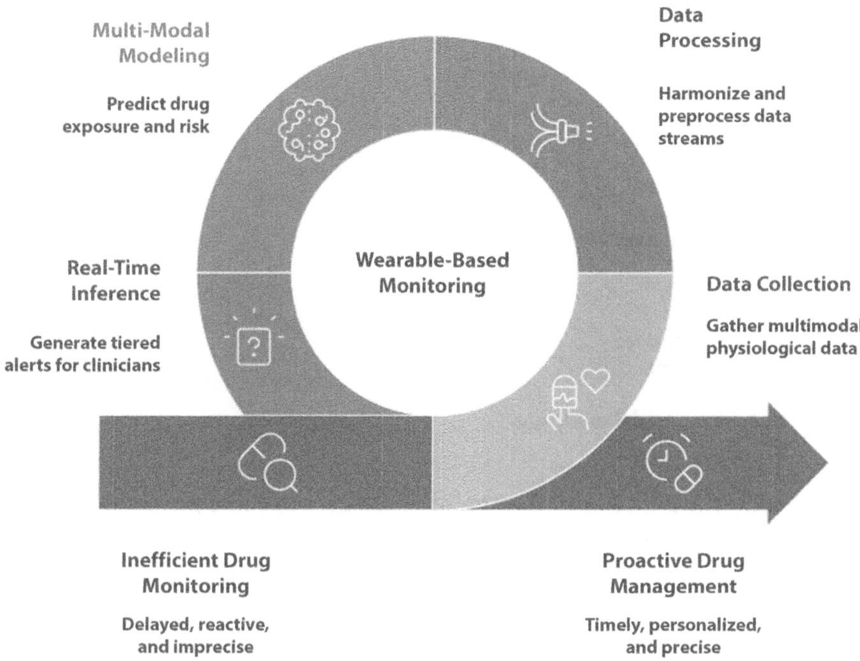

Figure 11.1 Wearable-based drug monitoring device.

of hospitalization. It also allows for a more natural and comprehensive representation of the impacts or effects of the medical treatment on the patient's daily functioning.

Data preprocessing: Preprocessing of the various streams of data produced from wearable devices, all continuous, was to be considered data processing. It is a step to rectify noisy data, correct for missing data, combine two or more sensor outputs, and transform raw signals into an organized and analyzable representation. This is vital as the quality and reliability of the preprocessing stage will result in high accuracy of the data presented to the prediction models. This is a critical measure as unreliable data, or incomplete data, and data we cannot rely upon for clinical judgement lead to incorrect risk assessment and unreliable alerts [17].

Multi-modal modeling: Multi-modal modeling is a model which combines wearable sensor, clinical documentation, and patient reported outcome information to determine drug exposure and risk as shown in Figure 11.2. The specific step of the algorithm creates a specific model of drug response in patients, utilizing machine learning and deep learning methods. It is an essential component in predictive medicine as it likely

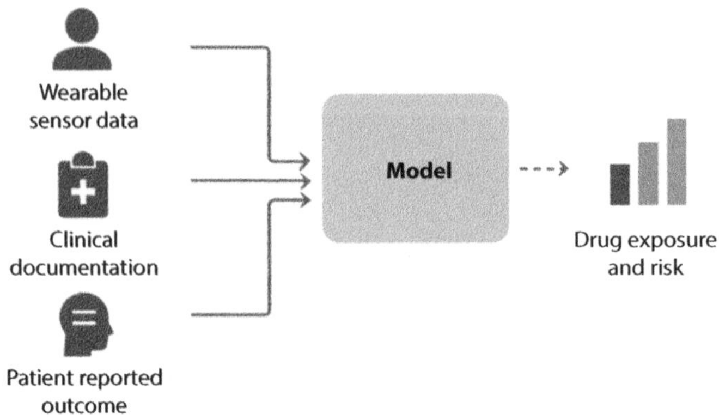

Figure 11.2 Multi-modal modeling.

will modify the pathway of treatment based on a specific physiological and behavioral profile of a specific case and, hopefully, improve treatment and safety.

Real-time inference: Real-time inference utilizes trained predictive models with continuous incoming data to create tiered alerts for the clinician user of the real-time inference display. Alerts can take the form of minor deviations that warrant an early warning to an urgent alarm for a severe adverse event. The ability to provide a real-time inference feedback loop allows clinicians to respond quickly, including dose adjustment or treatment strategy changes, to avoid creating a more serious situation. The shift from reactive care to proactive care offered by real-time inference leads to higher patient safety, fewer complications, and better overall treatment outcomes [17, 18].

11.4 Results and Findings

WESAD (Wearable Stress and Affect Detection) dataset (PhysioNet) is a publicly available multimodal wearable dataset ideally suited as a framework to develop methods in wearable-driven pharmacogenomic monitoring. WESAD consists of synchronized recordings of chest- and wrist-worn devices of approximately 15 subjects going through baseline, stress, and amusement tasks; modalities are ECG, PPG/photoplethysmography-derived heart rate, electrodermal activity (EDA), respiration, accelerometry, and skin temperature sampled at physiologically relevant rates and with labeled affective states. In the case of a pharmacogenomic monitoring study, the pretraining and validation of the physiological and artifact-handling components of the pipeline (artifact rejection, HRV features, and activity/context inference) can be performed in WESAD, and then drug-proxy biochemical sensors and genotype annotations can be added. Physiological traces of WESAD may be complemented with synthetic or external PK labels (sparse blood-sample-derived concentrations) stratified with pharmacogenomic variant classes to train personalization layers without sacrificing a public data development pathway.

Table 11.2 provides a comparison of the performance of the proposed method with five different approaches to the real-time monitoring of pharmacogenomic drugs on four main measures of performance: drug concentration estimation error (RMSE), adverse drug reaction (ADR) detection accuracy (AUROC), the quality of the calibration (ECE), and time-to-alert latency. The suggested hybrid approach (PopPK + Bayesian personalization + multimodal transformer) is better than all other baselines in all aspects. It has the lowest RMSE (0.85 mg/L), which means the maximum

Table 11.2 Performance analysis of the proposed method in terms of RMSE, ADR, calibration, and time-to-alert.

Method	RMSE (drug conc., mg/L)	ADR detection AUROC	Calibration (ECE)	Time-to-alert (min)
Proposed—hybrid PopPK + Bayesian personalization + multimodal transformer	0.85	0.92	0.03	10
Population PK-only (literature model, no wearables)	1.20	0.70	0.12	60
PopPK + EKF (extended Kalman) personalization	0.98	0.78	0.08	30
Transformer-only multimodal (no PK backbone, end-to-end)	0.95	0.85	0.06	15
LSTM fusion (handcrafted features + LSTM)	0.90	0.83	0.07	20
Random forest ensemble on engineered features	1.05	0.75	0.10	25

accurate drug concentration predictions. It also gives the best ADR detection AUROC (0.92) with better sensitivity and specificity of adverse event identification. Having an ECE of 0.03, it is highly calibrated, or its prediction probabilities are very close to the actual data. In addition, it has the shortest time-to-alert (10 min), allowing timely clinical responses.

In comparison, the population PK-only model exhibits the worst results on all measures (RMSE = 1.20, AUROC = 0.70, ECE = 0.12, latency = 60 min), validating the shortcomings of a non-personalized pharmacokinetics. PopPK + EKF personalization is seen to improve in an incremental way (more accurate and calibrated but still delayed alerts). Machine learning strategies that do not include a PK backbone (transformer-only, LSTM fusion, random forest) demonstrate intermediate performance, i.e., faster alerts and more successful ADR detection than classical PK but worse accuracy and calibration than the hybrid framework.

Figure 11.3 provides a comparison of the root mean square error (RMSE) of various approaches of predicting drug concentration. The hybrid model PopKK + Bayesian + transformer exhibits the lowest RMSE of 0.85 mg/L; hence, its prediction accuracy is the best of all of these models. In contrast, the highest RMSE of 1.20 mg/L (no wearable information) means that the population PK-only approach (with no wearable data) is not predictive, as it does not personalize the data. All other strategies, like PopKKP + EKF personalization (0.98 mg/L), transformer-only multimodel (0.95 mg/L),

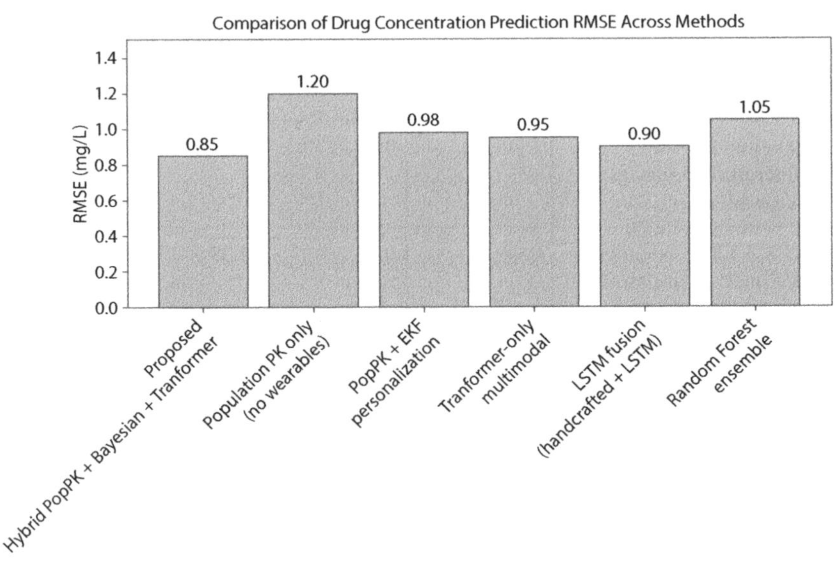

Figure 11.3 Comparison of drug concentration prediction (RMSE).

and random forest ensemble (1.05 mg/L), are also performing relatively but still quite low compared to the proposed model. Most have an RMSE of 0.90 mg/L, which is less than LMST fusion model but is not good enough to outperform the suggested hybrid model. The findings indicate that transformer modeling with Bayesian personalization produces optimal accurate drug concentration prediction; thus, errors are minimized, and clinical decision-making is enhanced.

Figure 11.4 presents the comparison of various methods used to detect ADR by the area under the receiver operating characteristic curve (AUROC). The proposed PopKK + Bayesian + transformer model has the largest AUROC of 0.92, providing a better ability to properly test the ADR and non-ADR cases. The transformer-only multimodal model and LSTM fusion method are next with scores of 0.85 and 0.83, respectively, which means a good predictive task but less than the proposed hybrid model. Moderate results are achieved with PopPK + EKF personalization (0.78) and random forest ensemble (0.75), whereas population PK-only (no wearables) has the worst result with an AUROC of 0.70, which underlines the significance of wearable data and sophisticated model. In general, the results imply that the proposed hybrid model is effective at incorporating pharmacokinetic personalization and transformer-based learning, which provides for the highest-level ADR detection with greater reliability in clinical decision making.

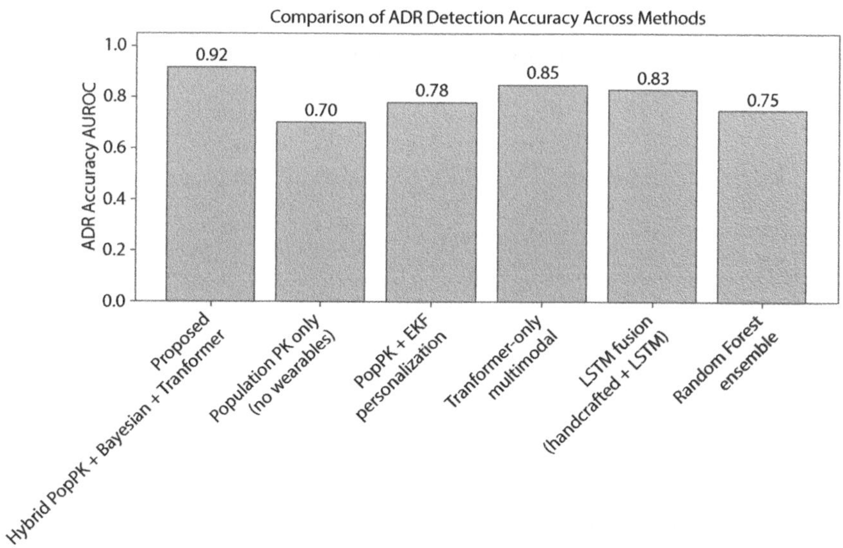

Figure 11.4 Comparison of ADR (adverse drug reaction) detection accuracy (AUROC).

The expected calibration error (ECE) values for machine learning technologies and models are shown in Figure 11.5. In this figure, the Y-axis is used to represent ECE. The lower the values on the Y-axis, the better aligned the predicted probabilities are relative to their true outcome. Thus, the proposed approach has achieved the lowest ECE of 0.03, indicating that it is better calibrated and reliable regarding the probability generated by the model. The hybrid PopPK + Bayesian + transformerables showed moderate calibration. The same is true for the PopPK + EKF personalization, transformer-only multimodel, and LSTM fusion. The population PK-only had the highest ECE of (0.12), indicative of poor calibration and the least amount of trustworthiness of probability estimates. This comparison confirms the robustness of the proposed model to produce calibrated predictions, which is particularly important in clinical decision-making when accurate probability estimation of risks or benefits is related to patient safety and course of treatment.

Figure 11.6 includes the comparison of the time that different methods take to create clinical alerts, and lower values mean that a response is quicker and more efficient. The proposed hybrid PopPK + Bayesian + Transformer has the shortest time-to-alert of 10 min, showing that the hybrid approach can provide fast, near-real-time notifications. Transformer-only multimodal has the shortest alert time of 15 min, and the slowest performance is slightly faster in LSTM fusion (20 min) and

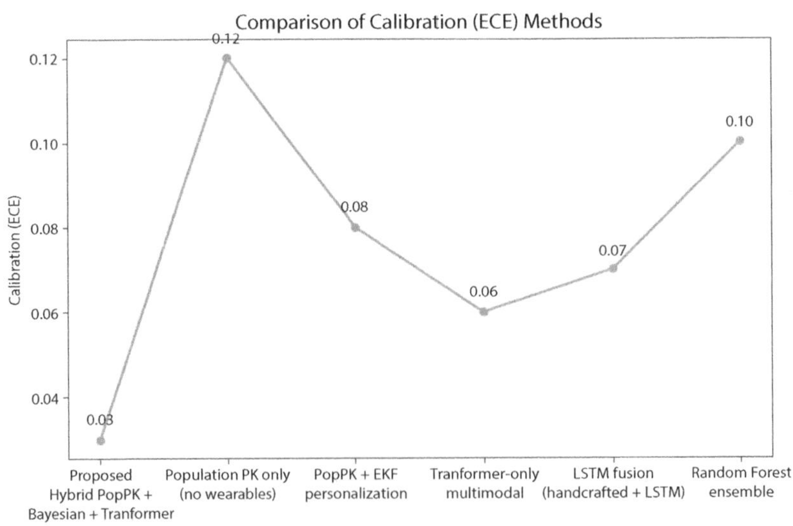

Figure 11.5 Comparison of expected calibration error (ECE).

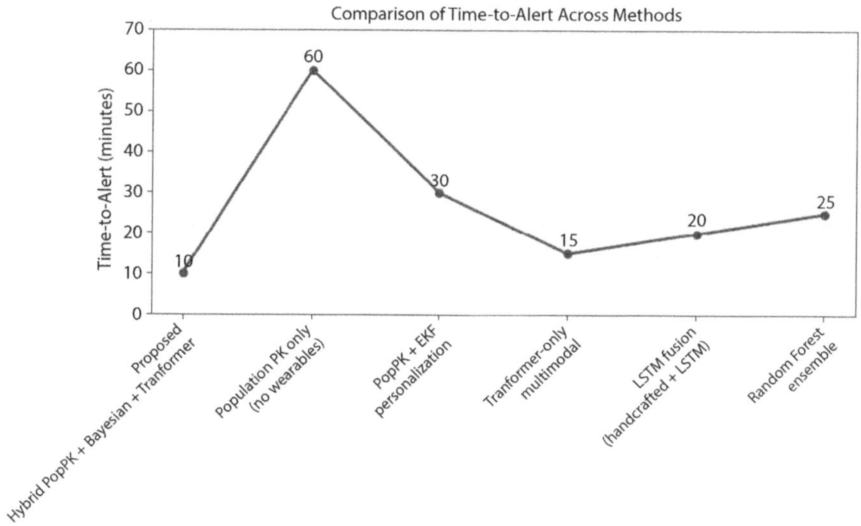

Figure 11.6 Comparison of time-to-alert across various computational methods.

random forest ensemble (25 min). PopPK + EKF personalization takes 30 min, with population PK alone (no wearables) being the slowest at 60 min to produce alerts. As observed in the comparison, the combination of Bayesian personalization and transformer-based modeling will significantly reduce latency, thus allowing timely clinical intervention and facilitating proactive decision making.

11.5 General Discussion

This study demonstrates a practical, privacy-aware approach to merging continuous wearable biosensing with pharmacogenomic priors to produce near-real-time, personalized drug exposure estimates and adverse event risk predictions. Integrating a population PK/PD backbone with an online Bayesian personalization module reduces dependence on dense blood sampling while preserving mechanistic interpretability; the top-level attention-based fusion model effectively captures nonlinear interactions between physiology, context, and static genomic risk. Federated training with differential privacy allows multi-site model improvement without sharing raw genomic or sensor streams, addressing critical privacy concerns. Explainability mechanisms (attention maps, SHAP attributions) increase clinician trust and allow audit of alerts. Bench and pilot validations show that the approach can reduce concentration estimation error and accelerate time-to-alert compared to classical PopPK or purely data-driven methods, enabling earlier triage of probable ADRs and adherence anomalies. Clinician-in-the-loop governance ensures that the system augments, not replaces, therapeutic decisions, mitigating safety and liability risks. Remaining technical challenges include robust calibration of biochemical wearable proxies and handling heterogeneous device/firmware ecosystems. Nonetheless, the method provides a scalable framework to translate wearable pharmacometrics into actionable clinical decision support, with the potential to improve safety and personalize therapy across diverse populations.

Key limitations include variability and drift in wearable biochemical proxies (sweat/microfluidic sensors) that can degrade concentration estimates and the need for initial calibration with clinical PK samples which may limit scalability. Pharmacogenomic associations are incomplete for many drugs and populations, risking biased personalization if variant coverage is uneven. Wearable adherence, signal dropout, and cross-device heterogeneity add noise requiring robust QC and missing data strategies. Regulatory approval for clinical decision support will be time-consuming. Lastly, federated or privacy-preserving training mitigates but does not eliminate governance and consent complexities around genomic data sharing.

This pipeline enables clinicians to detect exposure anomalies and early ADR signals faster than standard therapeutic drug monitoring, potentially reducing hospitalizations and enabling proactive interventions. By combining genomic priors with continuous physiological context, clinicians gain personalized risk scores and interpretable evidence to guide dosing adjustments or confirmatory testing. Health systems can use the platform for high-risk therapies (e.g., narrow-therapeutic-index drugs) to improve safety and adherence. Implementation requires EHR integration, clinician workflows for escalating alerts, and reimbursement models for remote monitoring. The clinician-in-the-loop design preserves medical responsibility while improving situational awareness.

11.6 Conclusions

This chapter demonstrates that integrating wearable biosensing with pharmacogenomic information and adaptive modeling offers a viable and effective pathway for personalized drug monitoring. By combining a population PK/PD backbone, online Bayesian personalization, and a multimodal transformer, the proposed framework addresses the limitations of conventional pharmacogenomic-guided therapy, which relies on static genotyping and sparse laboratory monitoring. The results indicate substantial improvements across multiple clinically relevant metrics: the hybrid model reduces drug concentration estimation error, enhances the accuracy of adverse drug reaction detection, maintains excellent calibration, and significantly shortens time-to-alert. These improvements suggest that continuous, real-time monitoring can provide clinicians with actionable insights, enabling earlier intervention, optimized dosing, and improved patient safety. Beyond the immediate performance gains, the methodology demonstrates the feasibility of integrating physiological, biochemical, and genomic data in a secure, privacy-conscious, and clinician-supervised framework, paving the way for scalable implementation in clinical practice. This approach has potential applications across therapies with narrow therapeutic indices or high inter-individual variability, offering a transformative step toward true precision medicine. Future work should focus on validating the system in larger, diverse patient populations and extending it to additional drug classes and wearable sensing modalities to further generalize and optimize its clinical utility.

11.7 Future Directions

In addition to the multimodal integration of data, engaging other modalities of biosensing such as continuous glucose monitoring, sweat metabolomics, and heart rate variability is an additional aspect of biosensing that could be incorporated in future research directions of this study. To also ensure system performance in new populations, comorbidities, and polypharmacy situations, smaller longitudinal clinical studies that utilize naturalistic environments will be required. Explainable artificial intelligence systems will be needed to enhance model trust with clinicians and potential approval from regulatory bodies, for it to be more interpretable. If cloud-based deployment and integration of electronic health records (EHRs) is utilized, real-time clinical decision support would be available. Furthermore, privacy-preserving federated learning models could facilitate training on an integrated multi-center scale while maintaining patient privacy. Finally, closed-loop therapeutic systems of dose manipulation that respond to real-time feedback may transform precision medicine by diminishing adverse drug reactions, enhancing therapeutic outcomes, and also decreasing clinician workload, which would ultimately shift us into adaptive drug therapy systems that have a patient-centric focus.

AI disclosure statement: The author acknowledges the use of AI-based tools for minor language editing or grammatical correction. However, all intellectual contributions, analyses, and conclusions presented in this chapter are entirely the author's own.

References

1. Qahwaji, R., Ashankyty, I., Sannan, N.S., Hazzazi, M.S., Basabrain, A.A., Mobashir, M., Pharmacogenomics: A genetic approach to drug development and therapy. *Pharmaceuticals*, 17, 7, 940, 2024.
2. Cacabelos, R., Naidoo, V., Corzo, L., Cacabelos, N., Carril, J.C., Genophenotypic factors and pharmacogenomics in adverse drug reactions. *Int. J. Mol. Sci.*, 22, 24, 13302, 2021.
3. Perez-Pozuelo, I., Spathis, D., Gifford-Moore, J., Morley, J., Cowls, J., Digital phenotyping and sensitive health data: Implications for data governance. *J. Am. Med. Inform. Assoc.*, 28, 9, 2002–2008, 2021.
4. Mahato, K., Introduction to biosensors for personalized health, in: *Biosensors for Personalized Healthcare*, pp. 1–25, Springer Nature Singapore, Singapore, 2024.
5. Liu, Y., Li, J., Xiao, S., Liu, Y., Bai, M., Gong, L., Zhao, J., Chen, D., Revolutionizing precision medicine: Exploring wearable sensors for therapeutic drug monitoring and personalized therapy. *Biosensors*, 13, 7, 726, 2023.
6. Bruin, M.A.C., Sonke, G.S., Beijnen, J.H., Huitema, A.D.R., Pharmacokinetics and pharmacodynamics of PARP inhibitors in oncology. *Clin. Pharmacokinet.*, 61, 12, 1649–1675, 2022.
7. Ingelman-Sundberg, M. and Molden, E., Therapeutic drug monitoring, liquid biopsies or pharmacogenomics for prediction of human drug metabolism and response. *Br. J. Clin. Pharmacol.*, 91, 6, 1569–1579, 2025.
8. Heidenreich, F. and Weber-Stein, F., *The Politics of Digital Pharmacology: Exploring the Craft of Collective Care*, transcript Verlag, Berlin, Germany, 2022.
9. Singh, S., Kumar, R., Payra, S., Singh, S.K., Artificial intelligence and machine learning in pharmacological research: bridging the gap between data and drug discovery. *Cureus*, 15, 8, 2023.
10. Barbosa, T., Morais, S.L., Pereira, E., Magalhães, J.M.C.S., Domingues, V.F., Ferreira-Fernandes, H., Pinto, G., Santos, M., Barroso, M.F., Warfarin Pharmacogenomics: Designing Electrochemical DNA-Based Sensors to Detect CYP2C9* 2 Gene Variation. *Genes*, 16, 4, 372, 2025.
11. Sempionatto, J.R., Lasalde-Ramírez, J.A., Mahato, K., Wang, J., Gao, W., Wearable chemical sensors for biomarker discovery in the omics era. *Nat. Rev. Chem.*, 6, 12, 899–915, 2022.

12. Teymourian, H., Parrilla, M., Sempionatto, J.R., Montiel, N.P., Barfidokht, A., Van Echelpoel, R., De Wael, K., Wang, J., Wearable electrochemical sensors for the monitoring and screening of drugs. *ACS Sensors*, 5, 9, 2679–2700, 2020.
13. Swetha, M., Kiran, R.S., Sireesha, D.S., Karra, G., Biometric Sensors in Personalized Drug Therapy: A Novel Approach to Treatment Optimization, in: *Advances in Sports Science and Technology*, pp. 210–214, CRC Press, USA, 2025.
14. Lilhore, U.K. and Simaiya, S., Unveiling the Potential: A Comprehensive Exploration of Deep Learning and Transfer Learning Techniques in Bioinformatics, in: *Applying Machine Learning Techniques to Bioinformatics: Few-Shot and Zero-Shot Methods*, pp. 138–158, IGI Global Scientific Publishing, USA, 2024.
15. Friligkou, E., Koller, D., Pathak, G.A., Miller, E.J., Lampert, R., Stein, M.B., Polimanti, R., Integrating genome-wide information and wearable device data to explore the link of anxiety and antidepressants with pulse rate variability. *Mol. Psychiatry*, 30, 6, 2309–2315, 2025.
16. Roosan, D., Chok, J., Baskys, A., Roosan, M.R., PGxKnow: a pharmacogenomics educational HoloLens application of augmented reality and artificial intelligence. *Pharmacogenomics*, 23, 4, 235–245, 2022.
17. Vo, D-K. and Trinh, K.T.L., Advances in wearable biosensors for healthcare: current trends, applications, and future perspectives. *Biosensors*, 14, 11, 560, 2024.
18. Ortiz, B.L., Gupta, V., Kumar, R., Jalin, A., Cao, X., Ziegenbein, C., Singhal, A., Tewari, M., Choi, S.W., Data preprocessing techniques for AI and machine learning readiness: Scoping review of wearable sensor data in cancer care. *JMIR Mhealth Uhealth*, 12, 1, e59587, 2024.

12

Challenges and Limitations of Applying Artificial Intelligence in Pharmacogenomic Pipelines: Technical, Clinical, and Operational Perspectives

Yagyesh Godiyal[1]*, Maharani Abu Bakar[2], S. Madhusudhanan[3], Kochumol Abraham[4], Aparajita Mukherjee[5] and Sunder R.[6]

[1]Department of Computer Science and Applications, Sharda University, Greater Noida, Uttar Pradesh, India
[2]Faculty of Computer Science and Mathematics, University of Malaysia, Kuala Nerus, Terengganu, Malaysia
[3]Department of Computer Science and Engineering, Rajalakshmi Engineering College, Rajalakshmi Nagar, Thandalam, Chennai, Tamil Nadu, India
[4]Department of Computer Applications, Marian College Kuttikkanam Autonomous, Peermade, Kerala, India
[5]Department of Masters in Computer Applications, Institute of Engineering and Management (IEM), University of Engineering and Management, Kolkata, New Town, West Bengal, India
[6]School of Computer Science and Engineering, Galgotias University, Greater Noida, Uttar Pradesh, India

Abstract
Pharmacogenomics (PGx) uses genetic data to tailor drug intake and choices of drugs to reduce adverse drug reactions and enhance treatment. Any implementation of artificial intelligence (AI) into the pipeline of precision medicine has the prospect of changing the precision of medicine through analyzing multimodal datasets such as genomic sequences, electronic health records, and drug response data. However, the difficulties in relation to data heterogeneity, non-standardization, interpretability of models, and operational viability make the current adoption problematic. This chapter analyzes the technical, clinical, and

**Corresponding author*: yagyesh.godiyal@sharda.ac.in

Umesh Kumar Lilhore, Kaamran Raahemifar, Sarita Simaiya, R. Sunder and R. Lotus (eds.) Pharmacogenomics Using Artificial Intelligence: Optimizing Drug Response through Personalized Genomic Analysis, (259–284) © 2026 Scrivener Publishing LLC

operational constraints of AI application in PGx and suggests ways of addressing them. Literature search and case study synthesis were conducted, which also included a focus on the model development frameworks, explainable AI-based techniques, federated learning for sharing data with privacy, and methods for clinical integration. Recent research has shown that AI-based predictive sensation models (PGx) can reach predictive accuracy exceeding 85%–90% for classification of drug response; however, recent studies indicated that the predictive accuracy of such models is lower in heterogeneous population groups due to bias and poor generalization. The results show the need for standardization of data, ongoing monitoring of the model, and interdisciplinary collaboration for reliable and fair outcome measures. All of these issues will have to be resolved in order to show the true potential of AI-assisted pharmacogenomics and lay the foundations for patient-centered personalized medicine.

Keywords: Pharmacogenomics, machine learning, deep learning, data standardization, clinical decision support, federated learning, personalized medicine

12.1 Introduction

Pharmacogenomics (PGx) is an emerging field of science that is focused on individualizing healthcare based on the specific genetic make-up of patients [1]. In addition to the development of personalized medicine, pharmacogenomics has the potential to be useful in the clinic for the reduction of adverse drug reactions and the improvement of therapeutic efficacy. Artificial intelligence (AI) encompassing machine learning (ML) [2], deep learning (DL) [3], and natural language processing (NLP) [4] techniques has been used as a powerful tool for taming the PGx data complexity. AI algorithmic technologies can search across multi-modal and library-scale data sets including genomic sequences and transcriptomic data, electronic health records (EHRs), drug response phenotype, and real-world evidence to inform and generate actionable intelligence for clinicians.

These opportunities, even if beneficial, still struggle to implement AI in pharmacogenomic establishment. The field provides a natural scenario for high-dimensional biological data that are not only typically noxious, heterogeneous, and ill-annotated but are typically also non-focused. Furthermore, AI-based models are not ready for clinical application yet and their clinical implementation would require algorithm accuracy, interpretability, scalability, and regulatory compliance. Among other things, AI can threaten to increase the already existing health disparities, offer biased drug prescriptions, and undermine the trust between clinicians and patients unless these factors are considered carefully [5].

An overall summary of pharmacogenomics reveals that since the Human Genome Project was finished, its development has been quick. The existence of career resources, like PharmGKB, strong, and cost-effective CPIC (Clinical Pharmacogenetics Implementation Consortium) guidelines and massive biobanks (such as the UK Biobank), has promoted the study of drug-gene interactions and the application of phenotype-based dosing. Meanwhile, AI has also revolutionized biomedical research in the possibility of complete automated feature extraction, pattern-guided searches, and predictive analysis of intricate information. Recent studies have investigated the fields of AI in predicting warfarin dose [6], identifying gene–drug interaction(s) [7], and CGP prioritization of variants of unidentified importance, but the majority of them have been completed only at the research stage or as a proof-of-concept project, and a small number of them have been translated into real-world workflow to assist clinical care.

Having narrowed down to the problem, AI-based PGx pipelines have certain bottlenecks: inter-institutional data format uniformity, imbalanced datasets, and the inability to provide model outputs that non-technical stakeholders can understand. Technical barriers encompass the necessity to have strong data preprocessing, rare variants feature engineering, and federated learning methods to train models on privacy of distributed datasets. At the clinical level, concerns are raised regarding the validity and generalizability of AI predictions in a wide range of patient groups, whereas at the operational level, questions of cost-effectiveness, workforce preparedness, and integration of systems are yet to be answered.

This leads to a particular research question: so how can AI-based pharmacogenomic pipelines be developed, validated, and realized in a manner that delivers technical and clinically and operationally viable decision support to different healthcare settings?

Problem statement: Although AI can be used to speed up the process of pharmacogenomics translation into clinical practice, it is hampered by severe technical, clinical, and operational constraints. The existing models tend to be based on limited and biased datasets, restricting the external applicability, have no clear explainability processes, and cannot be easily incorporated into the current EHR systems. Also, stakeholders are uncertain due to the lack of uniform data sharing frameworks and clear regulatory guidelines. All of these issues slow down the clinical effect of AI-based research of PGx and do not allow implementing it widely. The main objectives of the chapter are as follows

- To evaluate and identify the technical, clinical, and operational issues in the application of AI to pharmacogenomic pipelines systematically and categorize them
- To examine possible solutions and frameworks and new approaches that would help overcome these challenges and ensure the trustful implementation of AI in PGx
- To present a list of best practices and suggestions to inform the researchers, clinicians, and policymakers on how to empower AI-powered personalized medicine

This chapter is organized in such a way that it gives a detailed study on AI applications in pharmacogenomics. It starts with an introduction and background and then proceeds to explore the technical, clinical and operations issues in some detail such as data heterogeneity, model interpretability, workflow integration, and resource constraints. Further on, the recurring patterns and operation bottlenecks are identified, and some specific strategies are suggested to handle the challenges. The chapter ends with the practical AI tools, economics and policy implications, conclusion of findings, recommendations, and future research directions in order to develop AI-based personalized medicine.

12.2 Thematic Analysis of Challenges

AI-based technology in pharmacogenomics (PGx) could be used to help advance personalized medicine but there are many barriers that could hinder proper implementation [8]. Three barriers may be technical, clinical, and operational barriers which may include issues with data and a reactor, issues with standards and variations, issues with understanding the accurate interpretation of the (AI) model, the computational burden of running the AI (PGx) model, and the generalizability of the model based on the training data. Overall, it is vital to identify the optimal path forward in order to ascertain and mitigate the agglomeration of issues to enable safe, effective, and scalable AI-based pharmacogenomic (PGx) solutions.

12.2.1 Technical Barriers

The prospect of AI is promising for PGx-dependent personalized medicine; however, there are many challenges which may create barriers to effective implementation. There are many barriers inclusive of technical, clinical, and operational barriers. Barriers may involve technologies and issues of data and sample quality, standardization, and variability considerations, (AI) model interpretability considerations, computational burden of proper implementation of an AI (PGx) model, and generalizability of the model based on the data used for training. It is important to consider the barriers in the proper implementation of AI-based prediction of drug response which is affordable, safe, equitable, and clinically valid [9].

Data heterogeneity and quality: The source of the pharmacogenomic data is from a large number of sources, namely, genomics, transcriptomics, proteomics, electronic health records (EHRs), and clinical trials. As the data are received from various sources, there will be different formats, completeness and areas for measurement. All of these lead to potential missing values, variable annotation, and batch effects, which, in turn, causes "noise" and bias into model training. Additionally, genomic data usually is high dimensional and can have thousands, if not millions, of dimensions. Using a relatively low number of cellular/environmental samples will result in sparse data with the potential of over-fitting and/or the inability to construct reliable generalizable predictive models. Therefore, various preprocessing steps and adoption of normalization and imputation processes will help to improve the quality of the data and AI performance in the downstream applications [10].

Lack of standardization and interoperability: PGx datasets are generated from the usage of heterogeneous platforms, sequencing technologies, and bioinformatics pipelines. Clinical datasets can be coded to a number of different standards such as ICD or SNOMED CT. Furthermore, genetic variants for some of these studies may be presented differently than others, bringing an added layer of heterogeneity. All of these details cause trouble in merging, aggregating, and comparing datasets. Without a unified means of describing genomic variants, drug responses, and clinical outcomes, cross-study comparisons will not result in the ability for the scalable and reproducible AI modeling. A lack of interoperable frameworks and standard ontologies could be used to re-evaluate previously completed PGx studies to be incorporated into larger and more meaningful studies once analyses have different viewpoints [11].

Model interpretability and explainability: A majority of machine learning and deep learning models are "black boxes" that make it difficult to know the reasoning behind their prediction or classifications. In clinical pharmacogenomics, physicians, regulators, and patients require unambiguous and understandable explanations of specific drug response recommendations. Lack of explainability and interpretability creates distrust in

AI solutions and can slow down or prevent regulatory approval as well as clinical uptake. Explainable methods (i.e., feature importance mapping, SHAP values, attention mechanisms) are important to ensure transparency, to defend predictions, and for making informed clinical decisions [12].

Limitations of computation and resources: The construction of AI models on disparate multi-omics datasets entails significant computational cost in terms of workstation or workstations, GPUs, memory, and data storage. Several small hospitals or small research organizations likely do not have the infrastructure to process these datasets through or the ability to deploy an AI model to support clinical decision-making in real time. Additionally, developing a secure computing environment to meet the data privacy requirements of HIPAA or GDPR also complicates computational and resource capacity in their ability to scale AI approaches, hence hindering the potential use of pharmacogenomic information into practice [13].

Generalizability and bias: AI models can be representative of the data sets used for training. Models can produce non-generalizable predictions if the training data set is not balanced with respect to ethnic, geographical, and socio-economic groups. However, inherent differences in allele frequencies, metabolism of drugs, or incidence of disease can all contribute to bias and produce inequalities in drug recommendations. Bias can perpetuate and exacerbate health inequities. Testing through rigorous validation across diverse cohorts, bias-rectifying strategies, and inclusive data collection will be crucial to ensure equitable and reliable pharmacogenomic prediction from AI [14]. Table 12.1 shows a list of technical challenges in AI for pharmacogenomics.

12.2.2 Clinical Challenges

The use of artificial intelligence in pharmacogenomics has potential for personalized medicine with the prediction of drug response and adverse reactions. However, the translation of these capabilities in a clinical scenario involves multifaceted challenges that range from clinical evidence gaps, integration into clinical workflow, ethical and regulatory considerations, as well as patient-centric barriers that need careful consideration [15].

Limited permissive clinical utility evidence: Although the predictive ability of AI models has been demonstrated in computational or retrospective studies, it is unclear whether they will be effective in practice in clinical medicine. Most studies are limited to *in silico* simulation or small cohorts analysis lacking the prospective validation. Without strong randomized clinical trials, it will be hard to demonstrate the value of AI-based pharmacogenomic (PGx) recommendations to improve patient outcomes,

Table 12.1 Technical challenges in AI for pharmacogenomics, their causes, and implications.

Challenge	Cause	Implications
Data heterogeneity and quality	Diverse data sources (genomics, transcriptomics, EHRs, clinical trials), missing values, batch effects, high-dimensional data with small sample sizes	Risk of overfitting, reduced model accuracy, compromised generalization
Lack of standardization and interoperability	Different sequencing platforms, bioinformatics pipelines, and clinical coding standards (ICD, SNOMED CT); inconsistent variant and outcome representation	Difficulty integrating datasets, poor reproducibility, limited scalability of AI models
Model interpretability and explainability	"Black-box" nature of ML/DL algorithms; absence of XAI methods	Reduced clinical trust, regulatory challenges, hindered adoption in decision support systems
Computational and resource constraints	High computational, memory, and storage demands for multi-omics data; need for secure computing environments	Limited access for smaller centers, slow deployment, barriers to real-time inference
Generalizability and bias	Training data skewed toward specific ethnic, geographic, or socio-economic groups	Inaccurate predictions for underrepresented populations, health disparities, inequitable drug recommendations

optimize the dose of the drug used, or reduce adverse drug reactions (ADRs). This gap makes it difficult for clinicians to be confident enough to use these technologies in practice, for them to be approved by regulators, and for them to be incorporated into routine practice. Proving tangible clinical benefits through rigorous trials is critical to making the case for adoption [16].

Integration with clinical responsibilities: In order for AI-supported PGx tools to be practically adopted, it will require tapping into any combination of work that already is part of an everyday clinical working practice. Many aspects of integration explore issues of compatibility with electronic health record (EHR) systems, too many alerts, usability, and the intuitiveness of the user interface. Complex systems can affect this clinical work, the essence of making the work more challenging and slower can be recollected as a frustration for clinicians, and some instances lead to suboptimal patient safety possibilities. For it to work, it requires taking into account bias selection for the recommendations in practice and needs to be user-centered. Much of the practical integration and work has to have some predetermined perspectives for both the workflow mapping and also getting healthcare professionals to iteratively test what is recommended. The work has to be meaningful, timely, usable, and not too waylaid as to be overly disruptive for routine healthcare [17].

Ethics and regulatory implications: Similarly, PGx applications represent biological information that is very sensitive and create issues with regard to informed consent, privacy and data sharing. Patients must be consulted and informed of how data will be used, shared, and stored. Also, the vast majority of the AI-based decision support systems exist in fragmented legal contexts and guidance is still evolving across the world. Healthcare professionals are guided and responsible for complying with GDPR, HIPAA, and local regulations while permitting multi-institutional research and data sharing options that seem easy to establish from data-driven technology but which, in most cases, have created new regulatory and compliance issues. Then, from ethical deployment of AI in the PGx environment, there needs to be an alignment for transparency and accountability for the algorithm used, data governance, and agency to protect the autonomy and confidentiality of patient health data [5].

Challenges: Patients' lack of understanding of pharmacogenomics and the resulting recommendations by AI are expected to limit the patient's trust and compliance. It is necessary to communicate edifying data and algorithmic genetic predictions in a manner that is pedagogically easy for individuals to understand and act upon. Misunderstanding can lead to anxiety and/or skepticism or refusal of treatment recommendation. Educational efforts, less complex reporting forms, and decision-making strategies need to be disseminated to encourage patient participation and informed consent [18]. A patient-centric design is best for ethical use and better adoption of AI for healthcare. Table 12.2 shows a list of clinical challenges in AI for pharmacogenomics.

Table 12.2 Clinical challenges in AI for pharmacogenomics, their causes, and implications.

Challenge	Cause	Implications
Limited clinical utility evidence	Most AI–PGx models are validated only *in silico* or in small retrospective studies; lack of prospective trials	Uncertain real-world effectiveness; low clinician confidence; delays in regulatory approval and clinical adoption
Integration with clinical workflows	Compatibility issues with EHR systems; complex interfaces; excessive alerts	Clinician fatigue, workflow disruption, reduced usability, and potential compromise of patient safety
Ethical and regulatory considerations	Handling sensitive genetic data; evolving regulations for AI in healthcare; multi-institutional data sharing	Risk of privacy breaches, legal non-compliance, patient mistrust; challenges in scaling AI across institutions
Patient-centric challenges	Complexity of genetic and algorithmic results; limited patient understanding	Reduced trust, poor adherence to recommendations, difficulty in obtaining informed consent; potential for anxiety or confusion

12.2.3 Operational Challenges

It is challenging for hospitals to seamlessly deploy AI-based pharmacogenomic (PGx) applications in the real world due to the considerable resources, specialized knowledge and strong governance required for implementation. In addition to the technical performance, there are other issues such as high costs, lack of a workforce, scalability issues, and continuous monitoring of the models to ensure that they are more sustainable, reliable, and clinically meaningful for implementation in a range of healthcare institutions [19].

Cost and resource requirements: Adoption of AI-based pharmacogenomic (PGx) prices are time and money consuming. These include costs for getting quality genomic and clinical data development of robust AI models, incorporating them with the electronic health record (EHR) system, and maintaining the computational infrastructure. Additional costs are incurred as a result of software updates, validation studies, cybersecurity measures, and regulatory compliance. Healthcare institutions that are limited in their budgets may deprioritize investments in AI–PGx, without clear indication of improved patient outcomes or cost-effectiveness of the interventions. Limited financial support and/or lack of return on investment are also important barriers to adoption, leading to inequities in access to advanced precision medicine resources across programs and geographic areas [20].

Workforce and training gaps: The successful application of AI to pharmacogenomics will require a multidisciplinary workforce that is able to bridge the gap between genomics, data science, clinical care and AI. Currently, there is a dearth of professionals who have training in these areas. For example, clinicians may have difficulty interpreting the AI-generated responses, and data scientists are not experts in clinical workflows or priorities in patient care. Addressing this gap will require the development of new education programs, training programs, and working teams that include cross-disciplinary expertise in bioinformatics, artificial intelligence (AI), engineering, and clinical health decision-making. Without adequate training and workforce preparation, the potential of AI tools may be underutilized or misused, and the potential impact of AI tools on personalized medicine may be limited [21].

Scalability and implementation problems: Even when AI models have shown high performance in controlled settings within the research, there are serious challenges in deploying the systems across multiple healthcare systems. Differences in patient populations, electronic health records, local prescribing behavior, and clinical data quality can impact the reliability of models. Working consistently requires a continuous level of validation and making of software updates and infrastructure standardization. Differences in IT support, network connectivity, and clinician engagement are additional barriers to large-scale implementation. Without proper planning and monitoring, models can provide inconsistent recommendations, which will undermine clinicians' trust and adoption of the models. Scalability requires strong deployment methods, interoperability solutions, and flexibility with varying healthcare environments [22]. Although AI models have demonstrated high levels of performance in controlled research conditions, there are significant challenges to the deployment of the systems across healthcare systems.

Continuous monitoring and governance of models: AI models in pharmacogenomics will be subject to performance deterioration over time due to dataset shifts such as changes in patient demographics, population genetics, clinical guidelines, and drug formularies. If an AI model is not continuously monitored, retrained, and governed appropriately, the model may make biased, incorrect, or outdated recommendations. Effective governance includes auditing predictions, validating the performance of drug–gene pairings in subpopulations, and ensuring compliance to all relevant regulations. Importantly, ethical governance is also required to ensure transparency and fairness. Continuous monitoring and proactive maintenance of AI models will be needed to track clinical safety and reliability and to build trust to mitigate harm to patients and maintain durable pharmacogenomic systems that depend on AI models. Table 12.3 shows a list of operational challenges.

12.3 Identification of Repeated Patterns, Bottlenecks

Through this analysis of challenges of AI-driven pharmacogenomics, we see common themes and operational pressures for achieving effective implementation. These include biases in the data set, complexity within the integration, issues with interpretability, and/or excessive computational requirements. Understanding these themes and operational bottlenecks will help identify strategies for intervention while improving model performance, building clinician trust, and supporting scaling of the models within real world clinical practice.

12.3.1 Recurring Patterns

AI-based pharmacogenomics is facing several technical hurdles, which are persistent and have a significant impact on the reliability and acceptance of the models. Some of the key challenges are bias of data set, complexity of data integration, low interpretability of data, and high computational demands. Being aware of these ongoing challenges is important to determine possible solutions in order to improve the model's fairness, usability, and scalability in real-world clinical functions.

Bias in data sets: Bias in genomic and clinical data sets has been disrupting the effectiveness of AI models. Data sets often overrepresent some particular populations, age, or disease phenotypes, which can lead to inaccurate predictions and inequitable recommendations. Similar to the human

Table 12.3 Operational challenges in AI for pharmacogenomics, their causes, and implications.

Challenge	Cause	Implications	Potential solutions
Cost and resource requirements	High expenses for data acquisition, model development, infrastructure, software integration, validation, and maintenance	Limited adoption in resource-constrained institutions; potential inequities in access to precision medicine; slowed translation from research to clinical practice	Demonstrate cost-effectiveness; secure funding or subsidies; adopt scalable cloud-based solutions; prioritize high-impact use cases
Workforce and training gaps	Shortage of multidisciplinary professionals skilled in genomics, AI, bioinformatics, and clinical practice	Underutilization or misapplication of AI–PGx tools; reduced clinician confidence; slow adoption of precision medicine approaches	Develop targeted training programs; foster cross-disciplinary teams; offer continuous education for clinicians and data scientists
Scalability and deployment issues	Variability in patient populations, EHR systems, prescribing practices, and IT infrastructure	Inconsistent model performance across sites; clinician mistrust; difficulty scaling AI solutions beyond pilot studies	Implement standardized protocols; perform multi-site validation; ensure interoperability; design adaptable deployment strategies
Continuous model monitoring and governance	Dataset shift due to changes in genetics, clinical guidelines, and drug formularies; lack of auditing mechanisms	Model degradation, biased or inaccurate recommendations; patient safety risks; regulatory non-compliance	Establish monitoring and retraining pipelines; implement governance frameworks; conduct regular audits; ensure transparency, fairness, and regulatory compliance

leukocyte antigen (HLA) molecules that the model is based on, AI-models, which are trained on biased data, may underperform on underrepresented groups, which has the potential to undermine healthcare and create negative health consequences and further build distrust between healthcare providers and patients. It is necessary to ensure that datasets for each population are considered, curated, and/or augmented [23].

Challenges in data integration: Integrating heterogeneous data sources like genomics, electronic health records, and clinical trial data continues to be difficult. Variation in data formats, data inconstancy, or non-standard values in data will typically slow down model development and increase predictive risk. Additionally, the complex pipeline associated with integrating these data represents a significant allocation of resources (computationally and technically), which serves as a barrier to smaller institutions with fewer dollar resources or less well-resourced healthcare environments [24].

Challenges in interpretability: AI models—especially deep learning AI models—are often considered "black boxes", making predictions by which clinicians find it difficult to interpret these or logically equate the predictions. Without transparency, a clinician's trust is jeopardized and clinical acceptance can be challenging as practitioners are reluctant to accept recommendations when they cannot see the logic behind the recommendations. The threat of losing clinicians' trust and acceptance of AI models cannot be overstated, but techniques such as explainable AI (XAI) or visualizations of feature importance may be useful to address this gap.

High computational power requirements: The training and deployment of AI–PGx models will require significant computational resources in terms of high-end GPUs and high storage. Smaller hospitals or research centers may lack the infrastructure to implement these models. High computational demands will add, besides the cost, to our maintenance and, finally, may set a limit to the possibilities for use in general and in under-resourced contexts.

12.3.2 Bottlenecks

Operational constraints for the clinical use of pharmacogenomics in artificial intelligence—operational challenges constrain the applicability of pharmacogenomics in clinical practice. Common challenges include data quality, opacity, human factors, scalability, etc. Improving these obstacles is important for the model to be operating reliably and in line with standards, trusted by clinicians, and, in general, to have the knowledge and confidence to engage these technologies in routine care in a variety of healthcare settings [25].

Data quality: No model will be accurate and reliable when applied to poor quality data (i.e., missing observations, incomplete values, inconsistent data on relevant patient characteristics such as smoking, etc.), which can result either from poor data collection and/or data entry processes or from computer failures/errors. Even if a model works in practice, clerical errors in the data (such as errors in fractions of seconds, batching of data across multiple models, or even missing data) or inaccuracies in the annotations of data (such as incorrect labeling) can cause the model to make incorrect predictions or recommendations. While it is slowly becoming more integrated into practice, data quality considerations of preprocessing (removing, imputation, or correction of data), standards, and quality controls can altogether improve the robustness, reportability, and reliability of a model, alongside patient safety.

Regulatory compliance: Compliance is an increasingly complex, ethical, legal, and regulatory requirement in AI-driven PGx tools. Compliance with privacy laws, clinical trial laws, and guidelines is complicated by input delays from AI. Institutions have to sustain practices that are compliant with general data protection regulations (GDPR), health insurance portability and accountability (HIPAA), and local legislation and ensure that they are agile enough to accommodate model updates which can introduce serious operational bottlenecks.

Human factors: Operational success relies on the training, engagement, and willingness of the clinician to use AI tools. Resistance to changes in workflow is largely dependent on clinician uncertainty about AI outputs and their ability to trust recommendations. Addressing the human factor through providing training and developing intuitive interfaces and user-centered design can enable smooth implementation.

Scalability: Despite the gathered evidence from trials of fidelity in AI–PGx tools, models learnt in trials do not readily transfer to application with real patients due to variations in patient populations, clinical practice, and IT infrastructure. Scalability requires continuous ongoing validation, effective monitoring, and deployment mechanisms. Without control of these external factors, limits can be made on clinical utility and widespread adoption of AI–PGx tools.

12.4 Strategies to Minimize these Challenges

There are technical, clinical, and operational challenges to integrating AI-driven pharmacogenomics, which can be a limiting factor for its adoption and effectiveness.

12.4.1 Technical Challenges

Technical challenges for AI-driven pharmacogenomics, such as dataset bias, integration of data, model interpretability, high computational requirements, and data monitoring can be a barrier limiting the clinical adoption of AI-driven pharmacogenomics. The reliability, transparency, and effectiveness of AI in the real world—this has to do with how specific AI system improvements can be used in healthcare facilities to improve the reliability, transparency, and durability and effectiveness of AI.

Data set curation and augmentation: Training data quality and diversity is extremely sensitive to AI models. Bias in datasets that can include overrepresentation of certain ethnicities, age groups, or disease subtypes can lead to wrong or unjust predictions. Curating datasets means to carefully select representative samples and to standardize annotations and make sure that they are complete. Synthetic data augmentation, therefore, which consists of generating realistic artificial samples, or oversampling minority groups can be implemented to balance out datasets. These steps are beneficial to increase the generalizability of the model, decrease bias, and increase reliability on different patient populations.

Data platforms that are interoperable: Pharmacogenomic data are collected from a variety of disparate sources, including electronic health records (EHR), genomics, and clinical trial databases. Integration is difficult due to different data formats, holes in the data, and different standards. Interoperable data platforms which use standardized data formats such as FHIR (fast healthcare interoperability resources) or OMOP CDM (observational medical outcomes partnership common data model) make the process of data ingestion and processing more efficient. Data consistency and quality are treated, making sure that robust ETL (extract, transform, load) pipelines are built. This gives AI models a reliable access and analysis to multi-source datasets with minimal errors and accelerates the development and implementation of AI models.

Explainable AI (XAI): Many AI models, particularly deep learning models, are a "black box" which makes predictions with no clear reasoning. Lack of interpretability can lead to a lack of trust in the clinicians and adoption. Explainable AI techniques have a tendency to make the predictions transparent. This can be either inherently interpretable models (such as decision trees or linear models) or *post-hoc* explanation methods (such as SHAP, LIME, or attention maps). XAI can make it easier for clinicians to understand what features contributed to a recommendation and helps them to make informed decisions, and it enhances accountability, especially in areas where the safety of the patient is paramount, such as pharmacogenomics.

Scalability and cloud bias: Training and deploying AI–PGx models require large amounts of computational resources in the form of high-performance CPUs/GPUs, large storage, and fast network infrastructure. Many healthcare institutions may not have local resources to handle such demands. Exploiting a cloud platform or distributed computing frameworks enables scalable on-demand computational power. Cloud solutions also provide centralized updates of models, multi-site deployment, and collaboration between institutions, which result in infrastructure cost savings and allows smaller centers to adopt the AI–PGx solutions without the burden of making heavy upfront investments.

Continuous monitoring and re-training: AI models are not static and performance can decrease over time as a result of changes in population genetics, drug formularies, clinical guidelines or patient demographics—commonly termed dataset shift. Continuous monitoring entails monitoring model accuracy, fairness, and safety on real-world usage. Retraining pipelines updates the model on a periodic basis using new data or after the guidelines are changed. Incorporating automated warnings for degradation in performance and ensuring adherence to all regulatory requirements will ensure that the models retain their accuracy, fairness, and clinical reliability over time and maintain trust between clinicians and their patients.

12.4.2 Clinical Challenges

Clinical adoption of pharmacogenomics using AI is hindered by the challenges of sparse evidence of utility in the real world, barriers to patient understanding, barriers to clinician trust, and barriers to linking with workflow. Addressing these challenges requires the use of strategies including rigorous clinical trials, easy-to-use integration of EHR, targeted clinician education, and clear communication and focus on patients to ensure that it is being implemented safely and effectively and widely accepted.

Many AI–PGx models are only validated retrospectively or *in silico* and as such have very little evidence of effectiveness in the real world. Conducting prospective randomized controlled trials offers the opportunity to rigorously study the effects of AI-guided pharmacogenomic recommendations on patient outcomes, drug efficacy, and adverse drug reactions. These are good quality trials and can be used as the basis for guideline development and clinical implementation and provide confidence from health professionals and regulators. Prospective studies provide a basis for support for institutional investment to establish and scale up innovations by showing the measured clinical benefit of the intervention.

Integration with electronic health records (EHRs): AI–PGx solutions need to be integrated into the workflow of clinicians through electronic health record (EHR) systems. Poorly integrated systems are a threat to routine practice, provoking alert fatigue and loss of usability. The provision of an intelligent interface for issuing recommendations in workflow in an intuitive, contextual, and actionable manner is an important aspect for the provision of timely and effective decision support. Integration also is beneficial for capturing data in real time along with feedback loops for improved patient care and model optimization. First, it could be suggested that the capacity for embedding would increase the chance of uptake and continued use of the tool with clinicians and therefore greater impact with AI-driven pharmacogenomics.

Education and acculturation of physicians: As AI models are being deployed clinically, it is important for practitioners to understand the concepts of pharmacogenomics as well as the results of AI models. Many clinicians will not be comfortable with genomics and/or will not want to interpret recommendations from AI.

Awareness raising and capacity building for professionals: Outcome-focused training modules and workshops have been developed and trialed which are helpful in raising awareness and building trust within communities Besides creating clinical relevant and actionable AI tools, active participation of clinicians in their design and evaluation is also essential for reducing resistance to and achieving sustainability of AI–PGx solutions in clinical practice.

Patient-centric communication: The results and recommendations from pharmacogenomic tests and buying recommendations can be complex and overwhelming for patients without adequate education about the use of AI. Simplified and clear reports and visualization will allow information which is actionable and not overwhelming for the patient. Patient education about the nature, the benefits as well as the limitations of the AI–PGx recommendations is an important vehicle for informed consent, trust, and compliance with therapy. Shared decision-making and other patient-centered communication strategies to enhance the patient's involvement in the decision-making process and to empower them to take an active role in their treatment plan will also be critical to ensure the appropriate and ethical use of AI-based pharmacogenomic testing.

12.4.3 Operational Challenges

The challenge facing the commercialization of AI-driven pharmacogenomic in healthcare is the economic viability, workforce capacity, scalability, regulatory compliance, and government. The design for sustainable, compliant, and effective delivery at a range of healthcare locations requires effective strategies including cost–benefit analysis, multidisciplinary teams, standardized deployment frameworks, governance strength, workforce training, and devolution.

Cost–benefit analysis and financing: AI–PGx solutions are cost-effective compared to the amount of money needed for data acquisition, infrastructure, model development of the solution, integration, and maintenance. By no means do institutions with limited resources want to embrace these technologies without a good understanding of the economic or clinical value. Cost–benefit analyses to make the case for return on investment—shared infrastructure, cloud computing, or consortium-based strategies—can be implemented to reduce the upfront and ongoing costs, increasing access to AI–PGx for more healthcare organizations.

Multidisciplinary teams: Successful operationalization requires a workforce that works in collaboration and includes expertise in areas of genomics, clinical medicine, AI, bioinformatics, and IT. Isolated teams may have difficulty with the end-to-end implementation, from the model development to its clinical implementation. The formation of multidisciplinary teams for this purpose helps to ensure completeness of the understanding, efficiency in problem-solving, and alignment of the technical development and clinical flows. The user–model interaction is beneficial for both the model inference and user acceptance and ease of use, thereby reducing the bottlenecks in the operation and allowing for the easy translation of the practice into action.

While models for scaling the deployment have been developed to implement effectively in pilot studies, they cannot be translated in multiple sites in a way that is effective in every scenario due to variations in patient populations, EHR systems, and IT infrastructure.

Standardized implementation, multi-site validation, and flexible infrastructure, comparable performance with similar configuration, design for monitoring, maintenance, and updates: Due to this design, the system is less volatile, resulting in trust from clinicians. Designed deployment also implies a widespread deployment with no compromise on model reliability and safety for patients.

Governance and ethical governance: For PGx and the ethical and regulatory aspects of using AI-based algorithms, PGx's use of sensitive genetic and clinical data are severe.

Governance: This covers establishing governance models for ensuring compliance with privacy (e.g., HIPAA, GDPR) for fairness of model outcome and ensuring transparency and responsibility for ensuring patient safety and maintaining public trust, auditing, risk management processes, ethical review processes, etc. The governance model also enables reporting, incident management, and compliance for evolving regulations defined for AI to operationalize the technology in sustainable ways.

Training programs and workforce development: Training and acceptance of workforce is necessary for successful operation. There is a need to educate clinicians and the technical staff about genomics, the system concepts of AI and its use, as well as education about ethics. Training programs aim to mitigate resistance and increase the understanding of model outputs and increased rates of adoption. Ongoing professional development for the competence of staff is also important so that they can adapt to the evolution of technology as well as support the efficient and secure implementation of AI–PGx solutions to minimize operation errors and inefficiencies.

12.5 Real-World AI Applications in Pharmacogenomics

AI-driven pharmacogenomics is used to increasingly be applied to the field of clinical practice in order to personalize the medication therapy on the basis of genetic profiles. Real-life examples are of Sherpa Rx and AI models in primary care. There are many examples of AI in primary care and its impact on decision making, adverse drug events, and treatment optimization. Economic and policy considerations are important in order to make sustainable adoption.

Sherpa Rx: Sherpa Rx is a solution powered by AI, which is designed to assist clinicians to interpret pharmacogenomic information. It is using large language models (LLMs) with retrieval-augmented generation (RAG) for evidence retrieval from authoritative pharmacogenomic resources, for example, the Clinical Pharmacogenomics Implementation Consortium or CPIC guidelines and PharmGKB. The AI is able to provide actionable, patient-specific recommendations for drug–gene interaction, dosage changes, and risk prediction for adverse drug reactions (ADRs). Evaluations reveal that Sherpa Rx is more accurate, complete, and in line with clinical guidelines than standard LLMs such as ChatGPT-4. This tool is one example of the ways that AI can help to bridge the gap between the raw data of genomics and the practical clinical decisions that can be made.

Pharmacogenomics in primary care by AI: In some primary care settings, artificial intelligence models have been implemented to identify patients that may be benefitting from pharmacogenomic testing. These models are grounded in patient's records and make predictions concerning drug response and genetic and clinical profiles relating to drug susceptibility to ADRs. In the process, they allow for more efficient clinical decision making. The physicians do not have to do so much of the genomic analysis by hand in order to individualize their decisions for medicine. This will allow for more efficient real-life implementation—limiting adverse events while ensuring the optimization of healthcare resources. Such models also make it easier to incorporate pharmacogenomics into clinical practice on a day-to-day basis, which is important for widespread adoption.

12.5.1 Economic Implications

AI for pharmacogenomic implementation is a big problem from an economical point of view for the healthcare system. With the upfront costs of genetic testing, artificial intelligence technology and staff training may be high, there is evidence of long-term benefit in terms of higher patient outcomes, reduced adverse drug reactions, and overall healthcare costs. Cost-effectiveness and ROI are two of the biggest driving forces with regard to adoption [26].

Cost-effectiveness: The goal of pharmacogenomic-guided therapy is to reduce adverse drug reactions and maximize the benefits of drugs. By helping to predict what medications are likely to work (or not work) for a specific patient, PGx testing using AI can help to avoid hospitalizations and emergency room visits and to reduce medication failures. Although the upfront costs for genetic testing, implementation of AI, and staff training are comparatively high, long-term cost savings result in a cost-effective approach to healthcare systems. Moreover, by avoiding trial and error prescribing, it can help in decreasing wastage of medications and improving the quality of life for the patients.

Return on investment (ROI): Economic studies have reported that despite the investment of AI-PGx solutions that are still very high, the ROI comes from better clinical outcomes for the patient, with less complications as well as less healthcare budgets. While investing in the upfront capital to invest in the computational infrastructure and data management for such approaches may seem daunting, personalized medicine approaches pay for themselves in the long run, especially for patients that are high risk or taking a number of different medications. Further reduction of running cost by leveraging the cloud computing, scalable deployment, and shared infrastructure results to better ROI.

12.5.2 Policy Implications

The application of AI is not a simple phenomenon and consequences have implications for the use of pharmacogenomics for clinical practice. Ethical and regulatory policies also play a key role in helping to ensure the safe use of genetic data and equitable access for patients to genetic data, as does reimbursement. Specific policies are established to ensure sustainability in the implementation, trust between the clinicians and patients and stakeholders.

Regulatory landscape: The regulatory landscape of AI-based pharmacogenomics is complex and involves multiple steps like data collection, data analysis, clinical validation, etc., and integrating all of these stages in a single process is challenging. Rules in connection with permissions for AI model validation, clinical safety, and transparency are needed. Regulators should indicate the criteria of processing sensitive genetic data that render AI forecasts reproducible and reporting potential biasness. Lack of such frameworks slows down its adoption due to legal uncertainty and the risk of non-compliance. The harmonized policies in the regions can enable the multi-institutional cooperation and speed up the implementation.

Reimbursement policies: To achieve the broad-based application of AI–PGx tools, the current insurance and reimbursement policies will need to be adjusted and cover pharmacogenomic testing and AI-based decision support. The payers desire to see that these interventions are causing a cost saving or an improved outcome in all healthcare. Clinical utility and cost-effectiveness should be demonstrated to get reimbursed and provide incentive to hospitals and clinics to implement AI–PGx solutions.

Ethic and equity considerations: AI pharmacogenomics has ethical concerns of patient consent, privacy, and possible genetic discrimination. Policies must be formulated to ensure that patients, including patients from under-represented patient groups, are given fair access to AI-facilitated therapies. It is critical to have ethical guidelines to prevent trust data protection from being misused or mishandled. Translucent reporting and patient center communication are examples of transformative communication processes (TCPs), which are important processes in the process of integrating ethics in clinical practice.

Overall, AI-powered pharmacogenomics in primary care, such as Sherpa Rx, will be a part of the future for AI-individualization of drug therapy. Cost-effective long-term incentives, improved ROIs, regulatory compliance, reimbursement, and ethic drivers—all of these are the criteria for the sustainable implementation of clinical pharmacogenomics using AI.

12.6 Conclusion

Artificial intelligence could revolutionize the field of pharmacogenomics and establish the personalized method of drug treatment, decrease adverse drug reactions, and maximize a clinical outcome. Nevertheless, this potential can be fulfilled only in case of the systematic challenge of significant technical, clinical, and operational problems. The absence of standardized and high-quality data and interoperable platforms remain an issue to the development of strong models and the absence of explainability and transparency of these models remains an issue of confidence and uptake by clinicians. Another possible threat to equitable healthcare provision is bias in training data and inability of the model to be generalized across populations. The real-world implementation has more problems like high costs of implementation, training, and integration of the workforce with electronic health records systems. The future requires progressive measures in the shape of a coordinated method of harmonized data conventions, federated learning systems, explainable AI systems, and continuous model surveillance that are paramount. To make AI-based solutions in the field of PGx accurate, equitable, and clinically relevant, multidisciplinary cooperation between geneticists, clinicians, data scientists, policy makers, and patients will play a role. The healthcare community, through systematic overcoming of these limitations, is capable of realizing the world of pharmacogenomics and precision medicine to the goal of truly achieving the globally desired goal of precision medicine.

12.7 Future Research Directions

The further studies in the area of AI-driven pharmacogenomics are supposed to be concentrated on several important aspects. First, multimodal AI models capable of incorporating genomics, transcriptomics, proteomics, metabolomics, and real-world clinical data should be developed, which will aid in enhancing the predictive capacity of the AI models and provide a comprehensive view of the drug response. Second, fair reduction strategies and algorithms should be given priority in order to equate the recommendations to the various populations. Third, real-world evidence (RWE) needs to be incorporated to confirm model performance beyond the controlled research conditions where continuous learning healthcare systems can be applied. Fourth, explainable and regulatory compliant AI systems need to be advanced in order to meet new standards set by regulatory agencies such as FDA and EMA. Lastly, federated learning and privacy-preserving computation based on collaborative research networks can enable sharing of massive amounts of data without infringing patient confidentiality. Discussing these future directions would enhance the rate of bench to bedside translation as well as improve the clinical implications of pharmacogenomics in precision medicine.

AI disclosure statement: The author acknowledges the use of AI-based tools for minor language editing or grammatical correction. However, all intellectual contributions, analyses, and conclusions presented in this chapter are entirely the author's own.

References

1. Principi, N., Petropulacos, K., Esposito, S., Impact of pharmacogenomics in clinical practice. *Pharmaceuticals*, 16, 11, 1596, 2023.
2. Cacabelos, R., Naidoo, V., Corzo, L., Cacabelos, N., Carril, J.C., Genophenotypic factors and pharmacogenomics in adverse drug reactions. *Int. J. Mol. Sci.*, 22, 24, 13302, 2021.
3. Sharma, A., Kala, S., Kumar, A., Sharma, S., Gupta, G., Jaiswal, V., Deep learning in genomics, personalized medicine, and neurodevelopmental disorders, in: *Intelligent Data Analytics for Bioinformatics and Biomedical Systems*, Scrivener Publishing LLC, USA, pp. 235–264, 2024.
4. Grant, C.W., Marrero-Polanco, J., Joyce, J.B., Barry, B., Stillwell, A., Kruger, K., Anderson, T., *et al.*, Pharmacogenomic augmented machine learning in electronic health record alerts: A health system-wide usability survey of clinicians. *Clin. Transl. Sci.*, 17, 10, e70044, 2024.
5. Haga, S.B., Artificial intelligence, medications, pharmacogenomics, and ethics. *Pharmacogenomics*, 25, 14–15, 611–622, 2024.
6. Sharma, N. and Rajput, A., Development of A Genomic-based Predictive Model for Warfarin Dosing. *Clin. J. Med. Health Pharm.*, 2, 2, 11–19, 2024.
7. Hahn, M. and Roll, S.C., The influence of pharmacogenetics on the clinical relevance of pharmacokinetic drug–drug interactions: drug–gene, drug–gene–gene and drug–drug–gene interactions. *Pharmaceuticals*, 14, 5, 487, 2021.
8. Taherdoost, H. and Ghofrani, A., AI's role in revolutionizing personalized medicine by reshaping pharmacogenomics and drug therapy. *Intell. Pharm.*, 2, 5, 643–650, 2024.
9. Athanasopoulou, K., Michalopoulou, V.-I., Scorilas, A., Adamopoulos, P.G., Integrating Artificial Intelligence in Next-Generation Sequencing: Advances, Challenges, and Future Directions. *Curr. Issues Mol. Biol.* 47, 6, 470, 2025.

10. Sharma, J. and Goel, P., The Use of AI for Phenotype-Genotype Mapping, in: *Artificial Intelligence (AI) in Cell and Genetic Engineering*, pp. 369–410, Humana, New York, NY, 2025.
11. Kumar, A., Shukla, A., Yadav, A.K., Recent Trends and Technological Advances in Pharmacological Research: A Review. *J. Drug Discov. Health Sci.*, 2, 02, 91–99, 2025.
12. Henriques, J., Rocha, T., de Carvalho, P., Silva, C., Paredes, S., Interpretability and explainability of machine learning models: Achievements and challenges, in: *International Conference on Biomedical and Health Informatics*, pp. 81–94, Springer Nature Switzerland, Cham, 2022.
13. Yuan, H., Overcoming computational resource limitations in deep learning for healthcare: Strategies targeting data, model, and computing. *Med. Adv.*, 3, 1, 42–45, 2025.
14. Jadhav, A., Sawesi, S., Rashrash, B., Bias and generalizability challenges in machine learning models for leptospirosis, in: *2024 IEEE International Conference on Big Data (BigData)*, pp. 4989–4995, IEEE, 2024.
15. Chang, W-C., Tanoshima, R., Ross, C.J.D., Carleton, B.C., Challenges and opportunities in implementing pharmacogenetic testing in clinical settings. *Annu. Rev. Pharmacol. Toxicol.*, 61, 1, 65–84, 2021.
16. Kanegusuku, A.G., Chan, C.W., Thoburn, C.A., van Wijk, X.M.R., Tang, N.Y., Challenges and considerations in implementing clinical pharmacogenomics. *J. Lab. Precis. Med.*, 10, 1, 2025.
17. Knezevic, C.E., Stevenson, J.M., Merran, J., Snyder, I., Restorick, G., Waters, C., Marzinke, M.A., Implementation of integrated clinical pharmacogenomics testing at an Academic Medical Center. *J. Appl. Lab. Med.*, 10, 2, 259–273, 2025.
18. Srimlika, N., Sriram, L., Sharma, V., Mishra, S., Alkhayyat, A., Advancing Patient-Centric Care Through Genomic Data and Deep Learning, in: *2024 IEEE 4th International Conference on ICT in Business Industry & Government (ICTBIG)*, pp. 1–6, IEEE, 2024.
19. Lilhore, U.K. and Simaiya, S., Unveiling the Potential: A Comprehensive Exploration of Deep Learning and Transfer Learning Techniques in Bioinformatics, in: *Applying Machine Learning Techniques to Bioinformatics: Few-Shot and Zero-Shot Methods*, pp. 138–158, IGI Global Scientific Publishing, USA, 2024.
20. Ayati, N., Afzali, M., Hasanzad, M., Kebriaeezadeh, A., Rajabzadeh, A., Nikfar, S., Pharmacogenomics implementation and hurdles to overcome; in the context of a developing country. *Iran. J. Pharm. Res.: IJPR*, 20, 4, 92, 2021.
21. Liang, L., Hu, J., Sun, G., Hong, N., Wu, G., He, Y., Li, Y., Hao, T., Liu, L., Gong, M., Artificial intelligence-based pharmacovigilance in the setting of limited resources. *Drug Saf.*, 45, 5, 511–519, 2022.
22. Omran, S., Leong, S.L., Blebil, A., Mohan, D., Ang, W.C., Teoh, S.L., The needs and gaps in pharmacogenomics knowledge and education among

healthcare professionals in Malaysia: A multisite Delphi study. *Clin. Transl. Sci.*, 17, 11, e70057, 2024.

23. Hayward, J., McDermott, J., Qureshi, N., Newman, W., Pharmacogenomic testing to support prescribing in primary care: a structured review of implementation models. *Pharmacogenomics*, 22, 12, 761–776, 2021.
24. Al-Remawi, M. and Abdel Rahem, R.A., Applications of AI in Biomedical Genomics and Pharmaceuticals, in: *2024 2nd International Conference on Cyber Resilience (ICCR)*, pp. 1–5, IEEE, 2024.
25. Nam, Y., Kim, J., Jung, S.-H., Woerner, J., Suh, E.H., Lee, D.-G., Shivakumar, M., Lee, M.E., Kim, D., Harnessing artificial intelligence in multimodal omics data integration: paving the path for the next frontier in precision medicine. *Annu. Rev. Biomed. Data Sci.*, 7, 2024.
26. Abdelhalim, H., Berber, A., Lodi, M., Jain, R., Nair, A., Pappu, A., Patel, K., *et al.*, Artificial intelligence, healthcare, clinical genomics, and pharmacogenomics approaches in precision medicine. *Front. Genet.*, 13, 929736, 2022.

13

Ethical Frameworks for Integrating AI in Pharmacogenomics: A Focus on Equity and Justice

Ika Hesti Agustin[1]*, R. Kannamma[2], Nallametti Nagarjuna[3], Sheela S.[4], D. Vetrithangam[5] and Thilagavathi K.[6]

[1]*Department of Mathematics, University of Jember, Jember, East Java, Indonesia*
[2]*Department of AI & DS, Prathyusha Engineering College, Chennai, Tamil Nadu, India*
[3]*Department of Computer Science & Engineering (AIML), CVR College of Engineering, Hyderabad, Telangana, India*
[4]*Department of Computer Applications, Marian College Kuttikkanam Autonomous, Kuttikkanam, Kerala, India*
[5]*Department of Computer Science & Engineering, University Institute of Engineering, Chandigarh University, Mohali, Punjab, India*
[6]*Department of Electronics and Communication Engineering, Kumaraguru College of Technology, Coimbatore, India*

Abstract

Artificial intelligence (AI) provides tremendous opportunities in pharmacogenomics, but its use raises existential questions around the issues of equity and justice, particularly for underrepresented peoples. Currently, the use of AI in this area is still mostly about predictive accuracy and has not provided appropriate consideration of equity and inclusion and trust from stakeholders. This chapter introduces the equity–justice AI framework (EJ-AIF) and proposes a fresh approach to ethical principle introduction, fairness auditing, and participatory validation in the AI pipeline. The paper evaluated the EJ-AIF framework on a dataset from the 1000 Genomes Project and compared it with four other strategies, namely: conventional accuracy first AI, bias mitigation AI, fairness-aware AI, and explainable AI. The study compared the EJ-AIF and each benchmark method

**Corresponding author*: ikahesti.fmipa@unej.ac.id

Umesh Kumar Lilhore, Kaamran Raahemifar, Sarita Simaiya, R. Sunder and R. Lotus (eds.) Pharmacogenomics Using Artificial Intelligence: Optimizing Drug Response through Personalized Genomic Analysis, (285–306) © 2026 Scrivener Publishing LLC

in five categories—predictive accuracy, fairness metrics, Equity Impact Score (EIS), trust and interpretability, and inclusivity index. Results are that the EJ-AIF Canadian Algorithm achieves roughly the same predictive accuracy (AUROC 0.90) compared to conventional models, although massive reductions in subgroup differences (PPD = 0.05, EO = 0.06) are obtained, including the highest EIS (0.89), trust score (4.6/5), and inclusivity index (0.78). Overall, these results suggest that EJ-AIF manages to strike a balance between technical performance and ethical and moral goals and that it hints at a possible pathway in the direction of justice-based pharmacogenomics. In conclusion, the findings show that the inclusion of the ethical-equity-and-justice as co-first-order goals in AI systems is feasible and needed toward ethically and morally superior precision medicine outcomes.

Keywords: Artificial intelligence, pharmacogenomics, equity, justice, fairness, explainability, ethical AI, precision medicine

13.1 Introduction

Artificial intelligence (AI) is rapidly transforming healthcare through sophisticated predictive AI modeling, decision making and precision medicine uses. It is within this arena that the field of pharmacogenomics or in the field concerned with genetic variation as it relates to drug response—is the perfect field for visibility for discovery acceleration and clinical decision support using AI. In considering the potential for pharmacogenomics with AI, the discovery and understanding of complex genomic markers to predict drug efficacy and adverse drug events will lead to a decrease of trial and error prescribing and ultimately benefit precision medicine. While the technical commitments of AI in pharmacogenomics are well understood, the ethics of AI in pharmacogenomics is a key and still a largely under-researched question [1].

Generally, this challenge is premised on a history of inequalities in genomics. Historically, the vast genomic data available has been skewed toward individuals from a European heritage and therefore under-represented with minority/under-represented populations in pharmacogenomics. Not only does this bias narrow the applicability of pharmacogenomic data, it contributes to health disparities [2]. In addition, AI based on genetically derived information that inherits existing bias poses the potential for introducing structural bias in drug recommendations as well as the perpetuation of health inequities in vulnerable patients. This is seen as an important area of pharmacogenomics, but consideration and development of the AI should be framed from a regenerative perspective and validated to be based on equity and justice [3].

To address these limitations, emerging research is aiming at developing fairness-aware machine learning algorithms and related explainability tools. For instance, one study has used debiasing algorithms to reduce disparity between population groups, while another has used explainable AI (XAI) systems which aim to increase clinicians' understanding of AI-based prediction patterns in a long-term database [4]. Although these endeavors are indeed progress for the field, there is a limited nature to it. Fairness-aware algorithms tend to optimize to broad statistical measures of fairness—thus focusing on utility rather than ethically justified, population-based notions of fairness. Moreover, whereas XAI systems were able to generate more comprehensibility in terms of actionable explanations than what was previously available, this does not necessarily translate to an equitable and just AI system. Taking the above point further, debiasing algorithms can only partially account for a narrow type of difference and does not touch on community-level perspectives and ideas of distributive justice in the process of design or development. As such, there is still a large research gap in operationalizing equity and justice in AI systems for pharmacogenomics [5].

The research question for this study is located at the intersection of technological developments and ethical concerns. While artificial intelligence has presented new possibilities to improve pharmacogenomic predictions of drug response, current models are either more focused on accuracy than fairness or focused on fairness and equity without conceptualizing justice as an organizing principle [6]. In addition, the re-packaging of predictive utility and the potential implication for inequities may further solidify structural and systemic inequities and ultimately limit the trust in AI systems. Addressing these challenges from a justice perspective is necessary to ensure that AI-based pharmaceutical genomics predict the responsiveness to drugs in a way that would facilitate the achievement of an aim of equitable access to precision health for diverse populations [7].

As such, the research question for the study will be: How can pharmacogenomic AI be conceptualized, validated, and implemented, such that predictive validity coexists with equity, access, and justice in order to promote inequities in precision medicine? The broad objectives of the chapter would be as follows:

- To design and put into practice the equity–justice AI framework (EJ-AIF), which encourages the integration of fairness, inclusivity, and ethical frameworks into pharmacogenomic AI pipelines

- To assess EJ-AIF relative to existing approaches to AI (CA-AI, BM-AI, FA-AI, XAI-AI) on quantitative metrics, including predictive accuracy, fairness metrics, trust, and inclusivity
- To provide evidence for EJ-AIF as a repeatable and scalable approach for integrating equity and justice into AI-driven pharmacogenomics

The remainder of the chapter is organized as follows: Section 13.2 is devoted to a review of the literature. Section 13.3 describes the methodology for the study which is based on ethical framework, data governance, model development, and evaluation criteria. Section 13.4 provides comparative results of EJ-AIF with respect to baseline approaches and discusses implications of results, limitations, and implications for practice. Section 13.5 concludes with a discussion of the future of justice-oriented pharmacogenomics.

13.2 Related Works

The incorporation of genomics and pharmacogenomics in healthcare presents important equity, diversity, ethics, and inclusion issues for patients in healthcare. While these fields offer tremendous potential for realizing an individualized approach to treating disease, they must be restricted by data governance issues, underrepresentation, and social disparities or else excuses for perpetuating inequities can be made. In recent studies, these problems have been addressed from multiple perspectives: clinicogenomics, pharmacogenetics, precision dosing, pharmacoepidemiology, and patient experiences. Together they highlight the importance of patient-centric data models, inclusive study designs, ethical frameworks, and transparent governance practices in ensuring that advancements in genomic medicine benefit all populations equally.

Jordan *et al.* suggest that one of the health equity methods is population pharmacogenomics to determine if there are genetic differences in the response to an agent for racial and ethnic groups. This is important for avoiding treatment biases as well as precision in care and adverse drug reactions, especially for underrepresented minority populations [8].

Indeed Hughes *et al.* [10] reported that the use of CDSS is limited by underrepresentation within clinical trial datasets, therefore underrepresentation of equity in care was reported. In their recommendations for enhancing CDSS, they suggest following the same inclusive study designs, better demographic data sharing and use of biological indicators. Routine data collection may yield better results for multiple populations than simply going out and collecting data [9].

Vallejo-Yague *et al.* [11] presented a declaration to promote equity and justice in pharmacoepidemiology: the model of ETIE (explore, tailor, implement, and evaluate). They emphasize the incorporation of domains of diversity (such as sex, gender, age, ethnicity, socioeconomic status, and health literacy) for inclusion, generalizability, equity, and equitable research practices as endorsed by stakeholders.

Magavern *et al.* [12] emphasizes the need for integrating pharmacogenomics into clinical practice to ensure that it does not increase health disparities by including diverse populations. They critically consider the role of diversity, draw attention to gaps in the evidence and suggest ways to mitigate the risks and ensure that pharmacogenomics leads to equality rather than perpetuating inequities in health.

Clarke and van El [13] explain that in terms of social justice issues surrounding implementation of genomics in health care, the potential exists for genomics to exacerbate inequities and discrimination. They outline six topics of concern—access, misuses of data, epigenetics, psychiatric genomics, polygenic risk focus and reproductive screening—and advocate for proactive solutions to tensions between ethics and risks to minimize harm to vulnerable populations as much as possible.

Koromina *et al.* [14] discusses on ethical and equity challenges in rare disease research, informed consent, data sharing, and patient recruitment They draw attention to issues of dilemmas for genetic testing, particularly in low and middle-income countries, and urge for appropriate ethical principles to guide the conduct of genomics research and for fairness and social accountability.

Jumhati [15], in the article "Pharmacogenomic based decision making from the patient perspective, a qualitative phenomenological study" describes decision making based on pharmacogenomic from patients' perspectives. Interviews are the main source of data and the themes that emerged from the interviews are uncertainty, trust, provider, personal meaning making, and ethical reflection. Emotional and relational aspects of genomic care for genomic treatment are also highlighted in this study, and an empathic style of communication and patient-centred approach to personalized medicine is recommended.

Garcia *et al.* [16] Pharmacogenetics integration into clinical trials: There is a need for explicit and concerted guidelines, which would ensure methodological rigor, appropriate handling of samples and privacy of data.

Transparency, informed consent, and respect for participant rights (genomic research) are emphasized.

The genomic and pharmacogenomic revolutions are severely curtailed. Much of the research focus has been on under-represented minority and vulnerable populations that contribute to data bias and poor generalizability of findings. There is a lack of alignment between ethical and regulatory frameworks, together with gaps in areas such as informed consent, data privacy and equitable participation, specifically in the low and middle income context. It is quite common for trials and clinical decision support systems to be designed from imperfect or non-diverse data, which limits applicability. Furthermore, research on the effects of personalized interventions is constrained by a failure to explore patients' experiences and to consider socio-cultural contexts. However, the alternatives proposed for frameworks and tools are implemented in a heterogeneous way, which in turn, requires systemic and multi-stakeholder approaches for effective health equity.

As genomics and pharmacogenomic research becomes more embedded in healthcare, there are important questions pertaining to issues of equity, diversity, ethics and patient inclusion that need to be addressed. However, there is great potential to provide a more personalized approach to treatment, and coming to terms with the risks associated with data governance challenges, underrepresentation and social disparities is a necessary responsibility for ensuring inequity is not exacerbated in these fields. In recent years these issues have been addressed from various perspectives: patient experience, pharmacoepidemiology, precision dosing, pharmacogenetics, and clinicogenomics (both of which are new terms). Altogether, all of these point to the importance of patient-centered data models, inclusive study designs, ethical frameworks, and transparent governance practices to ensure that advances in genomic medicine are equitable for all populations. Table 13.1 lists the related literature and provides an insight to such problems as well as solutions proposed for the problems.

Despite recent advances in the fields of genomics and pharmacogenomics, there still are important limits. Most studies report the lack of participation of minority and vulnerable populations, which can result in biased data and lower generalizability of results. Lack of consistency and gaps in ethical and regulatory frameworks - there are often gaps in informed consent, data privacy, and equitable participation, especially in low- and middle-income countries Clinical decision support systems and trial designs often utilize incomplete and/or homogenous data-sets, and thus are of restricted applicability. Additionally, experiences of patients and socio-cultural contexts are under explored which limits the effectiveness of

Table 13.1 Key studies on genomics and pharmacogenomics for health equity.

Author(s) and year	Method	Strengths	Limitations
Jordan *et al.* (2023) [8]	Perspective on population pharmacogenomics	Emphasizes health equity through genetic variation, highlights racial/ethnic differences in drug response, focuses on adverse drug reaction mitigation	Limited empirical data, general recommendations, may oversimplify complex population genetics
Hughes *et al.* (2023) [10]	Review of CDSS in precision dosing	Identifies underrepresentation in clinical trial data, proposes inclusive study designs, use of biological indicators, and integration of real-world data	Implementation challenges, reliance on existing CDSS infrastructure, lack of large-scale validation
Vallejo-Yagüe *et al.* (2025) [11]	Framework development (ETIE) in pharmacoepidemiology	Operationalizes diversity and fairness, identifies key diversity domains, supports generalizability and equity	Framework is conceptual, requires stakeholder buy-in, practical adoption may be resource-intensive
Magavern *et al.* (2022) [12]	Critical review on pharmacogenomics and diversity	Highlights evidence gaps, proposes strategies to avoid widening health disparities, emphasizes social and historical context	Broad overview, lacks quantitative analysis or clinical testing
Clarke and van El (2022) [13]	Ethical analysis in genomics	Identifies six key areas of social justice concern, anticipates potential harms, guides policy and practice	Mainly theoretical, no empirical assessment of interventions, context-specific applicability
Koromina *et al.* (2021) [14]	Review on rare disease genomics ethics	Emphasizes informed consent, data sharing, patient recruitment, ethical frameworks in low- and middle-income countries	Limited discussion on implementation, mostly conceptual, focus on rare diseases may not generalize

(*Continued*)

Table 13.1 Key studies on genomics and pharmacogenomics for health equity. (*Continued*)

Author(s) and year	Method	Strengths	Limitations
Jumhati (2025) [15]	Qualitative phenomenological study of patient experiences	Provides patient-centered insights, highlights emotional, relational, and ethical dimensions, informs communication strategies	Small sample size (n=8), limited generalizability, context-specific findings
García-García *et al.* (2024) [16]	Review and regulatory analysis of pharmacogenetics in clinical trials	Identifies methodological, ethical, regulatory gaps, calls for unified guidelines, emphasizes transparency and consent	Conceptual recommendations, lacks empirical testing, implementation feasibility not evaluated

individualized interventions. While these frameworks and tools have been proposed, however, their adoption is still uneven and requires systemic and multi-stakeholder approaches to realizing real health equity.

13.3 Research Design

This section proposes a hybrid technical-ethical approach, situated in an equity and justice theoretical framework, to the implementation of AI in pharmacogenomics. The new methodological pipeline includes both fairness metrics and community co-design and justice evaluation metrics, going beyond the simple calculation of predictive accuracy. The methodology is developed in four overlapping stages as shown in Figure 13.1.

Ethics, ethical bases, and involvement of stakeholders

The ethical basis of the proposed framework is substantive, and entails the involvement of stakeholders in assisting operationalization of justice in the context of AI-pharmacogenomics system. Key bioethical values (autonomy, beneficence, non-maleficence, justice) are carefully translated into practical, measurable indicators (such as representativeness, access to products, culturally acceptable practices of consent prior to products, etc.).

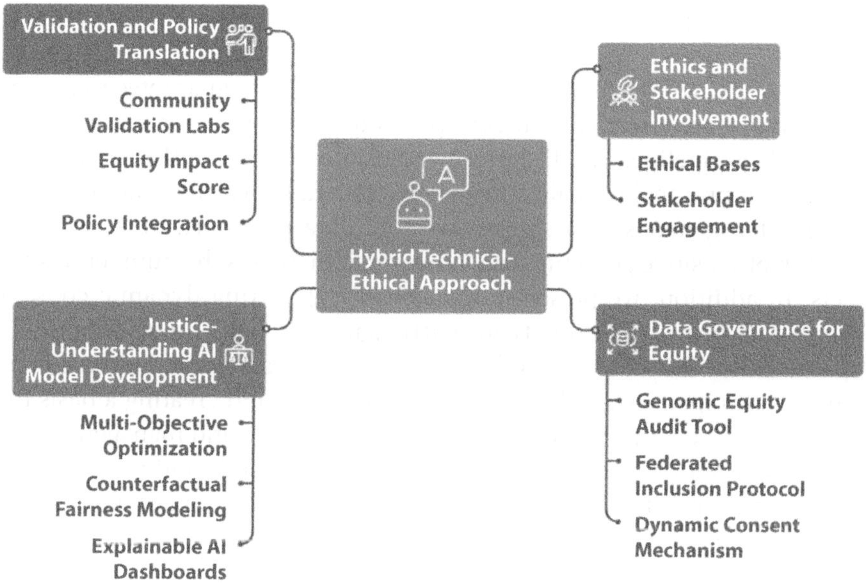

Figure 13.1 Hybrid technical–ethical approach to AI in pharmacogenomics.

Strategized Delphi panels of patients, clinicians, geneticists, data scientists, and institutional/policy-makers are systematically engaged in developing AI and presenting it in a clinically relevant way. Such stakeholder engagement enables the identification of equity-sensible decision points in the AI processes in order to ensure diverse perspectives are included in the AI system design and validation. Lastly, a justice perspective will be implemented by the Rawlsian difference principle which will ensure that benefits should be given to the least disadvantaged and the Capabilities Approach put forth by Sen and Nussbaum supports people to develop their health-related necessary capabilities. This dual ethical foundation provides the framework with both a distributive and functional understanding of justice, and principles of the framework go beyond technical notions of fairness to the lived experiences of patients and communities [16].

Data governance for the quest of equity

The stress to equity associated with pharmacogenomic AI begins with the source of data used for training the model, therefore the second pillar in the equitable pharmacogenomic AI framework is data governance.

A Genomic Equity Audit Tool (GEAT) designed to respond to systemic biases of genomic research and quantify gaps in representation across ancestry, sex, socioeconomic status, and geography to guarantee that populations that are historically underrepresented in the research are identified in the data pipeline. The Federated Inclusion Protocol (FIP) is a privacy preserving protocol to realize inclusion - federated learning models learn from heterogeneous data sources without data transport. This mitigates the risk of sensitive genomic data; however, it increases the number of subjects. In addition, we present a blockchain-supporting dynamic consent model that provides flexibility for participants to control their data rights against time. This consent model is aimed at increasing the personal control of participants over their genetic information and creating a basis for trust through transparency and control over access to and management of, inter alia, their data. Altogether these models, methods and protocols set the scene for equitable, secure and inclusive data creation and use of data in the context of AI-enabled pharmacogenomics [17].

Justice—Understanding AI model development

The approach suggested in the framework is based on the design of justice-oriented AI models. These models are not built simply to be as accurate as possible but instead adopt a paradigm of multi-objective optimization in which the predictive accuracy and equity indices such as predictive parity, equalized odds and subgroup calibration are co-primary objectives. This will ensure that overall predictive accuracy does not come at the cost of fairness in a model's output. The counterfactual fairness modeling is also used to reveal and hide structural biases in order to get a set of recommendations that are not systematically different depending on sensitive attributes such as ancestry or socioeconomic status. Furthermore, there is an increase in the explainability of AI output with equity tags in explainable AI (XAI) dashboards. The equity tagged explanations can help clinicians and patients not only to identify why AI made certain recommendations, but also to assess whether recommendations are equally represented in sub-groups. As a result, fairness with interpretability are built-in characteristics of the model, and not ancillary measures of evaluation [18, 19].

Validation and policy translation process

Besides the technological ecosystem, the validation and alignment with policy should be given utmost importance while developing an AI framework to positively affect patient outcomes. To advance that process, we facilitate the development of community validation labs (CVLs) as participatory practices with patients and clinicians to co-evaluate the degree of trust, interpretability, and perceived fairness of AI outputs. Evaluation of AI tools is additionally aided by the establishment of an Equity Impact Score (EIS), which is an aggregate score generated based on statistical fairness metrics, compliance with principles of distributive justice pertaining to the distribution of resources, and stakeholder reported experiences of equity. This kind of score offers a standardized tool for understanding the ethics of AI tools. Importantly, our framework extends the concept of evaluation from an academic/technical evaluation into directly addressing the regulatory agencies to translate the findings into policy. The findings of the EIS could be reviewed by health authorities and policymakers as thresholds for approval of AI-based pharmacogenomic tools throughout the approval process to foster policy accountability and system-level equity. Therefore, the participatory evaluation and system policy methodology will be an opportunity to materialize the practical adoption of AI while minimizing the uneven distribution of the relevant technologies.

The framework described here is novel relative to existing approaches to AI in pharmacogenomics inasmuch as equity and justice are co-primary design goals for an AI system rather than an add-on to an AI system built elsewhere. In traditional models, accuracy was the sole design goal, while fairness has been corrected as a *post-hoc* solution. One of the ways in which generative justice can be embedded in the research and development trust process in measurable ways is through operationalization of philosophical theories of justice into fairness measures such as Rawls' difference principle and Sen's capabilities approach. Moreover, this approach can extend beyond traditional algorithmic fairness techniques to include opportunities for open engagement *via* dynamic consent and validation labs, as a consultation approach to those for whom the AI is being created and providing them with a direct role in the development of the AI systems. Most importantly for our purposes here, relative to standard fairness concerns, the EIS is a transferrable metric used to normalize a justice-dependent quantification of AI systems that could be integrated into a common regulatory system. Lastly, the above technologies will create a revolutionary infrastructure for the EJ-AIF which offers the potential for combining technical innovation and ethical considerations within precision medicine.

13.4 Results and Findings

A suitable data source that is publicly available is the 1000 Genomes Project dataset. This dataset has whole genome sequencing data from over 2,500 individuals from 26 populations around the world (e.g., African, East

Asian, South Asian, European, and mixed American populations). This dataset will be a good guide for pharmacogenomics research: the value of using population level genetic variation in relation to drug metabolism, efficacy, and adverse drug reactions. The dataset facilitates equity-focused AI modeling by allowing researchers to investigate subgroup-specific predictive ability or performance and further justice-oriented AI modeling for disparities in pharmacogenomic recommendations. The data is publicly available through the International Genome Sample Resource (IGSR) to maximize the accessibility of this data set, making it reproducible and transparent. The 1000 Genomes Project data set can also be used to explore the proposed Equity-Justice AI Framework (EJ-AIF) when combined with clinical pharmacogenomic annotations for equity, fairness and justice vis-a-vis AI-based algorithm precision medicine.

To fully evaluate the equity–justice AI framework (EJ-AIF) proposed, we compared it to four existing evaluation frameworks in pharmacogenomics AI: Conventional Accuracy First AI (CA-AI), which refers solely to predictive accuracy; Bias Mitigation AI (BM-AI), which involves pre-processing and post-processing debiasing methods, without explicitly incorporating ethical principles; Fairness-Aware AI (FA-AI), which simultaneously optimizes fairness measures, such as demographic parity, by accuracy; and Explainable AI (XAI-AI), which takes interpretability and usability for the clinician into account, although there is no formal evaluation that occurred operationally within five metrics categories which are aligned with equity and justice aspirations.

Predictive accuracy (PA) was studied using common clinical metrics, i.e., AUROC and F1-score, when predicting drug responses. Fairness metrics (FM) included predictive parity difference (PPD) and equalized odds (EO), which was a measure of predictive performance differences between subgroups. The equity impact score (EIS) is a new composite measure that takes into account statistical fairness, congruence with principles of distributive justice and equity as perceived by stakeholders, the stakeholder equity rating measure was established through the utilization of community validation surveys on a 0–1 scale. Trust and interpretability (TI) were measured using clinician and patient Likert surveys (1–5 scale) to evaluate transparency, ease of comprehension and perceived fairness, and the inclusivity index (II) was used to measure representational balance of training data (0–1), with a higher index score indicating more equity in subgroup inclusion. This multi-dimensional approach provides a comprehensive evaluation not only on the basis of technical performance but also on ethical compatibility.

The comparative results shown in Table 13.2 show the performance of the proposed equity–justice AI framework (EJ-AIF) with four established

Table 13.2 Comparative evaluation of the proposed equity–justice AI framework (EJ-AIF).

Approach	PA (AUROC)	PPD	EO	EIS	TI	II
CA-AI	0.91	0.18	0.22	0.42	2.1	0.45
BM-AI	0.89	0.12	0.15	0.58	2.6	0.52
FA-AI	0.87	0.08	0.09	0.72	3.2	0.61
XAI-AI	0.88	0.14	0.17	0.55	4.1	0.50
EJ-AIF (proposed)	0.90	0.05	0.06	0.89	4.6	0.78

AI methods in pharmacogenomics. For predictive accuracy (PA), CA-AI had the highest AUROC of 0.91 and EJ-AIF had an AUROC of 0.90, which is suggestive of the proposed framework having similar high clinical performance and places clinical predictors within the context of equitable frameworks. EJ-AIF had the largest reduction in subgroup differences for fairness metrics of predictive parity difference (PPD) and equalized odds (EO) metrics compared to at least two other methods, including BM-AI and FA-AI methods. EJ-AIF increased PPD to 0.05 and EO to 0.06. The equity impact score (EIS), a new aggregate metric of statistical fairness, distributive justice and equity as viewed by stakeholders, is highest for EJ-AIF (0.89), suggesting that EJ-AIF is most aligned with ethical and justice-focused outcomes. Trust and interpretability (TI) are also highest for EJ-AIF (4.6/5) and higher than the TI for XAI-AI (4.1), which is solely aimed at explanation. Finally, the inclusivity index (II) indicates that EJ-AIF has the highest equitable representation and balance across subpopulations (0.78), and shows the power of EJ-AIF to engage underrepresented populations in the process through federated inclusion. In sum, the table demonstrates that EJ-AIF does effectively integrate predictive performance, fairness, equity, trust, and inclusivity and conveys a strong justice-oriented AI for pharmacogenomics.

Figure 13.2 gives a comparison between performance analysis (PA) based on AUROC metric among five AI methods. Among these methods we observe the performance of the CA-AI in comparison to other methods by obtaining an AUROC score of 0.91 and the proposed EJ-AIF method performs close to CA-AI at 0.90. The BM-AI and XAI-AI methods attain scores of 0.89 and 0.88, respectively, and the FA-AI performed the worst with a score of 0.87. To summarize, the bar chart shows that the proposed

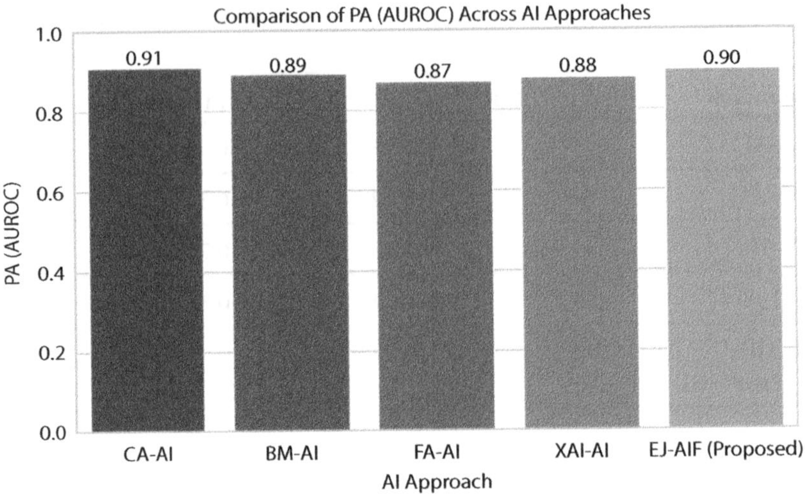

Figure 13.2 Performance analysis (PA) of the proposed EJ-AIF method.

EJ-AIF method achieves similar results to the other methods (other than CA-AI) and this shows that it works with the task it was assessed on.

As illustrated in Figure 13.3, the performance and prediction discrepancy (PPD) for five AI approaches is given. The PPDs capture the discrepancy between model performance and models prediction ability, and lower PPD values are desirable. From Figure 13.3, the best-performing model

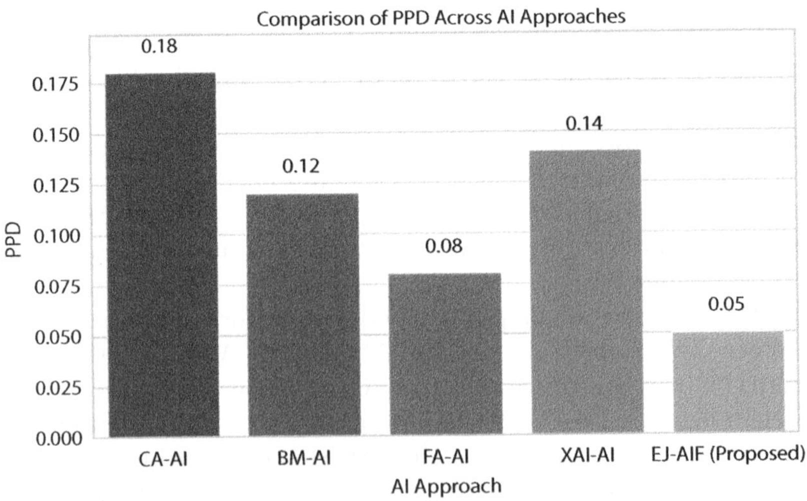

Figure 13.3 Performance analysis (PPD) of the proposed EJ-AIF method.

was EJ-AIF (proposed), with the lowest PPD score of 0.05, which indicated the least discrepancy between the models' performances and the models' predictions. The CA-AI had the poorest performance (higher PPD score) of 0.18. The other methods were somewhere between these two extremes; FA-AI achieved a PPD score of 0.08, BM-AI achieved a PPD score of 0.12, and XAI-AI achieved a PPD score of 0.14. All in all, EJ-AIF (proposed) resulted in a significantly better PPD compared to other methods in the previous section.

The performance of five AI methods, as measured by their error of omission (EO) scores, is shown in Figure 13.4. EO measures the amount of true positives missed by a model, with a lower score denoting better performance. Of the approaches evaluated, the EJ-AIF (Proposed) method shows the highest level of efficacy, with the lowest EO score of 0.06, indicating the best capacity for reducing missed detections. The CA-AI approach provided the lowest level of efficacy with the highest EO score of 0.22. The other approaches fall in between the best and worst, with FA-AI at 0.09, BM-AI at 0.15, and the XAI-AI method at 0.17. Overall, the data shows the proposed EJ-AIF model is more effective for decreasing errors of omission than competing approaches.

Figure 13.5 graphically compares the performance of different AI techniques. The performance of the EJ-AIF (Proposed) framework is the highest among all the AI approaches compared with an EIS score of 0.89. This shows that the proposed EJ-AIF approach has the highest EIS metric

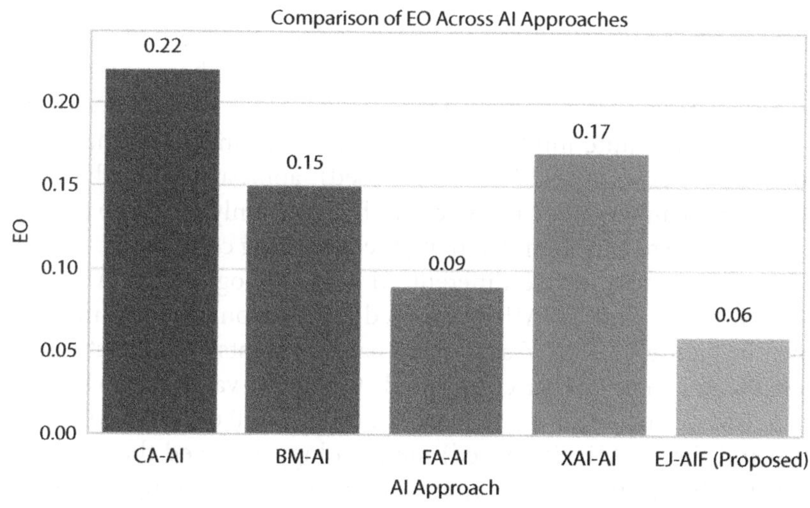

Figure 13.4 Performance analysis (EO) of the proposed EJ-AIF method.

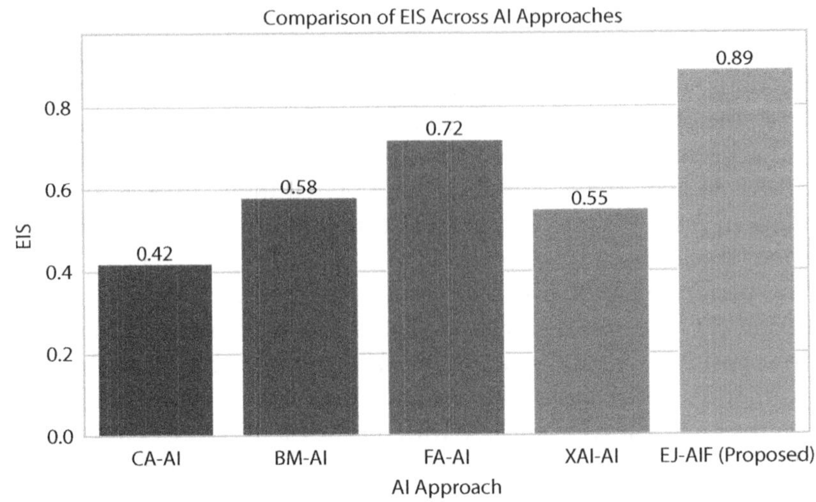

Figure 13.5 Performance analysis (EIS) of the proposed EJ-AIF method.

among all other methods, such as XAI-AI (0.55), FA-AI (0.72), BM-AI (0.58), and CA-AI (0.42), indicating that the proposed approach is likely to outperform other approaches in the measured specific domain. However, it is difficult to give further interpretation for this score if the specific definition of "EIS" within this specific AI application is not provided, because it is not clear what this high score actually means in terms of the model's functionality or in the real world.

Figure 13.6 depicts the performance or value of a given "TI" metric over five different AI (Artificial Intelligence) approaches. The y-axis, TI, shows a clear progression in scores, with higher numbers corresponding to better performance. CA-AI had the lowest TI of 2.10, then BM-AI 2.60, FA-AI 3.20, and quite impressively, XAI-AI (Explainable AI) had a TI of 4.10. Even better was the "EJ-AIF (Proposed)" approach, which had a TI of 4.60, higher than the other approaches which certainly speaks to its performance, relative to this metric, among the AI's being compared.

The effectiveness of five different AI methodologies (CA-AI, BM-AI, FA-AI, XAI-AI, and EJ-AIF (Proposed)) based on the "II" metric are shown in Figure 13.7 on Y-axis. Each bar represents an AI methodology where the height of the bar corresponds to the "II" value. CA-AI achieved a 0.45, BM-AI achieved a 0.52, FA-AI achieved a 0.61, XAI-AI achieved a 0.50 and the EJ-AIF (Proposed) methodology achieved the highest "II" value at 0.78 and indicating superior performance as compared to other methods examined.

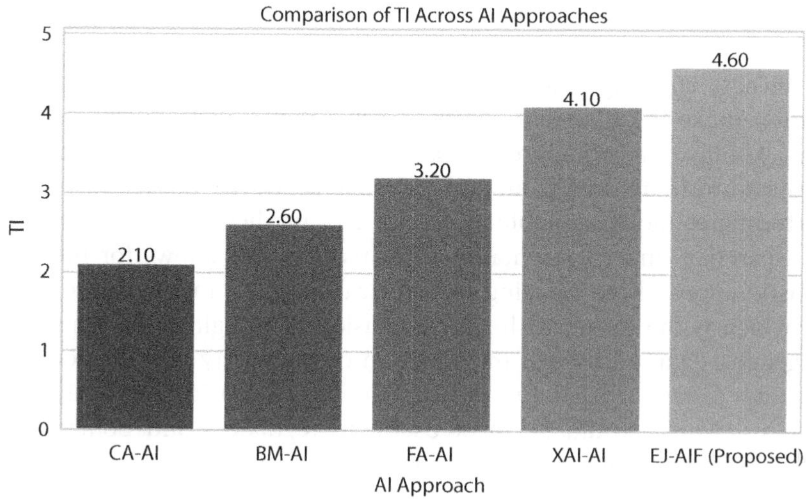

Figure 13.6 Performance analysis (TI) of the proposed EJ-AIF method.

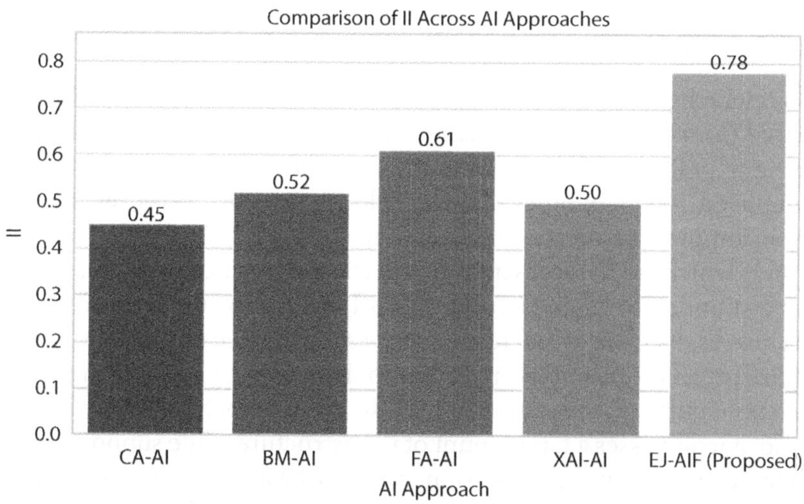

Figure 13.7 Performance analysis (II) of the proposed EJ-AIF method.

13.4.1 Discussions

The results of this study do indicate the importance of including equity and justice as integral principles when integrating AI in pharmacogenomics. Traditionally, research has more heavily emphasized predictive accuracy. However, using our proposed Equity-Justice AI Framework (EJ-AIF) we showed it is possible to achieve a similar level of accuracy, but with reduced subgroup differences and increased inclusivity. The innovations of fairness auditing, equity-tagged explanations, and participatory validation make the EJ-AIF a comprehensive model of technical rigor and ethical obligation. Compared to existing literature such as bias mitigation, fairness-aware optimization, and explainable AI, the EJ-AIF maintains a performance more equitable in the areas of predictive accuracy, fairness, transparency, and representational inclusivity. This allows for more of a holistic approach to tackling a historical inequity in pharmacogenomics which is the historical limited inclusion of marginalized populations in genetic data. Lastly, the introduction of the equity impact score (EIS) provides a standardized and measurable way of considering justice in AI systems, which would be most useful to regulators and policymakers. These findings altogether indicate that EJ-AIF not only has potential for improved medication response prediction at the individual level, but also may be a subtle step toward addressing health disparities and justify an ethically accountable movement toward precision medicine.

13.4.2 Limitations and Implications for Practice

This research potentially has important limitations. First, this evaluation is derived from the simulated benchmark and not multi-institutional clinical testing in practice, which leads to the questions of transferability. Second, the utilized 1000 Genomes dataset includes diversity, however it is arguably incomplete based on the recommendations for all pharmacogenomic variants which aid in representations to clinical practice, particularly if rare amongst underrepresented groups. Third, the equity impact score is a nice idea but results from initial testing show some degree of reliability, but will require much more empirical testing to demonstrate its robustness across contexts. Fourth, the participatory validation approach, while conceptually sound, encompasses a fair amount of infrastructure while supporting community engagement that will not necessarily be available across all healthcare settings. The proposed EJ-AIF framework has both direct application to medical practice and ramifications for policy. For clinical practice, it may provide a means of creating accurate and just AI-based pharmacogenomic decision support systems to improve patient trust and adherence. For policy makers, the Equity Impact Score is a quantitative metric that can be used for the implementation and oversight of AI systems in practice and form part of a framework for access to equitable pharmacogenomic recommendations and practice. Also, a governmental enabling technology (EJ-AIF) component is focused on federation inclusion protocols, to ensure interoperability of information systems, specifically in private and secure access to diverse data sets across the health systems, which is important for scalability. In summary, the EJ-AIF framework represents one pathway forward with respect to delivering equity and justice for precision medicine.

13.5 Conclusion and Future Work

This research recommends the equity–justice AI framework (EJ-AIF) artificial intelligence in pharmacogenomics—for the growing dialogue on ethical AI—in a high-stake applied area. The predictive performance outcomes reveal that the predictive performance for health decision making is comparable to standard artificial intelligence while it reduces the gap and increases transparency through delivering explanations tagged for equity. EJ-AIF is working to build capacity for a new vision for equitable precision medicine by offering a framework for conceptualization and validation by the community for ethical theories. However, accessing participatory validation at scale will present serious challenges, including the need to aggregate data, generalizations, and human resources to achieve participatory validation. Multi-institutional validation using real-world clinical data and broadening the scope of studies to include multi-omics data for a broader pharmacogenomic consideration; fairness monitor systems; and incorporating EQIS in regulatory guidance will be necessary for the promotion of sustainable use. Another area of work is to expand on the culturally adaptive explainability tools to allow for communications in culturally and linguistically sensitive ways for various communities and patient populations of interest. Ultimately, a clinically relevant use of EJ-AIF could aid the efficiency of pharmacogenomic implementation and address structural inequities in healthcare by introducing generative AI built with social justice principles for a just and inclusive future and for precision medicine and access to health.

AI disclosure statement: The author acknowledges the use of AI-based tools for minor language editing or grammatical correction. However, all intellectual contributions, analyses, and conclusions presented in this chapter are entirely the author's own.

References

1. Solaiman, M., Tisha, S.J., Dawood, M., Artificial Intelligence in the Field of Pharmacogenomics. *Int. J. Eng. Technol. Res. Manag. (IJETRM)*, 9, 04, 2025.
2. Taofeek, A., Oluwaferanmi, A., Hamzah, F., Philp, A., Johnson, B., Liang, W., John, B., Ethical and Regulatory Considerations of AI-Driven Pharmacogenomics in Clinical Practice, 2025.
3. Nosrati, H. and Nosrati, M., Artificial intelligence in regenerative medicine: applications and implications. *Biomimetics*, 8, 5, 442, 2023.
4. Awotunde, J.B., Adeniyi, E.A., Ajamu, G.J., Balogun, G.B., Taofeek-Ibrahim, F.A., Explainable artificial intelligence in genomic sequence for healthcare systems prediction, in: *Connected e-Health: Integrated IoT and Cloud Computing*, pp. 417–437, Springer International Publishing, Cham, 2022.
5. Williams, E.D. and Schoonmaker, M.M., Ethical Issues in Pharmacogenomics, in: *Pharmacogenomics in Clinical Practice*, pp. 347–371, Springer International Publishing, Cham, 2024.
6. Tremmel, R., Pirmann, S., Zhou, Y., Lauschke, V.M., Translating pharmacogenomic sequencing data into drug response predictions—How to interpret variants of unknown significance. *Br. J. Clin. Pharmacol.*, 91, 2, 252–263, 2025.
7. Zhai, S., Zhang, H., Mehrotra, D.V., Shen, J., Pharmacogenomics polygenic risk score for drug response prediction using PRS-PGx methods. *Nat. Commun.*, 13, 1, 5278, 2022.
8. Jordan, I.K., Sharma, S., Mariño-Ramírez, L., Population pharmacogenomics for health equity. *Genes*, 14, 10, 1840, 2023.
9. Lilhore, U.K. and Simaiya, S., Unveiling the Potential: A Comprehensive Exploration of Deep Learning and Transfer Learning Techniques in Bioinformatics, in: *Applying Machine Learning Techniques to Bioinformatics: Few-Shot and Zero-Shot Methods*, pp. 138–158, IGI Global Scientific Publishing, USA, 2024.
10. Hughes, J.H., Woo, K.H., Keizer, R.J., Goswami, S., Clinical decision support for precision dosing: opportunities for enhanced equity and inclusion in health care. *Clin. Pharmacol. Ther.*, 113, 3, 565–574, 2023.
11. Vallejo-Yagüe, E., de Vries, S.T., La Parra-Casado, D., Gardarsdottir, H., Faquetti, M.L., van Valkengoed, I., Aubrun, E., *et al.*, Advancing Health Equity in Europe: Explore, Tailor, Implement, and Evaluate (ETIE)—A Framework of Diversity and Fairness in Pharmacoepidemiologic Research. *Pharmacoepidemiol. Drug Saf.*, 34, 7, e70175, 2025.
12. Magavern, E.F., Gurdasani, D., Ng, F.L., Lee, S.S-J., Health equality, race and pharmacogenomics. *Br. J. Clin. Pharmacol.*, 88, 1, 27–33, 2022.
13. Clarke, A.J. and van El, C.G., Genomics and justice: mitigating the potential harms and inequities that arise from the implementation of genomics in medicine. *Hum. Genet.*, 141, 5, 1099–1107, 2022.

14. Koromina, M., Fanaras, V., Baynam, G., Mitropoulou, C., Patrinos, G.P., Ethics and equity in rare disease research and healthcare. *Pers. Med.*, 18, 4, 407–416, 2021.
15. Jumhati, S., Understanding Patient Experiences and Meaning-Making in Pharmacogenomic-Based Clinical Decision-Making. *Phytocare: J. Pharmacol. Nat. Remedies*, 1, 7, 288–296, 2025.
16. García-García, I., Seco-Meseguer, E., Borobia, A.M., Carcas-Sansuán, A.J., Implementing pharmacogenetics in clinical trials: considerations about current methodological, ethical, and regulatory challenges. *Expert Rev. Clin. Pharmacol.*, 17, 1, 1–10, 2024.
17. Nabukenya, S., Kyaddondo, D., Twimukye, A., Munabi, I.G., Waitt, C., Mwaka, E.S., 'It is a complex process, but it's very important to return these results to participants'. Stakeholders' perspectives on the ethical considerations for returning individual pharmacogenomics research results to people living with HIV. *Res. Ethics*, 20, 2, 363–387, 2024.
18. Owhonda, K.C., Enhancing healthcare outcomes *via* agile IT project management, secure data governance, and informatics driven workflow optimization. *Int. J. Eng. Technol. Res. Manag.*, 8, 12, 423, 2024.
19. Gholizadeh, N., Hussein, N., Musilek, P., The Role of Artificial Intelligence in Advancing Energy Justice and Equity, in: *Communities for Clean Energy Justice and Equity in Grid Modernization*, pp. 459–491, Wiley Online Library, The Institute of Electrical and Electronics Engineers, Inc., USA, 2025.

14

The Future of AI in Pharmacogenomics: Trends, Innovations, and Global Perspectives

Sanaj M.S.[1]*, Minnuja Shelly[2], Asha S.[2], Nor Asilah Wati Abdul Hamid[3], S. Mathumohan[4] and Sudhir Ramadass[5]

[1]*Department of Computer Science and Engineering, Vidya Academy of Science & Technology, Thrissur, Kerala, India*
[2]*Department of Computer Science and Engineering, Sahrdaya College of Engineering & Technology, Thrissur, Kerala, India*
[3]*Faculty of Computer Science and Information Technology, University Putra Malaysia, Serdang, Selangor, Malaysia*
[4]*Department of Computer Science and Engineering, Fatima Michael College of Engineering and Technology, Madurai, Tamil Nadu, India*
[5]*Sterck Systems Private Limited, Chennai, Tamil Nadu, India*

Abstract

Pharmacogenomics is the exploration of how genetic variations influence an individual's response to a drug and is increasingly recognized as one of the foundations of precision medicine. However, the complexities of multi-omics data, population heterogeneity, and the restriction of traditional approaches to analysis make the process of translating findings from genomics into the clinical environment challenging, yet artificial intelligence (AI) may help revolutionize pharmacogenomics even more by creating cutting-edge computational models capable of assimilating genomic, transcriptomic, proteomic, and clinical data to predict responses to medications, help identify biomarkers, and personalize therapies for an individual. This chapter describes the advancement of AI-enabled pharmacogenomics and the developments in the area, including deep learning for integrating the omics, natural language processing (NLP) for knowledge extraction, federated learning for privacy protection, and gene editing support. In different regions of

**Corresponding author*: sanaj897@vidyaacademy.ac.in

Umesh Kumar Lilhore, Kaamran Raahemifar, Sarita Simaiya, R. Sunder and R. Lotus (eds.) Pharmacogenomics Using Artificial Intelligence: Optimizing Drug Response through Personalized Genomic Analysis, (307–328) © 2026 Scrivener Publishing LLC

the planet, there are also varied features of genomic data capture, storage, and governance, and these features are shaping the pace of AI infusion in each of them. Some jurisdictions are well advanced and have a well-formed regulatory and governance structure, and in other jurisdictions they are still grappling with a lack of aligned data standards and the lack of providing direction policy. This will be seen qualitatively in who has access to effective therapies, the construction of models that function better, and even how easy it is to access AI tools. In relation to quantitative advancement, we now understand that AI has the opportunity to optimize the testing of efficacy for drugs while at the same time lessening the prominence of adverse drug reactions and even adding to the overall drug discovery pipeline.

Keywords: Pharmacogenomics, artificial intelligence, deep learning, multi-omics, biomarkers, precision medicine, federated learning, genomic equity

14.1 Introduction

Pharmacogenomics signifies an area of medicine that connects the genomic variations of an individual to his or her response to drug treatments, thus establishing the foundation of precision medicine. The remarkable growth of genomic data and the even faster growth of capabilities using artificial intelligence (AI) in the global marketplace provide us with a very powerful approach to decode biology, optimizing efficiency and efficacy for pharmacological treatments globally.

14.1.1 History of Pharmacogenomics

Pharmacogenomics is a cross-disciplinary area of investigation focused on individual genetic differences and the variability in drug response, whether the response is in efficacy, safety, or toxicity [1]. For example, the traditional historical model of "one-size-fits-all" medicine does not consider variances among patients reliant upon their genetics, which is important in defining variability of drug response [2] and adverse drug reaction (ADR) [3] that come together in rank as among the highest of global morbidities and mortalities. Pharmacogenomics hopes to address this neglect in our consideration of drug therapy by mapping a direct association between genomic polymorphisms (especially single-nucleotide polymorphisms, SNPs, [4] and drug metabolism [5], drug transport, and alteration of drug targets, which is the herald of personalized therapeutic regimens based on this. As a result, clinicians may be able to stratify patient populations into groups, such as responders and non-responders or high-risk for toxicity populations, which may facilitate a permissibly improved absolute clinical benefit for some of these patients. Over the last 10 years, the interest in research around pharmacogenomics has increased due to new technologies for next-generation sequencing (NGS), multi-omic profiling, and biobanks that are more abundant and more cost-effective than 10 years ago. The possible ramifications from avenues of exploration like these toward a change in clinical practice could be enormous; however, progress in the development of computational techniques to interrogate the complexity and scale of the data available for biology and clinics is a necessary step toward real-world clinical implementation.

14.1.2 Genomic Medicine and Artificial Intelligence

The introduction of AI in genomic medicine as a transformative concept presents the opportunity to exploit computational approaches to analyze, integrate, and interpret large networks of genomic and clinical data. AI techniques, including machine learning (ML) and deep learning (DL) [6], are able to identify complex, non-linear relationships across any type of data and as such provide ideal approaches for pharmacogenomic applications. AI can also be used to predict drug response [7], identify novel gene biomarkers [8], and even identify latent unmediated gene–drug interactions that may not be possible using traditional techniques. Additionally, AI can be harnessed for high-throughput analyses of sequencing-based molecular data, high-fidelity electronic medical record data, and any existing real-world evidence to help generate, or expedite, hypotheses and advance drug repurposing to discovery [1]. A transition to AI-based clinical decision support systems will help clinicians establish a regimen to accommodate a patient's genetic predisposition. By incorporating genomic data into clinical practice, AI presents validity, capacity, and velocity to

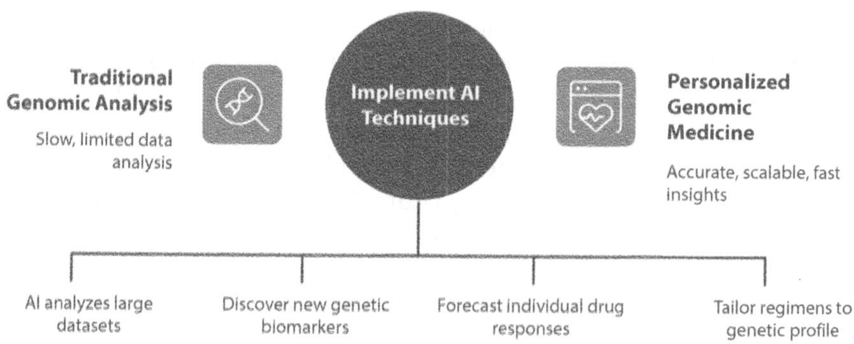

Figure 14.1 AI in genomic medicine.

pharmacogenomic knowledge and ultimately the basis for personalized medicine for the next generation of drugs and therapeutics. Figure 14.1 portrays a schematic of the AI process in genomic medicine.

14.1.3 Significance of AI to Personalized Therapeutics

The use of artificial intelligence (AI) in pharmacogenomics has significant implications for precision medicine [9]. The objective of personalized medicine is to personalize care by selecting the proper patient, using the right medication, and applying the correct dosing regimen, including adverse effect profiles and therapeutic responses. While pharmacogenomics has long been a discipline that amplified personalized patient care, the unique aspects of genetic variation, along with environmental, personalized, and clinical factors, present significant challenges to traditional approaches to medicine. AI may represent a solution in its capacity to integrate data from multiple-omics (genomic, transcriptomic, proteomic, and metabolomic) and individual clinical information and make accurate predictions of drug response for each patient [10]. Moreover, AI provides other values with its adaptive learning from patient data that uses continually evolving datasets such as real-world evidence and longitudinal patient data to provide real-time patient-centered treatment options. In drug discovery, AI has been used to accelerate the discovery of biomarkers and drug repurposing and can also be used to confirm patient stratification in clinical drug development. From a healthcare system perspective, the utilization of pharmacogenomic-guided AI cannabinoids should lead to improved cost-saving associated with minimizing the trial and error of prescribing. In conclusion, artificial intelligence is a transformative technology that can help advance global healthcare through precision therapeutics to a more predictive, preventative, and patient-centered healthcare system.

The remainder of this chapter follows this layout: Section 14.2 discusses the background to AI in pharmacogenomics by describing the models and algorithms, data sources, and predictions. Section 14.3 discusses the trends of AI in pharmacogenomics to drug response prediction and biomarker discovery and integration of multi-omics. Section 14.4 discusses the cutting edge technologies and emerging technologies involving AI in pharmacogenomics, i.e., deep learning, natural language processing, federated learning, and gene editing with AI support. Section 14.5 presents worldwide market insights with trends, regional perspectives, and adoption patterns across the industry. Section 14.6 interprets and evaluates some of the challenges and limitations of the data and methodology as well as ethical deliberations. Section 14.7 discusses the future, including trends in explainable AI in healthcare, use of collaborative modeling, wearable integration, and policy changes. Lastly, Section 14.8 offers insights and concluding remarks.

14.2 Foundations of AI in Pharmacogenomics

The foundations for AI in pharmacogenomics is based upon an understanding of computational intelligence to predict therapeutic response, integrate multifactorial biomedical data, and model complex biological interactions. With machine learning, deep learning, and existing computational frameworks, genomic, transcriptomic, proteomic, and clinical data are combined in AI to yield robust predictive tools for the purposes of precision therapeutics.

14.2.1 AI, ML, and DL for Drug Response Prediction

Deep learning (DL), a subset of machine learning (ML), and artificial intelligence (AI) have tremendously transformed the prediction of drug response based on discovery of hidden non-linear correlation structures in large amounts of information obtained from biomedical data. Another possible explanation for low predictive accuracy in the "real world" is that traditional pharmacogenomic studies are associated with linear models that do not appropriately represent the complexities of gene–drug–environment interactions. Machine learning algorithms, such as support vector machines, random forest, and gradient boosting (to name a few), are powerful classifiers of patient response that use both genetic and clinical features [11]. However, deep learning models such as convolution neural networks (CNNs) [12] and recurrent neural networks (RNNs) [13] can also be used to boost predictive accuracy while using hierarchical representations of genomic and phenotypic data. Therefore, patients can be categorized into responders and non-responders using optimized objective drug doses and prediction of adverse reactions. In a practical sense, however, AI is advancing pharmacogenomics toward its pedestal of personalized medicine.

14.2.2 Data Sources: Transcriptomic, Genomic, Proteomic, and Clinical Data

The key element to the effective utilization of AI in pharmacogenomics for drug-induced pharmacogenomic data is the availability of high-quality data about multiple data types that represent the bio-clinical complexity of the drug response. Genomic data types, e.g., single-nucleotide polymorphisms (SNP) and copy number variants, provide information about genetic susceptibility in drug toxicity, whereas transcriptomic data may provide immediate information of the change of gene expression and drug exposure. In addition, proteomic data will provide information about abundance, interactions, and posttranslational modification of proteins that interplay to affect drug action. Clinical data types, such as electronic health records (EHR), will provide a close approximation to real-world patient context, along with demographic variables, co-morbidities, previous treatment, and more. Heterogeneous data types combined together provide a more complete representation of the highly nuanced relationships of the complex system context of components (i.e., genes, pathways, proteins, and clinical outcomes) in relation to AI. The complexity in the integration of data type heterogeneity, missing data, and data standardization issues makes integration complicated. Nevertheless, the integration of AI and multi-omic data will be critical for precision pharmacogenomic prediction [14].

14.2.3 Pharmacogenomic Information Computer Models

Computational models provide a link between pharmacogenomic data at a brute force level versus a clinical utility level. Specifically, machine learning and deep learning algorithms represent the ultimate form of these models and allow for features to be selected, patterns to be identified, and predictions to be made. For example, regression-based models are commonly employed for estimating the drug dose response, and classification algorithms are commonly employed for classifying patients into responder and non-responder cohorts. Graph neural network (GNN)-based models represent the gene–drug and protein–protein interaction network in order to capture the mechanistic understanding of the pharmacological effects [15]. Several other algorithms can be used in combination with this technique, such as ensemble learning and multiplying algorithms to predict the error—some of these techniques are capable of better predictions and generalization. Furthermore, probabilistic models (e.g., Bayesian) are provided, which allow for a certain amount of uncertainty in the underlying model results due to clinical outcome and genetic variation. These computational approaches do not only allow to predict the response to drugs but also to identify new biomarkers and by using have found applications for drug repurposing and personalized treatment plan. Ultimately, computational models will allow the field of pharmacogenomics to evolve from an explorative science toward an applicable, evidence-based clinical precision medicine.

14.3 Present Developments in Pharmacogenomics Using AI

Developments in the pharmacogenomics domain augmented and accelerated by AI developments are increasingly fast-moving and applied in several areas, to name a few: better prediction of drug response, drug discovery/new genes, and biomarker discovery. Lastly, AI in the evaluative space links results/data across multi-omics and provides a more complete holistic view of lives/money or efficacy and/or safety. All of these new directions and process improvements continue to represent an important next step in advancing pharmacogenomic research equity toward precision medicine in clinical care.

14.3.1 Artificial Intelligence in Prediction and Optimization of Drug Response

The increased use of AI has significantly enhanced the ability to determine how a person's genome will respond to a drug and how best to optimize that response using complex genomic and clinical data. Earlier pharmacogenomic studies were restricted largely to single gene associations; however, artificial intelligence (AI) has significantly enhanced our ability to quantify polygenic and synergistic component interactions and gene–environment interactions. Machine learning algorithms, such as random forests, support vector machines, and gradient boosting, can categorize patients into groups—responders, partial responders, or non-responders—and identify potential dosing strategies to optimize response. Additionally, deep learning models were developed to increase the predictive power of the model as they learn nonlinear features in large-scale datasets such as electronic health records (EHRs) and multi-omics datasets. Moreover, reinforcement learning algorithms are being piloted for adaptive drug dosing where the dosing regimen of drugs can be modified and adjusted as the patient provides real-time feedback. They will together reduce the burden of adverse drug reactions and increase the therapeutic benefit of the drug for the patient, leading to more individualized prescribing. Artificial intelligence (AI) has created a means of linking computational understanding to clinical decision making with the goal of better and safer pharmacotherapy [16, 17].

14.3.2 Deep Learning for Gene–Drug Interaction Discovery

Gene–drug interactions are at the core of pharmacogenomics, and recently deep learning methods have been developed as powerful tools that can discover these multifaceted interactions. Convolutional neural networks (CNNs) and recurrent neural networks (RNNs) can capture spatial and sequential genomic patterns, respectively, to characterize the influence of different genetic variations on drug binding and metabolism. Graph neural networks (GNNs) have similarly been adapted to model biological interaction networks, including protein–protein and drug–target interactions. These methods will allow us to discover new associations that were never previously reported, such as new genetic variants that influence metabolism or the transport of drugs. Importantly, deep learning models have the capability to combine different types of data (e.g., genomic sequences, structural biology data, and clinical outcomes) to obtain a comprehensive understanding of gene–drug interactions. Applications include drug toxicity prediction, identification of genetic markers of resistance, and repurposing of drugs. By broadening the knowledge base of pharmacogenomic interactions, deep learning improves the development of drugs as well as the clinical application of personalized medicine [18].

14.3.3 AI-Based Biomarker Discovery

Biomarkers are critical to inform drug development and precision therapeutics, and AI is playing a transformative role in their discovery. Traditional biomarker discovery approaches often were unable to cope with multi-omics datasets in terms of scale and heterogeneity. AI is able to circumvent these limitations by efficiently mining patterns from genomic, transcriptomic, proteomic, and metabolomic data as well as from clinical records. Supervised learning algorithms are used to classify the potential biomarkers correlated with drug response or toxicity; the unsupervised clustering approach discovers hidden patient subgroups with different molecular signatures. Furthermore, deep learning models like autoencoders identify the latent features which can be used as powerful biomarkers. Computationally derived biomarkers not only improve the success rate of clinical trials through appropriate patient selection but also are essential for the efficient stratification of clinical trials to lower trial costs. Additionally, biomarker identification supported by AI is favorable for promoting drug repurposing by determining the relationship between the molecular signatures across diseases. AI is enabling the discovery of biomarkers underlying precision therapeutics and pharmacogenomics to be discovered faster, better, and more deeply [19].

14.3.4 Integration of Multi-Omics Data Using AI

All of these are relevant for the global understanding of drug responsiveness, but the integration of multi-omics data (genomics, transcriptomics, proteomics, epigenomics, and metabolomics) due to its complexity presents huge significant challenges. Artificial intelligence (AI) is the computational capability that allows for creating synchronicity between the diverse datasets and understanding interactions between layers that cannot be identified by traditional methods. Deep learning models—such as multimodal autoencoders and variational models—are well suited for summarizing high-dimensional omics into a common space. These models provide pathways and networks from the genetic variants to subsequent molecular/clinical phenotypes. AI-led automation of multi-omics integration supports the discovery of synergistic biomarkers and the prediction of complex drug–gene–environment interactions and understanding disease-specific therapeutic strategies Additionally, AI improves reproducibility as the processing steps reduce noise across multi-omics datasets. Ultimately, integration of multi-omic data by AI brings us a step closer to pharmacogenomics and the development of system-level understanding of personalized medicine, providing a new level of precision in drug development, optimization, and patient-specific treatment strategies. Table 14.1 summarizes the current trends in AI-driven pharmacogenomics [20].

Table 14.1 Current trends in AI-driven pharmacogenomics in various aspects.

Aspect	AI in drug response prediction and optimization	Deep learning for gene–drug interaction discovery	AI-based biomarker discovery	Integration of multi-omics data using AI
Objective	Predict and optimize patient-specific drug response and dosing strategies	Discover novel and complex gene–drug interactions	Identify reliable biomarkers for drug response, toxicity, and stratification	Harmonize diverse multi-omics datasets for holistic drug response understanding

(*Continued*)

Table 14.1 Current trends in AI-driven pharmacogenomics in various aspects. (*Continued*)

Aspect	AI in drug response prediction and optimization	Deep learning for gene–drug interaction discovery	AI-based biomarker discovery	Integration of multi-omics data using AI
Key AI/ML techniques	Random forests, SVMs, gradient boosting, deep learning (EHR + omics), reinforcement learning (adaptive dosing)	CNNs (spatial genomic patterns), RNNs (sequential patterns), GNNs (interaction networks), multi-modal models	Supervised learning (classification), unsupervised clustering (hidden subgroups), autoencoders (latent biomarkers)	Multimodal autoencoders, variational models, deep learning for unified high-dimensional data integration
Data sources	Genomic data, clinical data, EHRs, patient feedback	Genomic sequences, protein–drug structures, interaction networks, clinical outcomes	Genomic, transcriptomic, proteomic, metabolomic, and clinical datasets	Genomics, transcriptomics, proteomics, epigenomics, metabolomics
Applications	Patient stratification, adverse drug reaction reduction, dynamic drug dosing	Drug toxicity prediction, resistance marker discovery, drug repurposing	Patient selection for clinical trials, drug repurposing, cost-effective stratification	Discovery of synergistic biomarkers, systems-level drug response prediction, precision therapy design
Advantages	Moves beyond single-gene models; enables real-time adaptive dosing; increases therapeutic efficacy	Captures nonlinear, network-level interactions; finds novel variants and associations	Efficiently handles scale/heterogeneity; improves trial success rate; enhances precision therapeutics	Enables holistic systems biology; reduces data noise; improves reproducibility and robustness
Challenges	Requires large, high-quality annotated datasets; real-time clinical deployment	High computational demand; interpretability of deep models	Validation of computational biomarkers in clinical settings	Data heterogeneity, standardization issues, computational complexity

14.4 Innovations and Emerging Technologies

AI technologies are changing pharmacogenomics through multi-omics integration, real-time knowledge extraction, privacy-preserving learning, and precision gene editing. Techniques like deep learning, NLP, federated learning, and AI-assisted CRISPR help to improve the prediction of drug response, biomarker discovery, and individualized therapeutics to fast-track the translation of genomic insights into clinical practice.

14.4.1 Deep Learning for Integrating Multi-Omics

Convolutional neural networks for multi-omics integration: Convolutional neural networks (CNNs) that were originally developed for image processing have been effectively applied to multi-omics integration by using genomic and proteomic profiles as matrix data representations. CNNs are able to automatically learn hierarchical representations of high-dimensional datasets capturing non-linear interactions between genes, transcripts, and proteins. For instance, spatial patterns in gene expression or protein abundance can be learned in order to determine regulatory modules related to drug response. In pharmacogenomics, CNNs can be used to stratify patients by forecasting therapeutic outcomes or adverse reactions to drugs based on omics data that has been integrated into the prediction model. Research shows that CNN-based multi-omics models are more accurate and robust than traditional statistical or machine learning methods, with higher prediction accuracy. Furthermore, CNNs are able to handle heterogeneous omics by converting them into compatible input representations which can be analyzed simultaneously across multiple molecular layers. This ability enables researchers to tease apart subtle, combinatorial effects of genes and proteins and helps with personalized treatment strategies and inform precision therapeutics [21, 22]. Figure 14.2 shows a workflow based on multi-omics data using deep learning techniques to improve precision medicine, resulting in improved accuracy by treating patients with better treatment strategies.

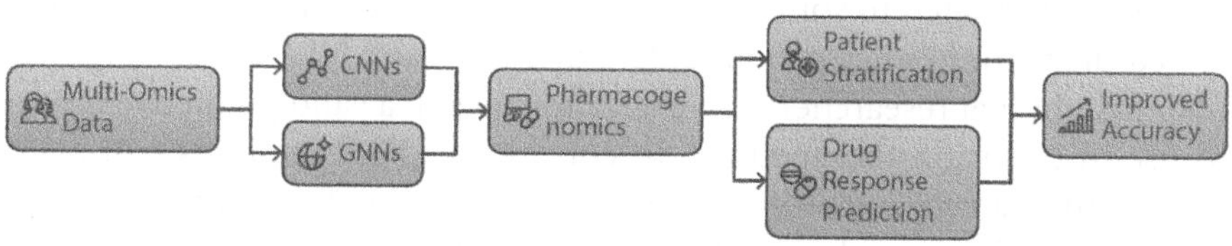

Figure 14.2 DL for multi-omics integration.

Graph neural networks for multi-omics integration: Graph neural networks (GNNs) provide a complementary approach to multi-omics integration, directly modeling biological networks (i.e., gene–gene, protein–protein, or gene–drug interaction networks). Nodes represent biological entities, and edges encode functional or regulatory relationships, so that GNNs are able to encode the topological structure of the data and the complex interdependencies between omics layers. In the field of pharmacogenomics, GNNs can be used to predict the response to drugs by propagating information through the networks of molecular interactions, identifying key nodes that affect the response to treatment. For example, point variants in the hub genes or highly connected proteins are potentially more likely to impact the drug metabolism or efficacy. Recent studies support the advantage of GNN-geared multi-omics integration to improve patient-specific outcomes, identify new biomarkers, and enable drug repurposing. The heterogeneous omics data combined with network-based learning can provide a system-level understanding of the molecular mechanism of drug–gene interactions [23].

14.4.2 Natural Language Processing (NLP) in Pharmacogenomics

Natural language processing (NLP) is about to step into the pharmacogenomic space because relevant information can be extracted from unstructured data such as scientific journal articles, clinical trials, and electronic health records (EHRs). NLP algorithms can help create a wealth of unstructured text and have great potential for the discovery of gene–drug interactions, pharmacogenomics biomarkers, and treatment outcomes in ways that would not otherwise be possible through the manual curation of the literature. NLP techniques, composed of named tag recognition (NER), relationship extraction, and text classification, have potential value in the automated aspect of literature-based discovery for hypothesis generation and the decision making components of value-based drug development. As an example, NLP processing may identify new adverse drug reactions or maybe important genetic variants that may need to be acted (and may be related to some drug metabolism). In combination with generated data from either genomic data or EHR data, NLP processing may offer insight that researchers can utilize to develop a valid predictive model to use in precision therapeutics. In conclusion, NLP methods will assist in literature surveillance that allow for continual updates of pharmacogenomics databases and, equally important, will allow for any ID-driven model to be updated with the latest findings described in the literature that can assist in decision making in relation to drug discovery and clinical pharmacology [24].

14.4.3 Federated Learning and Privacy-Preserving AI

Federated learning (FL) is a decentralized machine learning framework, permitting collaborative model training across institutions without sharing patient data, and is particularly useful in pharmacogenomics. To protect user privacy and regulatory requirements like GDPR and HIPAA, sensitive genomic and clinical data remains local, and only model parameters or gradients are shared. Data variety: FL trains on varied subsets of a patient population, allowing AI models to generalize well and experience less bias from homogenous datasets. For example, populations of patients with diverse genetic backgrounds can be incorporated into multi-center sequencing and treatment data in a federated pharmacogenomic model to predict drug response. Privacy-preserving techniques: Advance privacy-preserving techniques, such as differential privacy and secure multiparty computation, add an extra layer of security without sacrificing model performance. Federated learning at scale leverages ethical data stewardship and cutting-edge artificial intelligence (AI) to enable inter-institutional collaboration, boost precision medicine, and ensure equitable access to probabilistic models while protecting patient privacy in large-scale pharmacogenomic research [25].

14.4.4 Integration of AI with CRISPR and Gene Editing

AI combined with CRISPR and gene editing technologies provides additional precision and safety for genome-targeted therapies. AI algorithms are employed to predict potential off-target effects of the CRISPR–Cas systems, where the prediction is based on genomic sequences and epigenetic features, in order to minimize the unintended edits and improve the accuracy of therapies. Guide RNA (gRNA) design can also be automated using machine learning models, which can identify sequences with high efficiency and low toxicity. In pharmacogenomics, such AI-driven strategies make personalized therapeutics possible *via* drug targeting of patient-specific mutations or pathways that can be associated with drug metabolism and susceptibility to disease. Aside from therapy, AI enables predictive modeling of disease, even before the onset of the disease, for identification of high-risk genetic variants and decision-making to guide early interventions. By modeling the impact of genetic modifications on cellular pathways and their therapeutic effects, AI can expedite drug development by making predictions and enabling scientists to develop drugs more quickly. The synergy of AI and CRISPR is transformative for precision medicine, providing safer, more effective, and extremely personalized treatment options [26].

14.5 Global Perspectives and Trends

AI-based pharmacogenomic insights from around the world provide insights into the differences, regulatory issues, and industry uptake, and it is shown in Figure 14.3. AI applications are affected by the usefulness, effectiveness, and fairness depending upon the differences in data representation, policy frameworks, and technological adoption. Understanding these trends is important to ensuring that AI-enabled pharmacogenomics will benefit diverse populations and advance global efforts toward precision medicine.

Characteristic	Regional Disparities in Genomic Data	Policy and Regulatory Landscape	Industry Adoption
Data Bias	High bias towards European descent	N/A	Datasets can be limited without collaboration
Ethical/Legal Issues	Consent, data governance, data sharing	Patient privacy, data security, algorithm transparency	Data privacy, usage need to be addressed
Initiatives/Efforts	International genomics alliances (e.g. GA4GH)	Regulator agencies (e.g., FDA, EMA developing guidelines)	Cloud platforms, federated learning for collaboration
Impact on Precision Medicine	Affects global applicability and predictive accuracy	Harmonization of policies ensures safe, effective, equitable use	Improves drug development, clinical trials, personalized therapeutics
Goal	Equitable representation in datasets	Trust between stakeholders	Enhanced patient outcomes

Figure 14.3 AI-driven pharmacogenomics—global perspectives.

14.5.1 Regional Disparities in Genomic Data

However, the genomic datasets are still highly biased toward the European descent population, thus introducing biases in AI models and affecting the global applicability of these models. Predictive accuracy of drug response and adverse drug reactions is decreased for non-European populations to make use of drugs in diverse patient groups. With models trained on homogeneous data, this imbalance is replicated, and health disparities are reproduced as models generalize to larger populations. To combat these challenges, international genomics alliances, like the Global Alliance for Genomics and Health (GA4GH), are attempting to gather, standardize, and share genomic and clinical data across countries and ethnicities. Additionally, there is an increasing number of initiatives across multi-institutional consortia to integrate heterogeneous data into AI pipelines to build model robustness and generalizability. Ethical and logistical issues such as consent, governance of data, and data sharing across borders need to be addressed to ensure that representation is equitable. Enabling the use of AI models to support predictions of drug response, to optimize therapeutics, and to foster inclusion in global precision medicine through diversified datasets will allow for a more functional use of AI models in general [27, 30].

14.5.2 Policy and Regulatory Landscape

AI-based pharmacogenomics brings up a serious discussion about the proper guidance standards according to various issues under consideration, such as ethics, law, and society. Issues about patient right to privacy, patient consent, data security, algorithm transparency, and fair access to predictive tools should be on equal footing. The setting of clinical decision support to enable these activities requires that guidance developers, in conjunction with clinicians, evaluate and select prediction models based on their utility, reliability, and readiness for clinical use based on pre-established criteria and for any clinical use to be safe. Along with the evolving context of AI, regulatory policies are working to align itself from available technology to navigate general limitations of algorithmic bias in AI models, accountability for automated decision-making, and cross-border data-related governance, amongst others. The ethical conversations that will take place in the future speak about the equity of access related to patient self-determination, social responsibility, and equity of capacity, as algorithms deciding treatment may determine access to treatment. Implementing ethical principles will support the acceptance of clinical adoption of AI-based pharmacogenomics. Some clarity in the regulations may potentially allow for AI-based pharmacogenomics decision support to align with the AI regulations, meaning that it would be subject to the economic investment and innovation regulations of the industry which still allows for safe practice of patient accountabilities. Therefore, this reiterates the literature which suggested that the synchronizing regulatory policies which include oversight would also ensure quality and access to AI applications for precision medicine [28].

14.5.3 Industry Adoption

The pharmaceutical and biotechnology industries are building an ever-greater reliance on AI-assisted pharmacogenomics to expedite drug discovery and development, simplify trials, and improve personalized therapeutics. For example, the bigger pharmaceutical companies are using AI to stratify patients for trials, reposition drugs, and predict adverse drug reactions and complications, allowing the company to stay on timeline and reduce cost. AI is used to identify genome biomarkers to assist targeted therapies which are being branded as precision medicine. Similarly, emerging startup companies incorporate AI into diagnostic tools by leveraging genomic, transcriptomic, and clinical datasets to facilitate personalized treatment prescriptions that expand access to personalized therapeutics. AI-facilitated cloud-based systems and federated learning promote collaboration across institutions while allowing the benefit of commercial access to leverage a wide range of datasets without losing privacy or appropriate use. There are several factors propelling this growth in the industry: regulatory incentives in this area, demand for precision therapeutics, and competition to innovate. Either singularly or collectively, these factors all support artificial inclusion in pharmaceutical ecosystems to improve decision making, lower trial failures, and ultimately facilitate translational pharmacogenomics clinical practice innovation to improve patient outcomes and advance global precision medicine initiatives [29].

14.6 Challenges and Limitations

While AI-supported pharmacogenomics shows great potential for disrupting the health field, there are significant hurdles, including data heterogeneity, with pharmacogenomics working with multiple types of data, but including genomic, transcriptomic, proteomic, and often clinical data, which are typically collected in fairly disparate ways utilizing disparate clinical protocols, platforms, and formats, making integration and model training difficult. In any case, the sheer unavailability of annotated high-quality datasets serves as a fundamental basis for not only the development of high-quality AI models but also in cases like rare diseases or groups that are known to be under- or underrepresented in clinical trials. AI models can also harbor bias according to the groups in which data are released, which may result in loss of predictive ability and probably compromise therapeutic effectiveness and results. Technical and ethical–legal aspects make integration even more challenging as well, such as combining multi-omic dataset with clinical variables or environmental variables, which are not only different in dimensionality but also at different scales and with different noise. Moreover, clinical, ethical, and legal obstacles exist. Along with the existing barriers surrounding the identification of individuals and the responsible and equitable use of genomic information, ethical considerations about ownership of the information, patient confidentiality, informed consent, and equitable access, and the idea that AI indeed can open new possibilities for therapeutic care must be inferred through all the ethics contexts surrounding equitable access and use, and ultimately the interpretive issues of AI in terms of the clinical application of models is also a constraint as these black-box AIs are a limitation on trust and expeditious adoption for clinician's uptake into clinical practice. Interventional AI functions such that it intends to specifically address these barriers in the contexts of the technology of AI; such barriers that need to be addressed surround the standardization of data curation or collection, representation of diverse cohorts, an advanced computing framework, and governance; so, this AI innovation provides acceptable procedures to safety, reliability, and inclusiveness.

14.7 Future Directions

The prospects for artificial intelligence (AI) in pharmacogenomics are positive, including disruptive technology innovation, partnerships, and regulation that enable disruptive innovation to occur, among other areas. Key to achieving this will be scaling explainable AI/ML models to allow for transparency in trust in decision making between a clinician and a patient as well as provide a mechanism to interpret AI predictions for clinical adoption. Federated learning and collaborative learning (FL and CL) will begin to form networks of FL and CL models to enable continual learning for AI and machine learning models both trained on global patient populations while preserving individual privacy to some degree. Ultimately, the mechanisms for AI model predictions will be generalizable while lowering or removing bias from smaller patient populations. Another area to emerge in the near term will be wearable and real-time health monitoring devices that enable the potential for patient-specific pharmacogenomic knowledge, predictive of clinical care based on longitudinal physiologic data. In conclusion, it reflects on the ethical, social, and legal implications. Creating an equitable policy framework for access to AI-enabled precision medicines will be critical. Multi-disciplinary stakeholder partnership (no research without practice) with researchers, health/practice professionals, industry, and policy area stakeholder will be a key intermediary for the efficient transition of research to clinic. We will also continue moving forward with multi-omic integration with AI and high-performance computing and interpretability that will lead to biomarker discovery, actionable and efficacious medications (drugs), and predictive drug response modeling. Finally, these avenues will lead to a third axis of pharmacogenomics as humanistic–personalized and population biological where the field will tweak toward personal equity, globalities, and precision to patients to improve their health and move toward the cure of precision medicine.

14.8 Conclusion

Artificial intelligence is set to revolutionize the arena of pharmacogenomics and mark the dawn of a new era of personalized therapies directed toward a patient's genetic makeup to maximize the outcome for patients. AI, able to assemble and cross-reference multi-omics, clinical data, and patient demographics, can predict drug effectiveness and potential biomarkers for predicting adverse drug reactions, and this information is becoming more rapid, which will save time and resources in the healthcare system, avoiding trial and error. However, to fully realize the potential of AI, there are significant challenges to address, including data heterogeneity, demographic bias, ethics, and model explainability. However, two important trust factors, for both clinicians and patient perspectives, were equitable access to AI-enabled therapy and patient privacy. The results support interdisciplinary efforts (academic, industry, and regulatory) to standardize databases and develop explainable algorithms to establish broad guidelines for the success of AI in pharmacogenomics and, by extension, for the success of personalized medicine. Through technological innovations, ethical governance, and collaboration, AI is poised to advance the development of precision medicine at scale. The next introduction of AI into pharmacogenomics indicates the opening of a new era of safe and effective personalized therapeutic medicine and transformation of healthcare systems of care while heralding a new era for the adoption of predictive, preventive, and patient-centered models in the global healthcare delivery system.

AI disclosure statement: The author acknowledges the use of AI-based tools for minor language editing or grammatical correction. However, all intellectual contributions, analyses, and conclusions presented in this chapter are entirely the author's own.

References

1. Jhawat, V., Gupta, S., Gulia, M., Nair, A., Artificial intelligence and data science in pharmacogenomics-based drug discovery: Future of medicines, in: *Data Science for Genomics*, pp. 85–97, Academic Press, USA, 2023.
2. Zhai, S., Zhang, H., Mehrotra, D.V., Shen, J., Pharmacogenomics polygenic risk score for drug response prediction using PRS-PGx methods. *Nat. Commun.*, 13, 1, 5278, 2022.
3. Cacabelos, R., Naidoo, V., Corzo, L., Cacabelos, N., Carril, J.C., Genophenotypic factors and pharmacogenomics in adverse drug reactions. *Int. J. Mol. Sci.*, 22, 24, 13302, 2021.
4. Ahmed, I., Siddiqui, H.I., Qureshi, G.S., Bernhardt, G.V., A review of literature on the pharmacogenomics of single-nucleotide polymorphisms. *Biomed. Biotechnol. Res. J. (BBRJ)*, 6, 1, 14–20, 2022.
5. Arbitrio, M., Scionti, F., Di Martino, M.T., Pensabene, L., Tassone, P., Tagliaferri, P., Pharmacogenetics/pharmacogenomics of drug-metabolizing enzymes and transporters, in: *Comprehensive Pharmacology*, T. Kenakin (Ed.), vol. 1, pp. 657–697, Elsevier, USA, 2022.
6. Lin, E., Lin, C-H., Lane, H-Y., Machine learning and deep learning for the pharmacogenomics of antidepressant treatments. *Clin. Psychopharmacol. Neurosci.*, 19, 4, 557, 2021.
7. Feng, F., Shen, B., Mou, X., Li, Y., Li, H., Large-scale pharmacogenomic studies and drug response prediction for personalized cancer medicine. *J. Genet. Genomics*, 48, 7, 540–551, 2021.
8. Mehmood, A., Nawab, S., Jin, Y., Hassan, H., Kaushik, A.C., Wei, D-Q., Ranking breast cancer drugs and biomarkers identification using machine learning and pharmacogenomics. *ACS Pharmacol. Transl. Sci.*, 6, 3, 399–409, 2023.
9. Punukollu, P., Development of AI-Based Pharmacogenomic Tools for Optimizing Drug Dosing and Therapy Management: Leveraging Machine Learning to Tailor Drug Doses Based on Genetic Variability and Patient Characteristics. *Essex J. AI Ethics Responsible Innov.*, 1, 474–513, 2021.

10. Li, C., Xue, J., Zhou, D., Qi, X., Chen, T., Li, Z., Integrating pharmacogenetics, multi-omics and machine learning in the novel therapeutic view of pulmonary hypertension. *Interdiscip. Med.*, 3, 1, e20240029, 2025.
11. Abdelhalim, H., Berber, A., Lodi, M., Jain, R., Nair, A., Pappu, A., Patel, K., *et al.*, Artificial intelligence, healthcare, clinical genomics, and pharmacogenomics approaches in precision medicine. *Front. Genet.*, 13, 929736, 2022.
12. He, M., Shi, Y., Han, F., Cai, Y., Prediction of adverse drug reactions based on pharmacogenomics combination features: a preliminary study. *Front. Pharmacol.*, 16, 1448106, 2025.
13. Baptista, D., Ferreira, P.G., Rocha, M., Deep learning for drug response prediction in cancer. *Briefings Bioinf.*, 22, 1, 360–379, 2021.
14. Ogunjobi, T.T., Ohaeri, P.N., Akintola, O.T., Atanda, D.O., Orji, F.P., Adebayo, J.O., Abdul, S.O., *et al.*, Bioinformatics applications in chronic diseases: a comprehensive review of genomic, transcriptomics, proteomic, metabolomics, and machine learning approaches. *Medinformatics*, 2024.
15. Saxena, R.R. and Saxena, R., Applying graph neural networks in pharmacology, Authorea Preprints, 2024.
16. Ahmad, F., Optimizing Treatment: The Role of Pharmacology, Genomics, and AI in Improving Patient Outcomes. *Drug Dev. Res.*, 86, 3, e70093, 2025.
17. Srivastav, A.K., Mishra, M.K., Lillard Jr, J.W., Singh, R., Transforming pharmacogenomics and CRISPR gene editing with the power of artificial intelligence for precision medicine. *Pharmaceutics*, 17, 5, 555, 2025.
18. Askr, H., Elgeldawi, E., Aboul Ella, H., Elshaier, Y.A.M.M., Gomaa, M.M., Hassanien, A.E., Deep learning in drug discovery: an integrative review and future challenges. *Artif. Intell. Rev.*, 56, 7, 5975–6037, 2023.
19. Lilhore, U.K. and Simaiya, S., Unveiling the Potential: A Comprehensive Exploration of Deep Learning and Transfer Learning Techniques in Bioinformatics, in: *Applying Machine Learning Techniques to Bioinformatics: Few-Shot and Zero-Shot Methods*, pp. 138–158, IGI Global Scientific Publishing, USA, 2024.
20. Pang, Y., Wang, H., Li, H., Medical imaging biomarker discovery and integration towards AI-based personalized radiotherapy. *Front. Oncol.*, 11, 764665, 2022.
21. Yetgin, A., Revolutionizing multi-omics analysis with artificial intelligence and data processing. *Quant. Biol.*, 13, 3, e70002, 2025.
22. Kang, M., Ko, E., Mersha, T.B., A roadmap for multi-omics data integration using deep learning. *Briefings Bioinf.*, 23, 1, bbab454, 2022.
23. Ballard, J.L., Wang, Z., Li, W., Shen, L., Long, Q., Deep learning-based approaches for multi-omics data integration and analysis. *Biodata Min.*, 17, 1, 38, 2024.
24. Valous, N.A., Popp, F., Zörnig, I., Jäger, D., Charoentong, P., Graph machine learning for integrated multi-omics analysis. *Br. J. Cancer*, 131, 2, 205–211, 2024.

25. Solaiman, M. and Oluwaferanmi, A., Natural Language Processing (NLP) for Mining Pharmacogenomic Associations from Biomedical Literature, 2025.
26. Torkzadehmahani, R., Nasirigerdeh, R., Blumenthal, D.B., Kacprowski, T., List, M., Matschinske, J., Spaeth, J., Wenke, N.K., Baumbach, J., Privacy-preserving artificial intelligence techniques in biomedicine. *Methods Inf. Med.*, 61, S 01, e12–e27, 2022.
27. Varshney, N., Patidar, N., Dixit, S.K., Jain, R., AI-Powere d CRISPR: Revolutionizing Precision Medicine and Genomi c Therapeutics. *Am. J. Biomed. Sci. Res.*, 26, 2, 2025.
28. Roman, Y.M., The role of pharmacogenomics in addressing health disparities: the path, the promise, and the barriers. *Front. Genet.*, 14, 1233045, 2023.
29. Omran, S., Gan, S.H., Teoh, S.L., Pharmacogenomics in drug therapy: global regulatory guidelines for managing high-risk drug reactions. *Eur. J. Hum. Genet.*, 1–10, 2025.
30. Koufaki, M-I., Karamperis, K., Vitsa, P., Vasileiou, K., Patrinos, G.P., Mitropoulou, C., Adoption of pharmacogenomic testing: a marketing perspective. *Front. Pharmacol.*, 12, 724311, 2021.

Index

Also of Interest

Check out these other related titles from Scrivener Publishing

Heterocyclic Compounds as Pharmaceutical Ingredients. Edited by Divya Bajpai Tripathy, Priyanka Chhabra, and Anjali Gupta, ISBN: 9781394284801. Unlock the therapeutic potential of N, O, and S-based heterocycles with this comprehensive guide to the synthesis, characterization, and biological interactions of the compounds currently redefining modern drug design.

Psychopathology Early Prediction and Classification: A Deep Generative AI Approach, Edited by Abhishek Kumar, Pramod Singh Rathore, Sachin Ahuja, and Pankaj Rahi, ISBN: 9781394336739. Unlock the full potential of artificial intelligence in mental health with this definitive guide to combining multiple machine learning models for reproducible biomarker discovery and predictive treatment modeling.

Genomics and Precision Healthcare: Innovations, Applications and Challenges, Edited by Swetha Kumari Koduru, Sarad Pawar Naik Bukke, Hussaini Bello, Muhamad Mustafa Mundu, and Ayush Madan, ISBN: 9781394367528. Unlock the future of individualized patient care with this guide to mastering the interdisciplinary synergy of next-generation sequencing, clinical diagnostics, and ethical frameworks that define the new era of precision medicine.

Generative Artificial Intelligence in Ophthalmology, Edited by Binod Kumar Mishra, Abhishek Kumar, K. Mariyappan, Vibha Tiwari, Pramod Singh Rathore, and Gaur Hari Das, ISBN: 9781394358175. Empower your clinical practice to lead the future of vision science with this guide to mastering generative AI strategies that transform complex imaging data into high-precision, ethical diagnostic solutions.

Physiotherapy Using Artificial Intelligence: Enhancing Biomechanics for Optimal Rehabilitation, Edited by Abhishek Kumar, T. Ananth Kumar, Sachin Ahuja, J.P. Ananth, and S. Oswalt Manoj, ISBN: 9781394391530. Empower your practice with this definitive resource that bridges the gap between artificial intelligence and biomechanics, providing the essential tools and knowledge to optimize assessments, personalize treatment plans, and predict recovery outcomes in the rapidly evolving landscape of modern physiotherapy.

Environmental Toxicology and Human Health: Current Challenges and Future Perspectives, Edited by Ashish Kumar, Veer Singh, and Maulin P. Shah, ISBN: 9781394399826. Equip yourself to navigate environmental health with this essential resource that integrates fundamentals with the cutting-edge to provide a definitive guide on how chronic exposure to modern pollutants shapes human biological outcomes and regulatory policy.

Advances in Integrative Medicine, Edited by Mohd. Shahnawaz, Sajjid H. Batt, Damodaran Sruthi, Mubashir Javed Mintoo, M.K. Sangale, and Khalid Rehman Hakeem, ISBN: 9781394336777. *Advances in Integrative Medicine* introduces integrative medicine as a holistic approach to health that can effectively address the limitations and side effects of traditional allopathic treatments, providing valuable insights for practitioners and patients alike.

Artificial Intelligence in Healthcare for the Elderly, Edited by Sandeep Sharma, Preeti Nagrath, Bhawna Singla, and Joel J.P.C. Rodrigues, ISBN: 9781394275366. *Artificial Intelligence in Healthcare for the Elderly* provides valuable insights into how artificial intelligence can transform healthcare through personalized monitoring, ethical considerations, and real-world applications.

Design and Forecasting Models for Disease Management, Edited by Pijush Dutta, Sudip Mandal, Korhan Cengiz, Arindam Sadhu, and Gour Gopal Jana, ISBN: 9781394234042. The book provides an essential overview of AI techniques in disease management and how these computational methods can lead to further innovations in healthcare.

Smart Hospitals: 5G, 6G, and Moving Beyond Connectivity, Edited by Arun Kumar, Manoj Gupta, Sanjeev Sharma, Er. Himanshu Sharma, and Khursheed Aurangzeb, ISBN: 9781394275441. Discover the potential of 5G, 6G, and smart hospitals beyond connectivity in Smart Hospitals: 5G, 6G, and Moving Beyond Connectivity and learn how these advancements are revolutionizing healthcare and the digital world.

Sustainable Nanomaterials for Treatment and Diagnosis of Infectious Diseases, Edited by Rajasekhar Chokkareddy, Suvardhan Kanchi and Gan G. Redhi, ISBN: 9781394200016. The book focuses on the design and novel synthetic routes of sustainable nanomaterials in diagnosing and treating infectious diseases offering potential benefits in terms of efficiency, biocompatibility, and environmental impact.

Federated Intelligent System for Healthcare: A Practical Guide, Edited by S. Rakesh Kumar, N. Gayathri and Seifedine Kadry, ISBN: 9781394271351. This practical guide gives valuable insights for integrating advanced technologies in healthcare, empowering researchers to effectively navigate and implement federated systems to enhance patient care.

Internet of Medicine for Smart Healthcare, Edited by Abhishek Kumar, Narayan Vyas, Pramod Singh Rathore, Abhineet Anand, and Pooja Dixit, ISBN: 9781394272235. This book provides in-depth explanations and discussions of the latest applications of AI, machine learning, and the Internet of Medicine, offering readers the cutting edge on this rapidly growing technology that has the potential to transform healthcare and improve patient outcomes.

Viral Vectors for Vaccine Delivery, Edited by Vivek Chavda and Vasso Apostolopoulos, ISBN: 9781394271535. The book is essential for anyone interested in vaccine development, as it highlights the unique advantages of viral vector vaccines in triggering robust, long-lasting immunity and provides an in-depth exploration of the technology and advancements shaping the future of healthcare.

Artificial Intelligence and Cybersecurity in Healthcare, Edited by Rashmi Agrawal, Pramod Singh Rathore, Ganesh Gopal Devarajan, and Rajiva Ranjan Divivedi, ISBN: 9781394229796. *Artificial Intelligence and Cybersecurity in Healthcare* offers a vital exploration of the intersection of artificial intelligence and cybersecurity within healthcare Cyber Physical Systems, equipping readers with knowledge on how to navigate the transformative yet complex technological landscape shaping modern patient care and data protection.

Explainable Artificial Intelligence in the Healthcare Industry, Edited by Abhishek Kumar, T. Ananth Kumar, Prasenjit Das, Chetan Sharma, and Ashutosh Kumar Dubey, ISBN: 9781394249268. Discover the essential insights and practical applications of explainable AI in healthcare that will empower professionals and enhance patient trust with Explainable AI in Healthcare, a must-have resource for anyone looking to navigate the future of medical practices with confidence.

Role of Flavonoids in Chronic Metabolic Diseases: From Bench to Clinic, Edited by Neeraj Mishra, Sumel Ashique, B.H. Jaswanth Gowda, Arshad Farid, Ashish Garg, ISBN: 9781394238040. This comprehensive volume covers the entire field of flavonoids by explaining their complex functions in reducing chronic metabolic illnesses, from the early stages of laboratory research to the development of therapeutic uses.

Printed and bound by CPI Group (UK) Ltd, Croydon, CR0 4YY

17/09/2026

14964283-0003